Development and Treatment of PTSD

Robert W. Motta
Hofstra University, USA

IGI Global
Scientific Publishing
Publishing Tomorrow's Research Today

Vice President of Editorial Melissa Wagner
Managing Editor of Acquisitions Mikaela Felty
Managing Editor of Book Development Jocelynn Hessler
Production Manager Mike Brehm
Cover Design Phillip Shickler

Published in the United States of America by
IGI Global Scientific Publishing
701 East Chocolate Avenue
Hershey, PA, 17033, USA
Tel: 717-533-8845
Fax: 717-533-8661
Website: https://www.igi-global.com E-mail: cust@igi-global.com

Library of Congress Cataloging-in-Publication Data

Names: Motta, Robert W., editor.
Title: Development and treatment of PTSD / edited by Robert Motta.
Other titles: Development and treatment of Posttraumatic stress disorder
Description: Hershey, PA : IGI Global Scientific Publishing, [2025] | Includes bibliographical references and index. | Summary: "The principal objective of this book is to provide updated information on the development and treatment of PTSD"-- Provided by publisher.
Identifiers: LCCN 2024048490 (print) | LCCN 2024048491 (ebook) | ISBN 9798369320891 (h/c) | ISBN 9798369354537 (s/c) | ISBN 9798369320907 (eISBN)
Subjects: LCSH: Post-traumatic stress disorder--Treatment.
Classification: LCC RC552.P67 D488 2025 (print) | LCC RC552.P67 (ebook) | DDC 616.85/21061--dc23/eng/20250108
LC record available at https://lccn.loc.gov/2024048490
LC ebook record available at https://lccn.loc.gov/2024048491

British Cataloguing in Publication Data
A Cataloguing in Publication record for this book is available from the British Library.

Table of Contents

Detailed Table of Contents

A complicated and multidimensional psychological disorder, post-traumatic stress disorder (PTSD) has attracted a lot of interest in the realm of mental health. By analyzing PTSD from both behavioral and phenomenological angles, this chapter seeks to offer a thorough understanding of the condition. The first section of the chapter explores the behavioral components of PTSD. This covers an analysis of typical symptoms including hyperarousal, avoidance, and intrusive thoughts in addition to how trauma affects a person's relationships and day-to-day activities. This chapter also looks at the phenomenology aspect of PTSD. The purpose of this part is to shed light on the inner lives of persons afflicted with PTSD by exposing the profound and frequently hidden components of the condition. Understanding the relationship that exists between a person's lived experiences and their behavioral manifestations of PTSD can help with diagnosis, treatment, and support.

Diagnosis of PTSD. Posttraumatic stress disorder (PTSD) refers to long running disturbances in emotion, cognition, and behavior owing to having encountered frightening, disruptive, and often life-threatening experiences. These traumatic experiences are relived in such a way that the past, even a past that took place decades ago, is ever present. Common fear reactions often abate within brief periods of time. In contrast, PTSD is enduring and can sometimes last for as long as one lives. It is dysregulating across a wide variety of domains of functioning. PTSD can cause extreme fear reactions to common stressors; it can cause disruptions in one's memory and thinking process; it can cause startle reactions and sympathetic nervous system over-activation; can negatively alter one's mood; diminish one's sense of self; cause sleeplessness and nightmares, disrupt relationships, and cause an enduring distrust of the environment. To help in developing a perspective on PTSD, it is important to note that most people who encounter traumatic events do not develop PTSD.

Post-traumatic stress disorder (PTSD) is a well-known mental health condition that affects millions of people worldwide. PTSD is characterized by a spectrum of psycho-emotional and neurophysiological effects, such as re-experiencing the trauma in the form of vivid intrusive memories, flashbacks, or nightmares. These experiences often are followed by overwhelming fear and strong physical sensations. Neuroimaging studies in patients with PTSD as well as experimental studies show alterations in brain areas such as the amygdala, hippocampus and prefrontal cortex as well as in neurochemical stress response systems. Additionally, it is believed that the main neurochemical features of PTSD include abnormal regulation of catecholamines, monoamines, and opioid neurotransmitters among others, each of which is found in brain circuits that regulate/integrate stress and fear responses. This chapter will provide an overview on the recent pathophysiological mechanisms underlying the development of PTSD.

Post-Traumatic Stress Disorder (PTSD) stands as a complex and pervasive mental health challenge, woven into the fabric of individual and collective experiences. The chapter sheds light into the heart of PTSD, seeking to understand its multifaceted origins, and intricacies of its development focussing on psychological, neurological, and sociological influences playing roles in shaping PTSD trajectory. It covers holistic understanding of PTSD, from the profound impact of trauma on brain's architecture to cultural and environmental factors amplifying its effects, laying the groundwork for subtle analysis of disorder. It stresses on importance of tailored-treatment approaches that address the unique needs of individuals. Traditional therapies like cognitive-behavioral and exposure therapies are scrutinized alongside

This chapter presents Clinical Emotional Freedom Techniques (EFT) as a promising mind-body approach for treating post-traumatic stress disorder (PTSD). Through the compelling cases of Sarah and John, two individuals grappling with PTSD symptoms despite previous therapies, the chapter underscores the need for a more integrative treatment modality. It explores the foundations and principles of Clinical EFT, a technique that combines cognitive strategies with somatic acupressure point stimulation. The growing evidence base supporting EFT's efficacy is presented, and a detailed, step-by-step guide for clinicians is offered, including how clients can use at home, in and between sessions. Sarah and John's specific EFT protocol tailored to their cases is outlined, relating to repeated childhood trauma, and a single event military deployment trauma. With its emphasis on rapid symptom reduction, low dropout rates, and comparable efficacy to established therapies, Clinical EFT emerges as a valuable addition to the clinician's toolkit.

The chapter examines the role of spirituality and meaning in the aftermath of trauma. The chapter focuses on the variables that promote PTG and on the specific impact of spirituality and meaning. The chapter reviews PTG research results in multiple clinical settings, e.g., clinical psychotherapy centers and hospitals. The chapter conclude with a brief section on clinical applications. The goal of the chapter is to expand awareness of the necessity of spiritual resources into the assessment phase of treatment (e.g., assessment of client strengths and resources) and in the use of, whenever appropriate, a cognitive framework of spirituality in the treatment phase. Cognitive modification of posttraumatic expectations and infusion of meaning can support installation of hope in the face of trauma and tragedy.

Secondary trauma, once limited to therapists and first responders, is part of our everyday lives. Anyone with a phone and an account can talk about harrowing experiences sharing with the world at large. This creates social and psychological awareness but also trauma, inherited. We watched the murder of George Floyd,

Preface

In recent decades, our understanding of Post-Traumatic Stress Disorder (PTSD) has expanded dramatically, evolving from a concept closely associated with war-related trauma to a broader, more nuanced perspective that recognizes the wide variety of traumatic circumstances contributing to its development. As editor of *Development and Treatment of PTSD*, it is my hope that this book offers an up-to-date, comprehensive exploration of both the origins of PTSD and the diverse approaches to its treatment.

While the literature has traditionally emphasized trauma from warfare, it is now well understood that many other types of experiences—ranging from domestic abuse and emotional deprivation to racial trauma and social stigmatization—can lead to PTSD. These factors are equally significant in shaping both the onset and the course of this complex disorder. Intra- and interpersonal dynamics also play an integral role in the development of PTSD, further complicating the task of diagnosing and treating it. By examining these diverse influences, this book seeks to broaden our view of what PTSD entails, encouraging readers to consider a wider spectrum of traumatic experiences.

Treatment, too, has evolved. Cognitive Behavioral Therapy (CBT) and exposure therapy remain central to many approaches, but there is growing debate over their controversial emphasis on the importance of dysfunctional cognitions. Other non-traditional treatments such as yoga, meditation, Eye Movement Desensitization and Reprocessing (EMDR), acupuncture, and psychoactive drugs are shown to have a role in treating PTSD. This volume addresses the current controversies surrounding these treatments and aims to provide an evidence-based examination of how different therapeutic interventions can support recovery.

The objective of this book is twofold: first, to enhance understanding of the myriad factors that contribute to PTSD; and second, to explore the evolving landscape of treatments, including those that go beyond the standard CBT approach. While many existing resources focus on the immediate impacts of specific traumatic events, this book adds to the conversation by considering more complex, long-term contributors to PTSD, such as systemic abuse, emotional neglect, and violations of equity and inclusion. In doing so, it presents new research and theoretical perspectives alongside practical insights into therapeutic interventions.

This book is designed for professionals, but it is also written to be accessible to the informed public. The intended audience includes psychologists, psychiatrists, social workers, counselors, emergency responders, and medical personnel, among others—essentially anyone who works with individuals affected by trauma. It is my hope that the insights and knowledge provided here will empower those who are tasked with managing the emotional, cognitive, and behavioral impacts of PTSD to offer more informed, compassionate, and effective care.

ORGANIZATION OF THE BOOK

Chapter 1: Defining PTSD Both Behaviorally and Phenomenologically

This opening chapter delves into the multifaceted nature of post-traumatic stress disorder (PTSD), examining it from both behavioral and phenomenological perspectives. On the behavioral side, the chapter explores the key symptoms of PTSD, such as hyperarousal, avoidance, and intrusive thoughts, and how these symptoms manifest in everyday life and relationships. Complementing this is an immersion into the phenomenological aspect, which seeks to illuminate the internal, often hidden experiences of individuals with PTSD. By connecting these two dimensions, the chapter provides a comprehensive understanding of how lived trauma translates into behavioral patterns, aiding in better diagnosis, treatment, and support for those affected.

Chapter 2: Origins of PTSD and Overview of Treatments

This chapter presents a broad overview of PTSD, focusing on its origins and the spectrum of treatments available. PTSD is described as a long-lasting emotional, cognitive, and behavioral disturbance triggered by frightening, life-threatening experiences. Unlike common fear responses that fade, PTSD endures, disrupting multiple aspects of life, including memory, mood, sleep, and relationships. Importantly, not everyone exposed to trauma develops PTSD, which the chapter explores in the context of resilience and vulnerability. The discussion also covers traditional and emerging treatment strategies, aiming to provide readers with a foundational understanding of PTSD's complexities.

Chapter 3: The Neurobiological Basis of Post-Traumatic Stress Disorder: Insights into the Underlying Pathophysiological Mechanisms

This chapter examines the neurobiological mechanisms underlying PTSD, focusing on the brain structures and neurochemical systems involved. Through neuroimaging and experimental studies, the chapter highlights changes in key brain areas, including the amygdala, hippocampus, and prefrontal cortex, as well as alterations in neurochemical pathways, such as those involving catecholamines and opioids. By providing insight into how these systems regulate fear and stress responses, the chapter offers a detailed overview of the physiological basis of PTSD, setting the stage for a deeper understanding of the disorder's development and informing potential treatment approaches.

Chapter 4: Decoding PTSD and Paving the Way for Healing

This chapter takes a holistic approach to understanding PTSD, exploring its origins and the factors that shape its trajectory. It discusses the interplay of psychological, neurological, and sociological influences on PTSD development, offering a broad view of the disorder. Additionally, it evaluates traditional treatments like cognitive-behavioral therapy (CBT) and exposure therapy, alongside newer approaches such as technology-assisted, art, and nature-based interventions. The chapter also underscores the role of community in PTSD recovery and highlights emerging research that points toward innovative, personalized treatment methods, ensuring a thorough exploration of the pathways to healing.

Chapter 5: Unveiling the Path to Healing: A Comprehensive Examination of Current PTSD Treatment Strategies

This chapter provides an in-depth examination of current treatment strategies for PTSD, focusing on the individualized nature of care. It outlines common PTSD symptoms, such as intrusive memories and hyperarousal, and discusses the importance of personalized treatment plans that combine different approaches, including psychological, pharmacological, and alternative therapies. The chapter emphasizes the role of ongoing assessment and collaboration between mental health professionals and patients in refining treatment methods, and it highlights the evolving nature of PTSD treatment as new research and clinical practices emerge, offering hope for improved recovery outcomes.

Chapter 6: Exploring Diverse Interventions in Treating PTSD

Addressing the need for a multifaceted approach to PTSD treatment, this chapter explores non-traditional and innovative interventions. It covers a range of treatments, from yoga and meditation to more medical interventions such as stellate ganglion blocking and trans-cranial stimulation. The chapter also discusses the use of psychoactive substances and the potential benefits of outdoor environments for recovery. By examining the efficacy and mechanisms behind these diverse approaches, the chapter highlights the importance of expanding treatment options for individuals with PTSD.

Chapter 7: A Promising Mind-Body 4th Wave Approach to Treating PTSD: Clinical Emotional Freedom Techniques

In this chapter, Clinical Emotional Freedom Techniques (EFT) are introduced as an integrative mind-body therapy for PTSD. Through case studies of two individuals—one dealing with childhood trauma and another with military-related PTSD—the chapter demonstrates EFT's potential as a rapid and effective treatment. The technique combines cognitive therapy with acupressure, offering an innovative approach that reduces symptoms while maintaining low dropout rates. A detailed guide is provided for clinicians, along with suggestions for at-home use, positioning EFT as a valuable complement to established therapies.

Chapter 8: The Search for the Sacred in a Traumatized Population: An Investigation of the Impact of Spirituality on Posttraumatic Stress

This chapter explores the role of spirituality and meaning-making in the healing process for individuals with PTSD. It discusses how spiritual resources can foster post-traumatic growth (PTG) by helping individuals integrate their traumatic experiences into a larger existential framework. Drawing from research in clinical settings, the chapter offers practical applications for incorporating spirituality into PTSD treatment, advocating for the inclusion of these resources during both assessment and therapy phases. It highlights how cognitive reframing and spiritual guidance can instill hope and resilience in the aftermath of trauma.

Chapter 9: Social Media as a Conduit for Secondary Trauma

This chapter addresses the pervasive influence of social media in spreading secondary trauma. The ease of sharing harrowing events, from the murder of George Floyd to ongoing global conflicts, has exposed millions to trauma they may not have personally experienced but are now emotionally and psychologically affected by. The chapter discusses the impact of constant exposure to graphic violence and suffering through digital platforms, emphasizing the long-lasting effects this can have on individuals and society at large. Through a personal lens, the chapter highlights how social media can inadvertently become a source of secondary trauma, especially in an age of widespread digital consumption.

CONCLUSION

As we reach the conclusion of *Development and Treatment of PTSD*, it is important to reflect on the complexity of this disorder and the evolving landscape of its treatment. The chapters presented in this book have aimed to provide a comprehensive view of PTSD, going beyond the traditional focus on war trauma to encompass a wider range of contributing factors, from interpersonal abuse to systemic and racial trauma. These broader perspectives are essential if we are to fully understand the diverse ways in which trauma can manifest and impact individuals across different contexts and life experiences.

While the clinical community continues to rely on well-established therapeutic models like Cognitive Behavioral Therapy (CBT) and exposure therapy, this book has also highlighted the growing recognition of non-traditional treatments. Emerging therapies such as yoga, meditation, EMDR, and acupuncture have generated significant interest, and a more integrative approach to treatment holds great promise for those suffering from PTSD. By exploring both traditional and non-traditional methods, we can better appreciate the range of tools available to practitioners and the importance of tailoring treatment to the unique needs of each individual.

Ultimately, the aim of this book is to expand our understanding of PTSD, not only by shedding light on its development and treatment, but also by challenging existing assumptions and encouraging a more holistic view of trauma. As the field continues to grow, it is my hope that the research, theories, and practices shared within these pages will inspire ongoing dialogue, innovation, and, most importantly, effective interventions that bring healing and relief to those affected by trauma.

I extend my deepest thanks to the contributors, whose expertise and insights have made this book a valuable resource, and to the readers, whose dedication to understanding and treating PTSD will undoubtedly make a meaningful difference in the lives of many. I also wish to thank the personnel at IGI Global for their invaluable support in bringing this book to fruition.

Robert W. Motta
Editor

Chapter 1
Defining PTSD Both Behaviorally and Phenomenologically

Divya Surendran Nair
https://orcid.org/0000-0003-2353-3451
MIT Art, Design, and Technology University, India

ABSTRACT

A complicated and multidimensional psychological disorder, post-traumatic stress disorder (PTSD) has attracted a lot of interest in the realm of mental health. By analyzing PTSD from both behavioral and phenomenological angles, this chapter seeks to offer a thorough understanding of the condition. The first section of the chapter explores the behavioral components of PTSD. This covers an analysis of typical symptoms including hyperarousal, avoidance, and intrusive thoughts in addition to how trauma affects a person's relationships and day-to-day activities. This chapter also looks at the phenomenology aspect of PTSD. The purpose of this part is to shed light on the inner lives of persons afflicted with PTSD by exposing the profound and frequently hidden components of the condition. Understanding the relationship that exists between a person's lived experiences and their behavioral manifestations of PTSD can help with diagnosis, treatment, and support.

INTRODUCTION TO POST-TRAUMATIC STRESS DISORDER (PTSD)

In psychology, trauma is a fundamental concept that explores the deep impact of adverse experiences on mental well-being. Trauma can be defined as an event that overwhelms an individual's ability to cope, encompassing a wide range of

DOI: 10.4018/979-8-3693-2089-1.ch001

experiences such as natural disasters, accidents, and interpersonal violence. Key to understanding trauma is the stress response system, a basic mechanism designed to protect against harm by triggering a "fight or flight" response when faced with danger (Forkey, 2019). However, in situations of extreme danger or helplessness, this response can become disrupted, leading to a state of psychological numbness known as dissociation (Krüger, 2020). Following trauma, individuals may experience a variety of psychological symptoms, including intrusive thoughts, flashbacks, and heightened vigilance (Morina et al., 2018). These symptoms stem from the brain's efforts to process and integrate the traumatic experience, often impairing daily functioning and sense of safety.

Consider the case of Maya, a 40-year-old woman who experienced a harrowing incident of robbery at gunpoint while leaving her workplace late one evening. Despite escaping physically unharmed, the traumatic event left an indelible mark on Maya's psyche. She began experiencing intense fear and anxiety whenever she found herself in similar situations, avoiding certain routes and locations altogether. Sleep became elusive as she was plagued by vivid nightmares replaying the event. Maya's once vibrant personality dimmed as she withdrew from social interactions and struggled to concentrate at work. Though surrounded by supportive friends and family, she found it difficult to articulate the depth of her distress. The robbery may have been a singular event, unlike large-scale disasters seen on the news, but its impact on Maya's mental well-being was profound. As she grappled with the aftermath, Maya's experience mirrors the complex and debilitating effects of Post Traumatic Stress Disorder (PTSD), highlighting the enduring psychological toll of trauma, whether individual or collective.

Post-Traumatic Stress Disorder (PTSD) emerges as a significant concern after trauma, characterized by persistent and distressing symptoms. While not everyone exposed to trauma develops PTSD, those who do often face significant disruptions in daily life. Therefore, understanding the relationship between trauma and PTSD is crucial for providing effective support and interventions.

Post-Traumatic Stress Disorder (PTSD) is a psychiatric condition that typically arises following exposure to severe trauma, frequently involving violence and destruction (Bryant, 2019). According to the Diagnostic and Statistical Manual of Mental Disorders, Fourth Edition, Text Revision (DSM-IV-TR), diagnosing PTSD requires a documented history of such traumatic exposure. This exposure could take various forms, including personally experiencing the traumatic event, witnessing it, or being confronted with the aftermath of the event (Ehlers et al., 2004). Crucially, the traumatic event must have entailed actual or threatened death, serious injury, or a profound threat to the integrity of oneself or others. The diagnosis underwent a revision in 2013 with the release of the Diagnostic and Statistical Manual of Mental

Disorders (DSM) – V, transitioning it from being classified as an anxiety disorder to being categorized under trauma-associated disorders (Schrader & Ross, 2021).

Individuals who develop PTSD often experience a range of distressing symptoms, primarily characterized by feelings of fear, helplessness, and terror. These reactions can manifest in various ways, such as intrusive memories of the traumatic event, nightmares, and flashbacks (Bar-Haim et al., 2021). Additionally, individuals may exhibit avoidance behaviors, steering clear of reminders of the trauma, and may also struggle with negative changes in mood, cognition, and arousal (Saraiya & Lopez-Castro, 2016).

Post-Traumatic Stress Disorder (PTSD) presents with both behavioral and phenomenological aspects, each offering unique insights into the condition (Liberzon & Abelson, 2016). Behavioral aspects refer to observable actions, reactions, and behaviors exhibited by individuals. Phenomenological aspects, on the other hand, pertain to the subjective inner experiences and perceptions of individuals.

Let us now explore PTSD from both its behavioral and phenomenological components, elucidating how the disorder manifests in observable actions and inner experiences. We will commence our examination with the behavioral aspect of PTSD.

BEHAVIORAL COMPONENTS OF PTSD

Behavioral manifestations refer to observable actions, reactions, and patterns of behavior exhibited by individuals with PTSD as a direct result of their traumatic experiences. These manifestations encompass a wide range of symptoms that may manifest differently in each individual, reflecting the complex interplay between psychological, physiological, and environmental factors. Examples of such manifestations include intrusive memories, avoidance behaviors, negative alterations in mood and cognition, and heightened arousal responses (Holmes et al., 2005)

In individuals with PTSD, the traumatic memory persists and cannot be easily dismissed. Symptoms of intrusive recollection can manifest in various forms, from vivid flashbacks to haunting nightmares, or even intense anxiety triggered by seemingly innocuous stimuli (Trajkov, 2023). For instance, a survivor of a violent assault might experience overwhelming fear at the sight of a particular color reminiscent of the attacker's clothing.

A recent pilot study focusing on sensory symptoms in PTSD treatment found that survivors exhibit various sensory abnormalities, with differences based on the type of traumatic experience: Cluster 1, comprising child abuse and violence, showed hypersensitivity to auditory, tactile, and hyperarousal symptoms; Cluster 2, including natural disasters, accidents, and sexual assault, experienced vivid visual and olfactory flashbacks; Cluster 3, linked to multiple traumas, displayed dissociation symptoms, possibly indicating severe and repeated trauma from early childhood, particularly associated with taste (Aoki & Nozawa, 2024).

Moreover, individuals grappling with PTSD often exhibit a cluster of behavioral patterns. Efforts to suppress traumatic thoughts and emotions frequently prove futile, leading to a pervasive sense of emotional detachment and a diminished capacity for experiencing joy or affection. This emotional numbness may be likened to feeling as though one is watching life from behind a glass barrier, unable to fully engage. Consider, for instance, a veteran struggling to reconnect with loved ones after returning from war, feeling disconnected and unable to express love or affection as they once did.

Furthermore, memories of traumatic events can become fragmented or distorted, leaving significant gaps in one's recollection of the experience. Alongside this, there may be a profound sense of uncertainty about the future, making it difficult to envision a path forward filled with stability and fulfillment.

Additionally, individuals with PTSD often experience heightened arousal, characterized by difficulty sleeping, irritability, and an exaggerated startle response. For example, a survivor of a car accident might find themselves constantly on edge, unable to relax even in seemingly safe environments due to heightened vigilance and a persistent sense of danger.

The diagnosis of PTSD hinges on the endurance of these symptoms for at least a month, with some cases resolving relatively quickly while others become chronic, enduring for years or even a lifetime. Let us explore the behavioral symptoms of PTSD in more detail.

ANALYSIS OF TYPICAL BEHAVIORAL SYMPTOMS

Avoidance

Avoidance behavior is a hallmark symptom of Post-Traumatic Stress Disorder (PTSD) and plays a crucial role in how individuals cope with the aftermath of traumatic experiences (Monane et al., 2018). It encompasses a range of actions aimed at steering clear of anything that may remind the individual of the traumatic event they endured. This avoidance can extend to various aspects of their lives, including physical locations, specific people, activities, or even certain sensory stimuli that evoke distressing memories or emotions associated with the trauma.

The avoidance is driven by a deep-seated desire to sidestep the intense emotional distress and anxiety that often accompany recollections of the traumatic event. By actively avoiding triggers, individuals with PTSD attempt to shield themselves from the overwhelming flood of emotions, sensations, and memories that threaten to engulf them. This avoidance behavior becomes a coping mechanism, albeit a maladaptive one, as it provides temporary relief from distress but ultimately perpetuates the cycle of avoidance and emotional suppression (Yehuda et al., 2015).

For instance, someone who survived a car accident may avoid driving or even being near cars altogether to prevent triggering memories of the traumatic event. Similarly, a combat veteran might avoid crowded places or loud noises to avoid being reminded of their experiences in combat zones.

While avoidance behavior may offer temporary respite from distress, it can have profound and detrimental effects on the individual's life in the long term. When avoidance predominates as the primary coping mechanism, it significantly contributes to the onset and persistence of posttraumatic stress disorder (Coll et al., 2022). It can lead to social withdrawal, strained relationships, difficulty in maintaining employment, and a diminished quality of life.

A recent study, examined the gaze patterns of 159 participants, including those exposed to the 2015 Paris terrorist attacks and those who were not. Among the exposed participants, 52 were diagnosed with PTSD (PTSD+), while 51 did not develop PTSD (PTSD-). Results showed that PTSD+ individuals spent significantly less time looking at sad eyes compared to PTSD- and non-exposed individuals, a tendency that correlated with the severity of avoidance symptoms. No differences were observed in attention to neutral and happy faces. These findings suggest that maladaptive avoidance behaviors in PTSD extend to social processing, particularly in terms of reduced attention to others' emotions, unrelated to trauma (Coll et al., 2022).

Moreover, avoiding reminders of the trauma prevents the individual from processing and integrating the traumatic experience into their narrative, hindering the healing process.

Social Withdrawal

Social withdrawal is a prevalent and significant aspect of the experience of individuals living with Post-Traumatic Stress Disorder (PTSD) (Schweitzer et al., 2006). It manifests as a retreat from social interactions and relationships, stemming from a complex interplay of psychological and emotional factors deeply rooted in the aftermath of trauma.

A recent study investigated the connection between emotional suppression, rejection sensitivity, and social isolation in 300 veterans with PTSD. Results showed that emotional inhibition and sensitivity to rejection directly influenced social isolation among veterans with PTSD, with emotional inhibition indirectly affecting social isolation through rejection sensitivity (Eyni et al., 2024).

For those with PTSD, social withdrawal can become a pervasive pattern, characterized by a reluctance to engage with others, a sense of disconnection, and difficulties in trusting or feeling safe in interpersonal relationships (Lord, 2008). This withdrawal often arises from profound feelings of alienation and isolation, fueled by a sense of being fundamentally different from those around them. Individuals may struggle to relate to the experiences and concerns of others, feeling as though their own traumatic experiences set them apart from the rest of society. For example, a survivor of sexual assault might avoid social gatherings or intimate relationships out of fear of being vulnerable again.

At the core of social withdrawal in PTSD is a profound sense of mistrust and fear of vulnerability in social situations (Charuvastra & Cloitre, 2008). Having experienced the trauma, individuals may harbor deep-seated apprehensions about being hurt or betrayed again, leading them to erect emotional barriers and distance themselves from potential sources of emotional pain.

Moreover, the pervasive sense of loneliness and alienation that accompanies social withdrawal can exacerbate existing symptoms of PTSD, perpetuating a cycle of isolation and emotional distress.

Hyperarousal

It manifests as a persistent state of heightened physiological and psychological arousal, wherein individuals remain on high alert, perceiving threats in their environment even when none are present (Burback et al., 2024). For instance, a survivor of a natural disaster may become easily agitated by loud noises or sudden movements.

In a recent study on cognitive processing therapy (CPT) for active-duty service members with PTSD, researchers examined hyperarousal symptoms' responsiveness versus other clusters. Results showed that among improvers, hyperarousal persisted in 69% versus 49% for other symptoms. Among those recovered, 26% still had hyperarousal versus almost none for other clusters. These findings suggest the need for further targeted treatment for persistent hyperarousal symptoms post-CPT (Miles et al., 2023).

Physiologically, hyperarousal can manifest in various ways. Individuals may find themselves easily startled or jumpy, with even minor stimuli triggering exaggerated startle responses. This heightened reactivity stems from a primal instinct to react swiftly to potential danger, yet in the context of PTSD, it becomes maladaptive, causing distress and disrupting daily functioning. Furthermore, individuals may experience an increased heart rate, rapid breathing, muscle tension, and sweating, reflecting the body's heightened state of readiness to confront perceived threats (McCurry et al., 2020).

Psychologically, hyperarousal is accompanied by a persistent sense of unease and vigilance. Individuals with PTSD often exhibit hypervigilance, constantly scanning their surroundings for signs of danger. This hypervigilance is fueled by a deep-seated fear of re-experiencing the trauma or encountering situations reminiscent of the traumatic event. As a result, individuals may struggle to relax or let their guard down, leading to chronic feelings of anxiety, tension, and exhaustion.

Moreover, hyperarousal can profoundly impact cognitive functioning, impairing attention, concentration, and memory. Individuals may find it challenging to focus on tasks or engage in activities, as their attention is frequently drawn towards potential threats or triggers in their environment (Sadeghi et al., 2022). This cognitive fog further exacerbates feelings of frustration and helplessness, hindering the individual's ability to function effectively in their daily lives.

A research study investigated the relationship between childhood physical abuse, posttraumatic stress disorder (PTSD), depression, and suicidal ideation in PTSD patients using path analysis. A total of 114 PTSD patients completed psychological assessments, and structural equation modeling was utilized to analyze the data. Hyperarousal symptoms were found to specifically mediate the relationship between childhood physical abuse and suicidal ideation (Kwon et al., 2021).

Cumulative effects of hyperarousal can take a significant toll on individuals' overall well-being and quality of life.

Reckless or Self-Destructive Behavior

It encompasses a range of actions that disregard personal safety and well being, often driven by a desperate attempt to cope with the overwhelming emotional turmoil and distress stemming from the traumatic experience (Kerig, 2019).

Individuals with PTSD commonly engage in substance abuse as a reckless coping mechanism, using alcohol, drugs, or prescription medications to numb emotions and escape trauma memories. However, this fleeting relief can escalate into addiction, worsening symptoms and complicating recovery.

A research study aimed to assess the clinical significance of Criterion E2 ("reckless or self-destructive behavior") in the DSM-5 criteria for posttraumatic stress disorder (PTSD). Using data from the 2012–2013 National Epidemiologic Survey on Alcohol and Related Conditions, researchers examined the prevalence and associations of risky and unhealthy behaviors (RUBs) with Criterion E2 endorsement, as well as its associations with psychiatric conditions in trauma exposed adults. Results showed that all RUBs, except binge eating, were associated with Criterion E2 endorsement, with greater substance use being the most prevalent among those who endorsed E2. Additionally, Criterion E2 endorsement was linked to increased odds of PTSD, bipolar disorder, substance use disorders, and certain personality disorders, and decreased odds of major depressive disorder (Sommer et al., 2020).

A recent study investigated the relationships among different reckless behaviors and PTSD symptom clusters in a sample of 417 participants recruited from Amazon's Mechanical Turk. Results indicated strong associations within each construct (PTSD and reckless behaviors) and identified connections between PTSD clusters and reckless behaviors. Most reckless behavior items were directly linked to one or more PTSD symptom clusters (Armour et al., 2020).

Self-harm is another alarming expression of reckless behavior in individuals with PTSD. This may involve cutting, burning, or other forms of self-injury as a means of coping with emotional pain or regaining a sense of control over overwhelming feelings.

A study investigated the prevalence and factors associated with thoughts of suicide or self-harm among healthcare workers during the COVID-19 pandemic, as well as their help-seeking behaviors. Results showed that 10.5% of healthcare workers reported thoughts of suicide or self-harm over a 2-week period, with higher rates among those experiencing depression, anxiety, PTSD, and burnout (Bismark et al., 2022).

Despite offering temporary relief from distress, reckless or self-destructive behaviors ultimately perpetuate the cycle of trauma and exacerbate feelings of guilt, shame, and isolation.

Emotional Numbing

It manifests as a profound diminishment in the capacity to experience and express emotions, leaving individuals feeling detached or disconnected from their inner emotional landscape and external surroundings (Laws, 2019). Example, a person who witnessed a traumatic accident may find it difficult to feel happiness or enthusiasm about anything in their life.

Using data from two different sets of trauma-exposed individuals, a recent study evaluated the unique contribution of PTSD diagnosis and symptom severity to emotional numbing symptoms. Results showed that PTSD diagnosis contributed significantly to emotional numbing symptoms, even after accounting for MDD symptoms (Duek et al., 2023).

In PTSD, emotional numbing presents as a deep sense of emptiness or detachment, hindering connections with one's own emotions and others. This detachment acts as a protective barrier against overwhelming emotions tied to the trauma, like fear or sadness (Korem et al., 2022). Numbing emotions aims to create a buffer, offering temporary relief from emotional distress.

Emotional numbness, while offering temporary relief, hampers full engagement with life. It strains relationships, causing isolation, and prevents experiencing joy or fulfillment, leaving individuals feeling disconnected and adrift (Bryant, 2022).

Intrusive Memories: Flashbacks and Nightmares

They represent intrusive and distressing re-experiencing of the traumatic event, thrusting the individual back into the terrifying reality of their past trauma (Phelps et al., 2008).

Flashbacks are visceral and vivid recollections of the traumatic event that intrude upon the individual's consciousness with startling intensity (Bar-Haim et al., 2021). During a flashback, the individual may feel as though they are reliving the traumatic experience in real-time, complete with sensory details and overwhelming emotions.

A recent study explored the link between sleep duration on the first night after trauma and intrusive memories in the following week, and their connection to PTSD symptoms after 2 months. Patients from the emergency department documented their sleep and intrusive memories post-trauma. Results revealed a U-shaped pattern between sleep duration and intrusive memories, with both too little and too much sleep associated with more intrusive memories. Those meeting PTSD criteria at 2 months had notably more intrusive memories during the first post-trauma week (Porcheret et al., 2020). This suggests that keeping track of sleep and intrusive memories in the week following a traumatic event could help identify individuals who might be more likely to develop PTSD later on.

The involuntary re-enactment of the trauma can be triggered by various stimuli reminiscent of the traumatic event, such as sights, sounds, smells, or even specific thoughts or emotions. Regardless of the trigger, flashbacks plunge the individual into a state of acute distress and terror, disrupting their sense of time and reality and leaving them feeling utterly helpless and overwhelmed (Schäfer et al., 2023).

Nightmares, recurring dreams linked to trauma, disrupt sleep, depriving individuals of rest. For instance, a car accident survivor might relive the crash, feeling trapped in a nightmare. These vivid dreams replay the trauma, causing fear and panic upon waking, worsening exhaustion and distress.

A study investigated factors influencing posttrauma nightmares in 27 female college students with a history of sexual trauma. Participants recorded presleep cognitive arousal, sleep latency, and nightmares for six days. Results showed that both presleep cognitive arousal and sleep latency predicted nightmares. Presleep cognitive arousal also moderated the link between sleep latency and nightmares, highlighting its significance before sleep in triggering posttrauma nightmares (Youngren et al., 2020).

Flashbacks and nightmares relentlessly revive traumatic memories, fueling intense emotions like fear, anger, shame, and sadness. This cycle of intrusive memories and terrifying dreams can trap individuals in a perpetual state of terror, unable to break free from their past trauma (Lanctôt et al., 2020).

Aggression or Violence

PTSD can trigger aggression or violence due to intense anger, frustration, or fear (Novaco, 2010). It may be a misguided effort to assert control in overwhelming situations, stemming from feelings of powerlessness and vulnerability after trauma. For instance, a domestic abuse survivor might react aggressively during arguments, triggered by certain words or gestures.

A research study delved into how soldiers' experiences during deployment, such as exposure to violence and their own participation in it, affect their mental well-being afterward. The research found that soldiers who showed a strong desire for violence and experienced symptoms of posttraumatic stress disorder (PTSD), such as hyperarousal, were more likely to engage in violent acts during deployment. Furthermore, it revealed that these factors could create a cycle, where experiencing violence and trauma during deployment could lead to increased aggressive tendencies and PTSD symptoms afterward (Nandi et al., 2020).

Aggression in PTSD can be a misguided effort to regain control or power when faced with perceived threats or overwhelming situations (Wamser-Nanney et al., 2021). Stemming from a primal instinct for self-preservation, it can be distorted and exaggerated in this context.

During heightened arousal, individuals with PTSD may struggle to control their responses, resulting in verbal or physical outbursts towards themselves or others. These outbursts, from shouting matches to physical altercations, stem from a desperate attempt to relieve overwhelming distress (McRae et al., 2021).

The behavioral indicators of PTSD offer crucial insights into how trauma affects daily life and interactions, from avoidance behaviors to heightened arousal. However, alongside these, delving into the phenomenological indicators of the disorder is equally important.

PHENOMENOLOGICAL COMPONENTS OF PTSD

Shifting focus to the phenomenological aspects of PTSD means moving from observable behaviors to individuals' subjective experiences and internal processes. Phenomenology emphasizes each person's unique perspective, revealing the underlying structures and meanings in their subjective experiences. This approach explores the interplay between perception, interpretation, and meaning-making (Malaktaris & Lynn, 2019).

Phenomenology in psychology offers a valuable framework for exploring deeply personal and subjective phenomena like trauma, grief, identity, and existential concerns. Phenomenological aspects of PTSD cover subjective experiences not always visible in behaviors. These include changes in consciousness, disruptions in self-identity, existential questioning, and shifts in relationship to time and space (Perrotta, 2020). For example, those with PTSD may feel detached, experience unreality, or battle intrusive thoughts disrupting their sense of time continuity.

Phenomenological exploration reveals how trauma disrupts core beliefs about oneself and the world, leading to existential crises. Individuals question why it happened, its impact on identity, and its reconciliation with their worldview.

Moreover, phenomenological inquiry sheds light on the emotional landscape of PTSD beyond surface-level symptoms (Wilde, 2022). It explores the depth of emotional pain, despair, and existential angst that individuals may experience in the aftermath of trauma. This includes feelings of guilt, shame, anger, and profound sorrow that can permeate every aspect of one's being.

In the next section, we'll analyze key case studies by leading researchers to explore PTSD's phenomenological aspects. These studies provide insights into trauma, memory, and well-being, deepening our understanding of PTSD's effects.

NOTABLE CASE STUDIES

Anna Freud's Research on Child Psychoanalysis

An influential case study involves Anna Freud, daughter of Sigmund Freud, who explored the impact of trauma on child development. Her insights, drawn from her work with children during and after World War II, revealed the lasting effects of wartime experiences such as evacuations or loss of caregivers (Tyson, 2009). Working at the Hampstead War Nurseries in London, Anna Freud closely observed separated children, documenting their behaviors and emotional responses. She noted symptoms like anxiety, nightmares, behavioral issues, and attachment difficulties, highlighting the enduring psychological impact of such disruptions (Midgley, 2007).

Anna Freud observed intense anxiety as a prominent phenomenological symptom among children separated from their families. They displayed heightened vigilance and restlessness, even in the absence of immediate danger, indicating the lasting impact of trauma (Midgley, 2007). Nightmares were also prevalent, with children experiencing distressing dreams reliving traumatic events or themes of loss and danger, exacerbating their fear and helplessness. Additionally, behavioral disturbances, including aggression and withdrawal, were noted, with some children exhibiting regression or engaging in self-destructive behaviors as coping mechanisms (Midgley, 2007). Freud's case study underscored the complex relationship between traumatic experiences and phenomenological symptoms in childhood PTSD.

Bessel van der Kolk's Research

Bessel van der Kolk investigated the neurobiology of trauma, using advanced neuroimaging techniques like functional magnetic resonance imaging (fMRI) to uncover PTSD's neural correlates (Clark et al., 2022). His research revealed significant differences in brain activity patterns between individuals with and without PTSD, particularly in areas linked to emotional regulation, memory processing, and stress response. Van der Kolk noted heightened activity in regions associated with emotional reactivity and arousal, like the amygdala, suggesting a hypersensitivity to threat cues and contributing to characteristic hyperarousal and exaggerated startle responses in PTSD (Calinescu, 2023).

Van der Kolk's research revealed changes in brain regions linked to memory processing, like the hippocampus. Individuals with PTSD showed reduced hippocampal volume and impaired functioning, affecting the encoding and retrieval of traumatic memories (Reis & Ortega, 2021). These findings illuminate the persistent intrusion of traumatic memories and the challenges in processing and integrating them into coherent narratives. Van der Kolk's study offered vital insights into the intricate relationship between trauma and brain function.

Judith Herman's Research

Judith Herman's "Trauma and Recovery" significantly contributed to understanding PTSD's phenomenological aspects, especially in interpersonal trauma like domestic violence and sexual abuse. Her work revealed how traumatic experiences deeply affect survivors' identity, relationships, and self-perception (Zaleski et al., 2016).

Herman's work highlighted trauma's pervasive impact on survivors' sense of self, revealing how it fractures their life narrative and leads to identity fragmentation. Survivors struggle with disconnection from themselves, their emotions, and past experiences, finding it challenging to integrate trauma into their identity (DuBois, 2023). Additionally, Herman emphasized trauma's profound effect on survivors' self-perception and worldview, often resulting in shame, guilt, and self-blame. These negative self-appraisals intensify feelings of alienation and perpetuate cycles of distress (Mohammed, 2022).

Edward Tick's Research

Tick's research on collective trauma uncovered widespread psychological distress and cultural ruptures within affected communities (MacLeish, 2018). He documented high rates of anxiety, depression, and PTSD symptoms, alongside disturbances in interpersonal relationships and social dynamics (Temoney, 2021). Tick emphasized changes in cultural norms and the intergenerational transmission of trauma, highlighting the enduring legacy and long-term consequences of collective trauma (Hobbs, 2023).

Rachel Yehuda's Research

Yehuda's research on epigenetics and PTSD has shown how traumatic experiences can affect individuals and future generations (Bowers & Yehuda, 2016). She identified specific epigenetic changes linked to PTSD, including alterations in DNA methylation and histone modifications in genes related to stress response and emotional regulation (Carmi et al., 2023). These changes contribute to heightened stress reactivity and dysregulated emotional responses in PTSD. Yehuda also revealed transgenerational epigenetic inheritance, indicating trauma's effects can be passed down through non-genetic mechanisms.

Christine Courtois's Research

Christine Courtois's seminal work on Complex PTSD has significantly advanced our understanding of the unique challenges faced by individuals who have experienced prolonged, repeated trauma, often of an interpersonal nature. Through her research, Courtois has delved into the phenomenological aspects of complex trauma, shedding light on the intricate manifestations and symptoms associated with this condition (Brown et al., 2021).

Courtois's research highlights disruptions in self-organization in Complex PTSD, affecting identity, self-concept, and core beliefs. Individuals with this condition often struggle to maintain a cohesive sense of self, experiencing fragmentation, dissociation, and identity confusion due to trauma (Ford & Courtois, 2021). Affect dysregulation, studied by Courtois in Complex PTSD, involves difficulty regulating emotions, leading to mood swings, emotional numbing, and arousal challenges. This dysregulation can severely impact daily functioning, causing relationship issues, impulsivity, and self-destructive behaviors (Kumar et al., 2022).

COMPARING BEHAVIORAL AND PHENOMENOLOGICAL PERSPECTIVES

PTSD's behavioral symptoms, like avoidance, hypervigilance, and agitation, are evident to others, reflecting coping efforts post-trauma. In contrast, its phenomenological aspects explore inner experiences like consciousness alterations and identity disruptions, less observable but deeply felt by the individual (Palgi et al., 2021).

Behavioral symptoms of PTSD are overt and observable, while phenomenological aspects are covert and subjective, delving into the individual's thoughts, emotions, and perceptions of themselves and the world. Assessing these aspects often requires nuanced methods like qualitative interviews or narrative analysis (Jones et al., 2022). Both dimensions significantly impact daily functioning and quality of life, serving as adaptive or maladaptive coping mechanisms post-trauma, affecting work, relationships, and overall well-being.

Behavioral symptoms and psychological experiences in PTSD are intertwined. For instance, avoidance behaviors may stem from intrusive thoughts, while disruptions in self-identity may lead to social withdrawal or recklessness (Ophir & Jacoby, 2020). Understanding this connection is vital for effective PTSD assessment and treatment.

TREATMENT OF PTSD

The behavioral and phenomenological aspects of PTSD are pivotal in diagnosis, treatment, and support for affected individuals. While behavioral symptoms are central to diagnosis, understanding phenomenological aspects is equally vital. Delving into subjective experiences aids accurate diagnosis and treatment planning. Let's examine popular PTSD treatment strategies.

Exposure therapy

Exposure therapy is a well-established and highly effective treatment for PTSD that aims to reduce avoidance behaviors and alleviate the distress associated with traumatic memories. It operates on the principle of habituation, where repeated exposure to distressing stimuli leads to a reduction in the emotional response over time (McLean et al., 2022).

A recent meta-analysis investigated the effectiveness of exposure therapy for posttraumatic stress disorder (PTSD) compared to various control conditions. After screening 934 abstracts, 65 articles (comprising 4929 patients) were included. Exposure therapy showed significant benefits compared to waitlist and treatment-as-usual conditions, moderate benefits over medication at follow-up, and similar effectiveness to other exposure-based treatments. Moderator analyses revealed that exposure therapy was more effective in studies with fewer sessions, younger participants, and those with fewer individuals diagnosed with substance use disorder or on psychiatric medication. Additionally, it was more effective in studies of refugees and civilians, as well as in individual therapy compared to group therapy (McLean et al., 2022).

Another study explored the effectiveness of exposure therapy for posttraumatic stress disorder (PTSD) in military populations, compared to various control conditions. Nineteen randomized controlled trials involving Veterans and active duty military personnel were included in the meta-analysis, with a total of 2905 participants. Exposure therapy demonstrated medium to large effects compared to waitlist and treatment-as-usual conditions, a small effect compared to non-trauma-focused therapy, and no significant effect relative to other trauma-focused therapies. The effectiveness of exposure therapy was consistent both immediately after treatment and at follow-up. The study found that exposure therapy was more effective in studies with younger participants, more women, fewer individuals with comorbid major depression, and fewer participants taking psychiatric medication (McLean et al., 2022).

In exposure therapy, individuals collaborate with a therapist to create an anxiety hierarchy related to their trauma. This ranges from mild to intense triggers, with each step ensuring safety. Sessions involve gradual exposure to distressing stimuli through techniques like imaginal, in vivo, or virtual reality exposure.

During exposure, individuals are urged to confront their thoughts, emotions, and bodily sensations without avoiding or using safety behaviors. Repeatedly facing feared stimuli gradually reduces distress intensity. Through desensitization, exposure therapy aids in reprocessing traumatic memories, fostering emotional processing and mastery. This approach reduces symptoms of avoidance, numbing, and hyperarousal linked to PTSD (Bourassa et al., 2020).

Cognitive-Behavioral Therapy

CBT for PTSD combines cognitive restructuring with behavioral techniques to address cognitive and emotional aspects of the disorder. Traumatic experiences can distort thoughts, beliefs, and perceptions, leading to maladaptive coping and distress. In therapy, individuals and therapists collaboratively identify and challenge maladaptive thought patterns like catastrophizing, personalization, and overgeneralization (Shubina, 2015)

Through cognitive restructuring techniques, individuals learn to examine the evidence for and against their negative thoughts and beliefs, as well as to develop more balanced and realistic perspectives. This process involves identifying cognitive distortions, challenging their accuracy and validity, and replacing them with more adaptive and balanced interpretations of the traumatic event and its aftermath (Trottier & Monson, 2021).

Reframing negative thoughts and replacing them with adaptive ones reduces feelings of guilt, shame, or self-blame associated with PTSD. Individuals learn that their thoughts aren't always accurate reflections of reality but are shaped by past experiences, beliefs, and perceptions.

CBT for PTSD also includes behavioural interventions like relaxation techniques to manage hyperarousal and reactivity symptoms.

Overall, CBT for PTSD provides individuals with a structured and systematic approach to address the cognitive and behavioral aspects of the disorder. By challenging maladaptive thought patterns and equipping individuals with coping strategies, it empowers them to regain a sense of control over their thoughts, emotions, and behaviors, ultimately promoting recovery and resilience in the face of trauma (McGeary et al., 2022).

Narrative Therapy

Unlike traditional therapeutic models that focus solely on symptom reduction, narrative therapy emphasizes collaboration between the therapist and client to co-create a new understanding of one's experiences (Cloitre et al., 2017).

Central to narrative therapy is the concept of externalizing problems. Therapists encourage clients to view their traumatic experiences as separate from themselves, reframing them as external entities that can be explored and understood. This separation allows individuals to gain a sense of agency and control over their experiences, shifting from a position of helplessness to one of empowerment.

A study examined cognitive-narrative therapy's effectiveness in treating depression, PTSD, CPTSD, and borderline symptoms in women who've experienced intimate partner violence (IPV). It involved a longitudinal randomized controlled trial with 19 participants, comparing outcomes between control and treatment groups. Measures like the Patient Health Questionnaire, International Trauma Questionnaire, and Diagnostic Interview Schedule for PTSD and CPTSD were used. The treatment group received a four-session cognitive-narrative intervention. While no significant differences were found at baseline and follow-up, positive effect sizes were noted for depression, PTSD, and borderline symptoms, suggesting potential benefits (Moreira et al., 2022).

Therapists guide clients in constructing a new narrative that highlights their strengths, values, and aspirations, thereby diminishing the overwhelming impact of the trauma on their identity and sense of self (Raghuraman et al., 2021).

The process of narrative therapy involves engaging in a collaborative and reflective dialogue between the therapist and client. Through open-ended questions, active listening, and empathic understanding, therapists create a safe and supportive environment for clients to explore and make sense of their experiences. By sharing their stories and reflecting on their journey, individuals can begin to reclaim ownership of their narrative and reshape their understanding of themselves in relation to their trauma.

Importantly, narrative therapy fosters a sense of agency and self-determination, empowering individuals to take an active role in shaping their lives beyond the constraints of their past traumas. By reframing their experiences within a broader context of resilience and growth, individuals can integrate the trauma into their life narrative in a way that promotes healing and transformation.

Mindfulness Based Approaches

Mindfulness-based approaches, including mindfulness-based stress reduction (MBSR) and mindfulness-based cognitive therapy (MBCT), offer individuals with PTSD a transformative path towards healing by fostering present-moment awareness and non-judgmental acceptance of their experiences (Boyd et al., 2018).

Central to mindfulness-based interventions is the cultivation of mindfulness, which involves intentionally paying attention to the present moment with openness, curiosity, and acceptance. Through mindfulness practices such as meditation, breath awareness, and body scanning, individuals learn to observe their thoughts, emotions, and bodily sensations without getting caught up in them or reacting impulsively (Williston et al., 2021).

For individuals with PTSD, mindfulness practices can be particularly beneficial in several ways. A recent review examined the use of mindfulness-based interventions (MBIs) among military Veterans over the past five years to inform clinical care and future research. A systematic literature review identified 27 articles meeting inclusion criteria, with most employing quantitative methods. MBIs showed potential as adjunctive interventions for Veterans with PTSD and other psychiatric disorders (Marchand et al., 2021).

Rumination, or repetitive thinking about past traumatic events, is a common symptom of PTSD that can exacerbate distress and impair functioning. Mindfulness practices encourage individuals to observe their thoughts without getting entangled in them, breaking the cycle of rumination and creating space for more adaptive cognitive processing (Szoke et al., 2021). By cultivating a non-judgmental attitude towards their thoughts, individuals can reduce the grip of intrusive memories and gradually disengage from the cycle of rumination.

Mindfulness equips individuals with a toolkit of coping skills that they can draw upon to navigate the challenges of PTSD.

RECENT RESEARCHES ON TREATMENT STRATEGIES OF PTSD

Shared Decision Making and Collaborative Care

Shared Decision Making (SDM) involves healthcare providers and patients working together to make decisions about treatment. It emphasizes the importance of considering both the healthcare provider's expertise and the patient's preferences, values, and goals. Collaborative Care, on the other hand, is a model of healthcare delivery that involves multiple healthcare professionals (such as primary care physicians, mental health specialists, nurses, etc.) working together to provide comprehensive and coordinated care to patients. It often includes elements like care coordination, communication between providers, and integration of mental health services into primary care settings. In the context of treating PTSD, Shared Decision Making and Collaborative Care can involve discussing treatment options with the patient, considering their preferences and needs, and coordinating care between different healthcare professionals to provide holistic and effective treatment. This have been recognized as highly recommended treatment approaches for PTSD (Schrader & Ross, 2021), (US Preventive Services Task Force, 2022),

Trauma-focused therapies

Trauma-focused therapies, such as Cognitive Processing Therapy (CPT) and Prolonged Exposure (PE), are among the most widely researched and effective treatments for PTSD (Post-Traumatic Stress Disorder). These therapies are specifically designed to address the symptoms and underlying causes of PTSD resulting from traumatic experiences (Rutt et al., 2018), (Goetter et al., 2021), (Jericho et al., 2022), (Schnurr et al., 2022).

Cognitive Processing Therapy focuses on helping individuals understand and change unhelpful beliefs and thoughts related to their traumatic experience. It typically involves structured sessions where the therapist helps the individual identify and challenge maladaptive beliefs about themselves, others, and the world that may have developed as a result of the trauma.

Prolonged Exposure (PE) aims to reduce symptoms of PTSD by helping individuals confront and process traumatic memories and situations that they have been avoiding. This therapy involves gradually and systematically exposing the individual to trauma-related memories, thoughts, and situations in a safe and controlled environment. Through repeated exposure, individuals learn that their anxiety and distress decrease over time, leading to habituation and decreased avoidance of trauma-related stimuli. PE also includes elements of imaginal exposure, where individuals vividly recount their traumatic experiences, and in vivo exposure, where they gradually approach real-life situations that they have been avoiding.

In a randomized clinical trial by Schnurr et al. (2022) involving 916 veterans, two evidence-based psychotherapies were compared for treating PTSD. Both treatment groups showed improvements in PTSD symptoms. However, Prolonged Exposure was found to be more effective than Cognitive Processing Therapy in reducing PTSD symptoms.

In a study conducted by Rutt et al. (2018), 750 veterans from 10 U.S. states who underwent individual psychotherapy with either cognitive processing therapy or prolonged exposure were included. Among them, 376 participants received cognitive processing therapy, and 374 received prolonged exposure. The study utilized multilevel modeling to assess the absolute and relative effectiveness of both treatments and examine the association between patient-level variables and total Posttraumatic Stress Disorder Checklist scores during treatment. Cognitive processing therapy and prolonged exposure were found to be effective in real-world clinical settings and with a diverse sample of veterans.

Lewis et al. (2020) conducted a systematic review to assess the effect sizes of manualized therapies for post-traumatic stress disorder (PTSD). The study suggests that recent research supports CBT with a trauma focus and EMDR as first-line treatments for PTSD, with CPT, CT, and PE being preferred options among the CBT therapies.

Both CPT and PE are typically delivered over a series of sessions by trained mental health professionals. These therapies have been extensively researched and have demonstrated effectiveness in reducing PTSD symptoms, improving overall functioning, and enhancing quality of life for individuals who have experienced trauma. Additionally, they are recommended as first-line treatments for PTSD by organizations such as the American Psychological Association and the Department of Veterans Affairs (Schrader & Ross, 2021).

Van Minnen et al., 2020, explored the impact of treatment sequence on the effectiveness of two trauma-focused therapies, Prolonged Exposure (PE) and Eye Movement Desensitization and Reprocessing (EMDR), for PTSD. The study found that administering PE sessions before EMDR sessions resulted in better treatment outcomes and subjective patient evaluations compared to the reverse sequence.

Eye Movement Desensitization and Reprocessing (EMDR), has gained recognition as a first-line treatment for PTSD, particularly in cases where traditional psychotherapies may not be feasible or preferred by the patient (Al Jowf et al., 2023). It is supported by over 30 published randomized controlled trials (RCTs) showcasing its effectiveness in treating posttraumatic stress disorder (PTSD), both in adults and children (de Jongh et al., 2024). EMDR involves the patient recalling distressing memories while simultaneously undergoing bilateral sensory stimulation, such as following the therapist's hand movements with their eyes. This process aims to help the individual reprocess traumatic memories and alleviate associated distress and symptoms (Scelles & Bulnes, 2021).

CONCLUSION

In this chapter, the exploration of both behavioral and phenomenological perspectives sheds light on the multifaceted nature of Post-Traumatic Stress Disorder (PTSD) and its significance in understanding individuals' experiences of trauma. Beginning with an introduction to PTSD, the chapter highlights the profound impact this disorder has on individuals' lives, particularly in today's context where mental health awareness is growing.

By analyzing typical behavioral symptoms, the chapter provides a framework for recognizing and addressing observable manifestations of PTSD. This discussion emphasizes the importance of identifying outward signs that individuals may exhibit in response to trauma.

Simultaneously, the exploration of phenomenological components emphasizes the significance of understanding the internal experiences and subjective realities of those grappling with PTSD. This perspective highlights the importance of acknowledging the diverse ways in which individuals experience and cope with trauma.

The inclusion of notable case studies humanizes the discussions, illustrating the various ways in which PTSD can manifest in individuals' lives. These case studies serve as reminders of the complexities and nuances inherent in the experience of trauma.

Comparing behavioral and phenomenological perspectives allows for a holistic understanding of PTSD, emphasizing the interconnectedness of observable behaviors and internal experiences. This integrated approach is particularly relevant in today's context, where mental health care is increasingly focused on providing personalized and comprehensive support to individuals affected by trauma.

Finally, the exploration of treatment modalities underscores the importance of implementing evidence-based interventions that address both the behavioral and phenomenological aspects of PTSD. By integrating diverse therapeutic approaches, individuals can receive more effective support on their journey towards healing and recovery in today's complex world.

In summary, the discussions within this chapter highlight the importance of taking a holistic and compassionate approach to understanding and addressing PTSD. By embracing both behavioral and phenomenological perspectives, clinicians and support systems can provide more effective care and support to individuals affected by trauma, ultimately fostering resilience and promoting healing.

REFERENCES

Al Jowf, G. I., Ahmed, Z. T., Reijnders, R. A., de Nijs, L., & Eijssen, L. M. T. (2023). To Predict, Prevent, and Manage Post-Traumatic Stress Disorder (PTSD): A Review of Pathophysiology, Treatment, and Biomarkers. *International Journal of Molecular Sciences*, 24(6), 6. Advance online publication. DOI: 10.3390/ijms24065238 PMID: 36982313

Aoki, S., & Nozawa, E. (2024). Pilot Study on Classification of Sensory Symptoms in PTSD. *Journal of Child & Adolescent Trauma*, 17(2), 283–293. Advance online publication. DOI: 10.1007/s40653-023-00602-5 PMID: 38938954

Armour, C., Greene, T., Contractor, A. A., Weiss, N., Dixon-Gordon, K., & Ross, J. (2020). Posttraumatic Stress Disorder Symptoms and Reckless Behaviors: A Network Analysis Approach. *Journal of Traumatic Stress*, 33(1), 29–40. DOI: 10.1002/jts.22487 PMID: 32086982

Bar-Haim, Y., Stein, M. B., Bryant, R. A., Bliese, P. D., Ben Yehuda, A., Kringelbach, M. L., Jain, S., Dan, O., Lazarov, A., Wald, I., Levi, O., Neria, Y., & Pine, D. S. (2021). Intrusive Traumatic Reexperiencing: Pathognomonic of the Psychological Response to Traumatic Stress. *The American Journal of Psychiatry*, 178(2), 119–122. DOI: 10.1176/appi.ajp.2020.19121231 PMID: 33517759

Bismark, M., Scurrah, K., Pascoe, A., Willis, K., Jain, R., & Smallwood, N. (2022). Thoughts of suicide or self-harm among Australian healthcare workers during the COVID-19 pandemic. *The Australian and New Zealand Journal of Psychiatry*, 56(12), 1555–1565. DOI: 10.1177/00048674221075540 PMID: 35128948

Bourassa, K. J., Smolenski, D. J., Edwards-Stewart, A., Campbell, S. B., Reger, G. M., & Norr, A. M. (2020). The impact of prolonged exposure therapy on social support and PTSD symptoms. *Journal of Affective Disorders*, 260, 410–417. DOI: 10.1016/j.jad.2019.09.036 PMID: 31539674

Bowers, M. E., & Yehuda, R. (2016). Intergenerational Effects of PTSD on Offspring Glucocorticoid Receptor Methylation. In Spengler, D., & Binder, E. (Eds.), *Epigenetics and Neuroendocrinology: Clinical Focus on Psychiatry* (Vol. 2, pp. 141–155). Springer International Publishing., DOI: 10.1007/978-3-319-29901-3_6

Boyd, J. E., Lanius, R. A., & McKinnon, M. C. (2018). Mindfulness-based treatments for posttraumatic stress disorder: A review of the treatment literature and neurobiological evidence. *Journal of Psychiatry & Neuroscience*, 43(1), 7–25. DOI: 10.1503/jpn.170021 PMID: 29252162

Brown, S. L., Wanamaker, K. A., Greiner, L., Scott, T., & Skilling, T. A. (2021). Complex Trauma and Criminogenic Needs in a Youth Justice Sample: A Gender-Informed Latent Profile Analysis. *Criminal Justice and Behavior*, 48(2), 175–194. DOI: 10.1177/0093854820964513

Bryant, R. A. (2019). Post-traumatic stress disorder: A state-of-the-art review of evidence and challenges. *World Psychiatry; Official Journal of the World Psychiatric Association (WPA)*, 18(3), 259–269. DOI: 10.1002/wps.20656 PMID: 31496089

Bryant, R. A. (2022). The nature of posttraumatic stress disorder in treatment-seeking first responders. *European Journal of Psychotraumatology*, 13(1), 2011602. DOI: 10.1080/20008198.2021.2011602 PMID: 35096284

Burback, L., Brult-Phillips, S., Nijdam, M. J., McFarlane, A., & Vermetten, E. (2024). Treatment of Posttraumatic Stress Disorder: A State-of-the-art Review. *Current Neuropharmacology*, 22(4), 557–635. DOI: 10.2174/1570159X21666230428091433 PMID: 37132142

Calinescu, A. (2023). The Many Worlds of Trauma: An Interdisciplinary Perspective. *Border Crossing*, 13(2), 2. Advance online publication. DOI: 10.33182/bc.v13i2.2843

Carmi, L., Zohar, J., Juven-Wetzler, A., Desarnaud, F., Makotkine, L., Bierer, L. M., Cohen, H., & Yehuda, R. (2023). Promoter methylation of the glucocorticoid receptor following trauma may be associated with subsequent development of PTSD. *The World Journal of Biological Psychiatry*, 24(7), 578–586. DOI: 10.1080/15622975.2023.2177342 PMID: 36748398

Charuvastra, A., & Cloitre, M. (2008). Social Bonds and Posttraumatic Stress Disorder. *Annual Review of Psychology*, 59(1), 301–328. DOI: 10.1146/annurev.psych.58.110405.085650 PMID: 17883334

Clark, T. J., Conrad, C. G., Cummings, A. D. P., & Johnson, A. D. (2022). Trauma-Informed Policing: The Impact of Adult and Childhood Trauma on Law Enforcement Officers. *Case Western Reserve Law Review*, 73, 843. https://heinonline.org/HOL/Page?handle=hein.journals/cwrlrv73&id=880&div=&collection=

Cloitre, M., Garvert, D. W., & Weiss, B. J. (2017). Depression as a moderator of STAIR Narrative Therapy for women with post-traumatic stress disorder related to childhood abuse. *European Journal of Psychotraumatology*, 8(1), 1377028. DOI: 10.1080/20008198.2017.1377028 PMID: 29038682

Coll, S. Y., Eustache, F., Doidy, F., Fraisse, F., Peschanski, D., Dayan, J., Gagnepain, P., & Laisney, M. (2022). Avoidance behaviour generalizes to eye processing in posttraumatic stress disorder. *European Journal of Psychotraumatology*, 13(1), 2044661. DOI: 10.1080/20008198.2022.2044661 PMID: 35479300

Contractor, A. A., Weiss, N. H., Dolan, M., & Mota, N. (2020). Examination of the structural relations between posttraumatic stress disorder symptoms and reckless/self-destructive behaviors. *International Journal of Stress Management*, 27(1), 35–44. DOI: 10.1037/str0000133 PMID: 33776397

Davidson, K. W., Mangione, C. M., Barry, M. J., Nicholson, W. K., Cabana, M. D., Caughey, A. B., Davis, E. M., Donahue, K. E., Doubeni, C. A., Kubik, M., Li, L., Ogedegbe, G., Pbert, L., Silverstein, M., Stevermer, J., Tseng, C.-W., & Wong, J. B.US Preventive Services Task Force. (2022). Collaboration and Shared Decision-Making Between Patients and Clinicians in Preventive Health Care Decisions and US Preventive Services Task Force Recommendations. *Journal of the American Medical Association*, 327(12), 1171–1176. DOI: 10.1001/jama.2022.3267 PMID: 35315879

de Jongh, A., de Roos, C., & El-Leithy, S. (2024). State of the science: Eye movement desensitization and reprocessing (EMDR) therapy. *Journal of Traumatic Stress*, 37(2), 205–216. DOI: 10.1002/jts.23012 PMID: 38282286

DuBois, H. M. (2023). Empowerment and Transformation: Correlating John of the Cross and Judith Herman for Trauma Healing. *International Journal of Practical Theology*, 27(1), 99–113. DOI: 10.1515/ijpt-2022-0013

Duek, O., Seidemann, R., Pietrzak, R. H., & Harpaz-Rotem, I. (2023). Distinguishing emotional numbing symptoms of posttraumatic stress disorder from major depressive disorder. *Journal of Affective Disorders*, 324, 294–299. DOI: 10.1016/j.jad.2022.12.105 PMID: 36586605

Ehlers, A., Hackmann, A., & Michael, T. (2004). Intrusive re-experiencing in posttraumatic stress disorder: Phenomenology, theory, and therapy. *Memory (Hove, England)*, 12(4), 403–415. DOI: 10.1080/09658210444000025 PMID: 15487537

Eyni, S., & Musavi, S. E. (2024). Social Isolation of War Veterans with Post-Traumatic Stress Disorder Based on Emotional Inhibition: The Mediating Role of Rejection Sensitivity. *We are a service founded by Vietnam Veterans, now for all veterans and families., 32*(1).

Ford, J. D., & Courtois, C. A. (2021). Complex PTSD and borderline personality disorder. *Borderline Personality Disorder and Emotion Dysregulation*, 8(1), 16. DOI: 10.1186/s40479-021-00155-9 PMID: 33958001

Forkey, H. (2019). Putting Your Trauma Lens On. *Pediatric Annals*, 48(7), e269–e273. DOI: 10.3928/19382359-20190618-01 PMID: 31305944

Goetter, E. M., Blackburn, A. M., Stasko, C., Han, Y., Brenner, L. H., Lejeune, S., Tanev, K. S., Spencer, T. J., & Wright, E. C. (2021). Comparative effectiveness of prolonged exposure and cognitive processing therapy for military service members in an intensive treatment program. *Psychological Trauma: Theory, Research, Practice, and Policy*, 13(6), 632–640. DOI: 10.1037/tra0000956 PMID: 32915044

Hobbs, M. M. (2023). Healing Journeys: Veterans, Trauma, and the Return to Vietnam. *The Journal of American History*, 110(1), 82–107. DOI: 10.1093/jahist/jaad094

Holmes, E. A., Grey, N., & Young, K. A. D. (2005). Intrusive images and "hotspots" of trauma memories in Posttraumatic Stress Disorder: An exploratory investigation of emotions and cognitive themes. *Journal of Behavior Therapy and Experimental Psychiatry*, 36(1), 3–17. DOI: 10.1016/j.jbtep.2004.11.002 PMID: 15687006

Jericho, B., Luo, A., & Berle, D. (2022). Trauma-focused psychotherapies for post-traumatic stress disorder: A systematic review and network meta-analysis. *Acta Psychiatrica Scandinavica*, 145(2), 132–155. DOI: 10.1111/acps.13366 PMID: 34473342

Jones, M. B., Agrawal, R., Sharafkhaneh, A., Kunik, M. E., Jorge, R. E., & Marsh, L. (2022). Dream Enactment Behaviors Associated With Posttraumatic Stress Disorder. *The Journal of Neuropsychiatry and Clinical Neurosciences*, 34(2), 124–131. DOI: 10.1176/appi.neuropsych.21050115 PMID: 34763524

Kerig, P. K. (2019). Linking childhood trauma exposure to adolescent justice involvement: The concept of posttraumatic risk-seeking. *Clinical Psychology : a Publication of the Division of Clinical Psychology of the American Psychological Association*, 26(3), e12280. DOI: 10.1111/cpsp.12280

Korem, N., Duek, O., Ben-Zion, Z., Kaczkurkin, A. N., Lissek, S., Orederu, T., Schiller, D., Harpaz-Rotem, I., & Levy, I. (2022). Emotional numbing in PTSD is associated with lower amygdala reactivity to pain. *Neuropsychopharmacology*, 47(11), 1913–1921. DOI: 10.1038/s41386-022-01405-2 PMID: 35945274

Krüger, C. (2020). Culture, trauma and dissociation: A broadening perspective for our field. *Journal of Trauma & Dissociation*, 21(1), 1–13. DOI: 10.1080/15299732.2020.1675134 PMID: 31891334

Kumar, S. A., Brand, B. L., & Courtois, C. A. (2022). The need for trauma training: Clinicians' reactions to training on complex trauma. *Psychological Trauma: Theory, Research, Practice, and Policy*, 14(8), 1387–1394. DOI: 10.1037/tra0000515 PMID: 31580137

Kwon, A., Lee, H. S., & Lee, S.-H. (2021). The Mediation Effect of Hyperarousal Symptoms on the Relationship Between Childhood Physical Abuse and Suicidal Ideation of Patients With PTSD. *Frontiers in Psychiatry*, 12, 613735. Advance online publication. DOI: 10.3389/fpsyt.2021.613735 PMID: 33841200

Lanctôt, N., Reid, J. A., & Laurier, C. (2020). Nightmares and flashbacks: The impact of commercial sexual exploitation of children among female adolescents placed in residential care. *Child Abuse & Neglect*, 100, 104195. DOI: 10.1016/j.chiabu.2019.104195 PMID: 31582275

Laws, B. (2019). The return of the suppressed: Exploring how emotional suppression reappears as violence and pain among male and female prisoners. *Punishment & Society*, 21(5), 560–577. DOI: 10.1177/1462474518805071

Lewis, C., Roberts, N. P., Andrew, M., Starling, E., & Bisson, J. I. (2020). Psychological therapies for post-traumatic stress disorder in adults: Systematic review and meta-analysis. *European Journal of Psychotraumatology*, 11(1), 1729633. DOI: 10.1080/20008198.2020.1729633 PMID: 32284821

Liberzon, I., & Abelson, J. L. (2016). Context Processing and the Neurobiology of Post-Traumatic Stress Disorder. *Neuron*, 92(1), 14–30. DOI: 10.1016/j.neuron.2016.09.039 PMID: 27710783

Lord, S. A. (2008). Therapeutic Work with Trauma, Revictimization, and Perpetration: Bearing Witness, Offering Hope, Embracing Despair. *Psychoanalytic Social Work*, 15(2), 110–131. DOI: 10.1080/15228870802103671

MacLeish, K. (2018). On 'moral injury': Psychic fringes and war violence. *History of the Human Sciences*, 31(2), 128–146. DOI: 10.1177/0952695117750342

Malaktaris, A. L., & Lynn, S. J. (2019). The Phenomenology and Correlates of Flashbacks in Individuals With Posttraumatic Stress Symptoms. *Clinical Psychological Science*, 7(2), 249–264. DOI: 10.1177/2167702618805081

Marchand, W. R., Sandoval, K., Lackner, R., Parker, S. C., Herrmann, T., Yabko, B., Velasquez, T., Lewis, L., & Butler, J. (2021). Mindfulness-based interventions for military veterans: A systematic review and analysis of the literature. *Complementary Therapies in Clinical Practice*, 42, 101274. DOI: 10.1016/j.ctcp.2020.101274 PMID: 33276226

McCurry, K. L., Frueh, B. C., Chiu, P. H., & King-Casas, B. (2020). Opponent Effects of Hyperarousal and Re-experiencing on Affective Habituation in Posttraumatic Stress Disorder. *Biological Psychiatry: Cognitive Neuroscience and Neuroimaging*, 5(2), 203–212. DOI: 10.1016/j.bpsc.2019.09.006 PMID: 31759868

McGeary, D. D., Resick, P. A., Penzien, D. B., McGeary, C. A., Houle, T. T., Eapen, B. C., Jaramillo, C. A., Nabity, P. S., Reed, D. E.II, Moring, J. C., Bira, L. M., Hansen, H. R., Young-McCaughan, S., Cobos, B. A., Mintz, J., Keane, T. M., & Peterson, A. L. (2022). Cognitive Behavioral Therapy for Veterans With Comorbid Posttraumatic Headache and Posttraumatic Stress Disorder Symptoms: A Randomized Clinical Trial. *JAMA Neurology*, 79(8), 746–757. DOI: 10.1001/jamaneurol.2022.1567 PMID: 35759281

McLean, C. P., Levy, H. C., Miller, M. L., & Tolin, D. F. (2022). Exposure therapy for PTSD: A meta-analysis. *Clinical Psychology Review*, 91, 102115. DOI: 10.1016/j.cpr.2021.102115 PMID: 34954460

McLean, C. P., Levy, H. C., Miller, M. L., & Tolin, D. F. (2022). Exposure therapy for PTSD in military populations: A systematic review and meta-analysis of randomized clinical trials. *Journal of Anxiety Disorders*, 90, 102607. DOI: 10.1016/j.janxdis.2022.102607 PMID: 35926254

McRae, E. M., Stoppelbein, L., O'Kelley, S. E., Fite, P., & Smith, S. B. (2021). An Examination of Post-Traumatic Stress Symptoms and Aggression among Children with a History of Adverse Childhood Experiences. *Journal of Psychopathology and Behavioral Assessment*, 43(3), 657–670. DOI: 10.1007/s10862-021-09884-1

Midgley, N. (2007). Anna Freud: The Hampstead War Nurseries and the role of the direct observation of children for psychoanalysis. *The International Journal of Psycho-Analysis*, 88(4), 939–959. DOI: 10.1516/V28R-J334-6182-524H PMID: 17681901

Miles, S. R., Hale, W. J., Mintz, J., Wachen, J. S., Litz, B. T., Dondanville, K. A., Yarvis, J. S., Hembree, E. A., Young-McCaughan, S., Peterson, A. L., & Resick, P. A. (2023). Hyperarousal symptoms linger after successful PTSD treatment in active duty military. *Psychological Trauma: Theory, Research, Practice, and Policy*, 15(8), 1398–1405. DOI: 10.1037/tra0001292 PMID: 35901423

Mohammed, A. A. (2022). Trauma and Recovery: A Psychoanalytic Study of Gharbi Mustafa's When Mountains Weep. *Journal of University of Human Development*, 8(2), 2. Advance online publication. DOI: 10.21928/juhd.v8n2y2022.pp28-36

Monane, R., Sanchez, G. J., Kronish, I. M., Edmondson, D., & Diaz, K. M. (2018). Post-traumatic stress disorder symptoms and aversive cognitions regarding physical activity in patients evaluated for acute coronary syndrome. *European Journal of Preventive Cardiology*, 25(4), 402–403. DOI: 10.1177/2047487317746255 PMID: 29198138

Moreira, A., Moreira, A. C., & Rocha, J. C. (2022). Randomized Controlled Trial: Cognitive-Narrative Therapy for IPV Victims. *Journal of Interpersonal Violence*, 37(5–6), NP2998–NP3014. DOI: 10.1177/0886260520943719 PMID: 32755265

Morina, N., Schnyder, U., Klaghofer, R., Müller, J., & Martin-Soelch, C. (2018). Trauma exposure and the mediating role of posttraumatic stress on somatic symptoms in civilian war victims. *BMC Psychiatry*, 18(1), 92. DOI: 10.1186/s12888-018-1680-4 PMID: 29631551

Nandi, C., Crombach, A., Elbert, T., Bambonye, M., Pryss, R., Schobel, J., & Weierstall-Pust, R. (2020). The cycle of violence as a function of PTSD and appetitive aggression: A longitudinal study with Burundian soldiers. *Aggressive Behavior*, 46(5), 391–399. DOI: 10.1002/ab.21895 PMID: 32363661

Novaco, R. W. (2010). Anger and Psychopathology. In Potegal, M., Stemmler, G., & Spielberger, C. (Eds.), *International Handbook of Anger: Constituent and Concomitant Biological, Psychological, and Social Processes* (pp. 465–497). Springer., DOI: 10.1007/978-0-387-89676-2_27

Ophir, I., & Jacoby, R. (2020). "Sparks that became a little light over time": A qualitative investigation of musicking as a means of coping in adults with PTSD. *PLoS One*, 15(1), e0228050. DOI: 10.1371/journal.pone.0228050 PMID: 31999728

Palgi, Y., Karatzias, T., Hyland, P., Shevlin, M., & Ben-Ezra, M. (2021). Can subjective perceptions of trauma differentiate between ICD-11 PTSD and complex PTSD? A cross-cultural comparison of three African countries. *Psychological Trauma: Theory, Research, Practice, and Policy*, 13(2), 142–148. DOI: 10.1037/tra0000966 PMID: 32940522

Perrotta, G. (2020). The state of consciousness: From perceptual alterations to dissociative forms. Analysis of neurobiological and clinical profiles. *Journal of Neurology, Neurological Science and Disorders, 7*(1), 006–018. https://doi.org/ DOI: 10.17352/jnnsd.000042

Phelps, A. J., Forbes, D., & Creamer, M. (2008). Understanding posttraumatic nightmares: An empirical and conceptual review. *Clinical Psychology Review*, 28(2), 338–355. DOI: 10.1016/j.cpr.2007.06.001 PMID: 17629384

Porcheret, K., Iyadurai, L., Bonsall, M. B., Goodwin, G. M., Beer, S. A., Darwent, M., & Holmes, E. A. (2020). Sleep and intrusive memories immediately after a traumatic event in emergency department patients. *Sleep (Basel)*, 43(8), zsaa033. Advance online publication. DOI: 10.1093/sleep/zsaa033 PMID: 32133531

Raghuraman, S., Stuttard, N., & Hunt, N. (2021). Evaluating narrative exposure therapy for post-traumatic stress disorder and depression symptoms: A meta-analysis of the evidence base. *Clinical Psychology & Psychotherapy*, 28(1), 1–23. DOI: 10.1002/cpp.2486 PMID: 32525597

Reis, R., & Ortega, F. (2021). Neuroscientific perspectives for a theory of trauma: A critical review of integrative models of biology and culture. *Cadernos de Saude Publica*, 37, e00352820. DOI: 10.1590/0102-311x00352820 PMID: 34495102

Rutt, B. T., Oehlert, M. E., Krieshok, T. S., & Lichtenberg, J. W. (2018). Effectiveness of Cognitive Processing Therapy and Prolonged Exposure in the Department of Veterans Affairs. *Psychological Reports*, 121(2), 282–302. DOI: 10.1177/0033294117727746 PMID: 28886664

Sadeghi, M., McDonald, A. D., & Sasangohar, F. (2022). Posttraumatic stress disorder hyperarousal event detection using smartwatch physiological and activity data. *PLoS One*, 17(5), e0267749. DOI: 10.1371/journal.pone.0267749 PMID: 35584096

Saraiya, T., & Lopez-Castro, T. (2016). Ashamed and Afraid: A Scoping Review of the Role of Shame in Post-Traumatic Stress Disorder (PTSD). *Journal of Clinical Medicine*, 5(11), 11. Advance online publication. DOI: 10.3390/jcm5110094 PMID: 27809274

Scelles, C., & Bulnes, L. C. (2021). EMDR as Treatment Option for Conditions Other Than PTSD: A Systematic Review. *Frontiers in Psychology*, 12, 644369. Advance online publication. DOI: 10.3389/fpsyg.2021.644369 PMID: 34616328

Schäfer, S. K., Lüder, C. C., Porcheret, K., Hu, X., Margraf, J., Michael, T., Holmes, E. A., Werner, G. G., Wilhelm, I., Woud, M. L., Zeng, S., Friesen, E., Haim-Nachum, S., Lass-Hennemann, J., Lieb, K., Kunzler, A. M., Wirth, B. E., & Sopp, M. R. (2023). To sleep or not to sleep, that is the question: A systematic review and meta-analysis on the effect of post-trauma sleep on intrusive memories of analog trauma. *Behaviour Research and Therapy*, 167, 104359. DOI: 10.1016/j.brat.2023.104359 PMID: 37422952

Schnurr, P. P., Chard, K. M., Ruzek, J. I., Chow, B. K., Resick, P. A., Foa, E. B., Marx, B. P., Friedman, M. J., Bovin, M. J., Caudle, K. L., Castillo, D., Curry, K. T., Hollifield, M., Huang, G. D., Chee, C. L., Astin, M. C., Dickstein, B., Renner, K., Clancy, C. P., & Shih, M.-C. (2022). Comparison of Prolonged Exposure vs Cognitive Processing Therapy for Treatment of Posttraumatic Stress Disorder Among US Veterans: A Randomized Clinical Trial. *JAMA Network Open*, 5(1), e2136921. DOI: 10.1001/jamanetworkopen.2021.36921 PMID: 35044471

Schrader, C., & Ross, A. (2021). A Review of PTSD and Current Treatment Strategies. *Missouri Medicine*, 118(6), 546–551. PMID: 34924624

Schweitzer, R., Melville, F., Steel, Z., & Lacherez, P. (2006). Trauma, Post-Migration Living Difficulties, and Social Support as Predictors of Psychological Adjustment in Resettled Sudanese Refugees. *The Australian and New Zealand Journal of Psychiatry*, 40(2), 179–187. DOI: 10.1080/j.1440-1614.2006.01766.x PMID: 16476137

Shubina, I. (2015). Cognitive-behavioral Therapy of Patients with PTSD: Literature Review. *Procedia: Social and Behavioral Sciences*, 165, 208–216. DOI: 10.1016/j.sbspro.2014.12.624

Sommer, J. L., El-Gabalawy, R., Contractor, A. A., Weiss, N. H., & Mota, N. (2020). PTSD's risky behavior criterion: Associated risky and unhealthy behaviors and psychiatric correlates in a nationally representative sample. *Journal of Anxiety Disorders*, 73, 102247. DOI: 10.1016/j.janxdis.2020.102247 PMID: 32502805

Szoke, D., Putnam, A., & Hazlett-Stevens, H. (2021). Mindfulness-Based Interventions for Traumatic Stress. In Hazlett-Stevens, H. (Ed.), *Biopsychosocial Factors of Stress, and Mindfulness for Stress Reduction* (pp. 177–200). Springer International Publishing., DOI: 10.1007/978-3-030-81245-4_8

Temoney, K. E. (2021). The War Came Alive Inside of Them. *The Journal of Religious Ethics*, 49(3), 479–494. DOI: 10.1111/jore.12366

Trajkov, I. (2023). Stress, Trauma and Post-Traumatic Stress Disorder (PTSD). *The Annual of the Faculty of Philosophy in Skopje*, 76, 629–639. DOI: 10.37510/godzbo2376629t

Trottier, K., & Monson, C. M. (2021). Integrating cognitive processing therapy for posttraumatic stress disorder with cognitive behavioral therapy for eating disorders in PROJECT RECOVER. *Eating Disorders*, 29(3), 307–325. DOI: 10.1080/10640266.2021.1891372 PMID: 33656976

Tyson, P. (2009). Child Development and Child Psychoanalysis: Research and Education. *Journal of the American Psychoanalytic Association*, 57(4), 871–879. DOI: 10.1177/0003065109342097 PMID: 19724068

Van Minnen, A., Voorendonk, E. M., Rozendaal, L., & de Jongh, A. (2020). Sequence matters: Combining Prolonged Exposure and EMDR therapy for PTSD. *Psychiatry Research*, 290, 113032. DOI: 10.1016/j.psychres.2020.113032 PMID: 32454314

Wamser-Nanney, R., Walker, H. E., & Nanney, J. T. (2021). Trauma Exposure, Posttraumatic Stress Disorder, and Aggression Among Civilian Females. *Journal of Interpersonal Violence*, 36(17–18), NP9649–NP9669. DOI: 10.1177/0886260519860894 PMID: 31286814

Wilde, L. (2022). Trauma: Phenomenological causality and implication. *Phenomenology and the Cognitive Sciences*, 21(3), 689–705. DOI: 10.1007/s11097-020-09725-8

Williston, S. K., Grossman, D., Mori, D. L., & Niles, B. L. (2021). Mindfulness interventions in the treatment of posttraumatic stress disorder. *Professional Psychology, Research and Practice*, 52(1), 46–57. DOI: 10.1037/pro0000363

Yehuda, R., Hoge, C. W., McFarlane, A. C., Vermetten, E., Lanius, R. A., Nievergelt, C. M., Hobfoll, S. E., Koenen, K. C., Neylan, T. C., & Hyman, S. E. (2015). Post-traumatic stress disorder. *Nature Reviews. Disease Primers*, 1(1), 1–22. DOI: 10.1038/nrdp.2015.57 PMID: 27189040

Youngren, W. A., Hamilton, N. A., & Preacher, K. (2020). Assessing Triggers of Posttrauma Nightmares. *Journal of Traumatic Stress*, 33(4), 511–520. DOI: 10.1002/jts.22532 PMID: 32521086

Zaleski, K. L., Johnson, D. K., & Klein, J. T. (2016). Grounding Judith Herman's Trauma Theory within Interpersonal Neuroscience and Evidence-Based Practice Modalities for Trauma Treatment. *Smith College Studies in Social Work*, 86(4), 377–393. DOI: 10.1080/00377317.2016.1222110

KEY TERMS AND DEFINITIONS

Behavioral manifestations of PTSD: It refers to observable actions, reactions, and patterns of behavior exhibited by individuals with PTSD as a direct result of their traumatic experiences.

Phenomenological aspects of PTSD: It encompasses a wide range of subjective experiences that may not be readily apparent in behavioral observations.

Post-Traumatic Stress Disorder (PTSD): It is a psychiatric condition that typically arises following exposure to severe trauma, frequently involving violence and destruction.

Chapter 2
Origins of PTSD and Overview of Treatments

Robert W. Motta
Hofstra University, USA

ABSTRACT

Diagnosis of PTSD. Posttraumatic stress disorder (PTSD) refers to long running disturbances in emotion, cognition, and behavior owing to having encountered frightening, disruptive, and often life-threatening experiences. These traumatic experiences are relived in such a way that the past, even a past that took place decades ago, is ever present. Common fear reactions often abate within brief periods of time. In contrast, PTSD is enduring and can sometimes last for as long as one lives. It is dysregulating across a wide variety of domains of functioning. PTSD can cause extreme fear reactions to common stressors; it can cause disruptions in one's memory and thinking process; it can cause startle reactions and sympathetic nervous system over-activation; can negatively alter one's mood; diminish one's sense of self; cause sleeplessness and nightmares, disrupt relationships, and cause an enduring distrust of the environment. To help in developing a perspective on PTSD, it is important to note that most people who encounter traumatic events do not develop PTSD.

INTRODUCTION

Diagnosis of PTSD. Posttraumatic stress disorder (PTSD) refers to long running disturbances in emotion, cognition, and behavior owing to having encountered frightening, disruptive, and often life-threatening experiences. These traumatic experiences are relived in such a way that the past, even a past that took place decades ago, is ever present. Common fear reactions often abate within brief periods

DOI: 10.4018/979-8-3693-2089-1.ch002

of time. In contrast, PTSD is enduring and can sometimes last for as long as one lives. It is dysregulating across a wide variety of domains of functioning. PTSD can cause extreme fear reactions to common stressors; it can cause disruptions in one's memory and thinking process; it can cause startle reactions and sympathetic nervous system over-activation; can negatively alter one's mood; diminish one's sense of self; cause sleeplessness and nightmares, disrupt relationships, and cause an enduring distrust of the environment. To help in developing a perspective on PTSD, it is important to note that most people who encounter traumatic events do not develop PTSD. According to Breslau (2009), 7% of those in the general population who encounter traumatic experiences develop PTSD. These rates are far higher for rape victims, victims of torture, military combatants, and other traumatized groups.

The diagnostic term of "posttraumatic stress disorder" did not officially exist until 1980 when it was incorporated into the third edition of the diagnostic compendium of mental disorders, the Diagnostic and Statistical Manual of the American Psychiatric Association, the DSM (*third ed.* [*DSM-III*]; American Psychiatric Association, 1980). The stimulus for the inclusion of PTSD into the DSM was the large number of trauma cases that resulted from participation in the Vietnam war. The *DSM-III* "alluded to traumatic events that were beyond the range of normal human experience" (Motta, 2013, p.6). The issue of an event being "beyond the range" was dropped in later iterations of the DSM when it was realized that many experiences can eventuate in PTSD and that it was difficult to define what was "beyond the range."

While the initial inclusion of PTSD in the *DSM III* (1980) may have been brought about by observations of mental health professionals dealing with veteran returnees from the Vietnam War, the range of PTSD stressors has expanded markedly because of research studies into this disorder. A partial list of stressors leading to PTSD includes natural disasters, serious illnesses, car accidents, assaults of various kinds, neglect, maltreatment, minority status within a society, poverty, having addicted and abusive or neglectful parents, socioeconomic stressors, marital abuse and neglect, and many others.

Complicating matters still further is the fact that individuals differ in their propensity for developing PTSD. Some are more vulnerable than others. In general, younger people are more likely to develop PTSD than older people. Females are more vulnerable than males. Those who have experienced adjustment disorders, anxiety, or depression prior to being traumatized are more likely to develop PTSD than those who were well adjusted prior to the traumatic event. The less one feels in control of the trauma situation the more likely it is that PTSD will develop. Introverts are reportedly more likely to develop PTSD than extroverts (Waters, 2018).

The current iteration of the DSM is DSM-5 (*fifth ed.* [*DSM*-5]; American Psychiatric Association, 2013) differs from prior versions regarding PTSD in that PTSD is now listed under the category of trauma related disorders rather than anxiety disorders, and it includes disturbances in cognition and mood among the diagnostic criteria. Diagnostic criteria for PTSD now include the following symptom clusters:

- ***Re-experiencing the event*** — Recurrent memories of the event, traumatic nightmares, dissociative reactions, prolonged psychological distress
- ***Alterations in arousal*** — Aggressive, reckless, or self-destructive behavior, sleep disturbances, hypervigilance
- ***Avoidance*** — Distressing memories, thoughts, or reminders of the event are consciously or unconsciously pushed away.
- ***Negative alterations in cognition and mood*** — Persistent negative beliefs, distorted blame, or trauma-related emotions; feelings of alienation and diminished interest in life.

The Felt Experience of PTSD. While the PTSD sufferer certainly does endure the behaviors and emotions described above, the *DSM-5* clusters and criteria cannot convey the felt experience of PTSD. When interviewed, those suffering from PTSD often report that they have been altered in some way by a traumatic experience or experiences. These self-alterations often include the feeling of being vulnerable, threatened, weary, and a belief that the environment can be harmful and is not to be trusted. Traumatized individuals often report an almost animal-like weariness and fear of the environment. They often see themselves as two people (van der Kolk, 2014). One is the person that is presented to society – the accountant, the construction worker, the teacher, etc. The other is an anxious and often frightened being that is constantly scanning the environment for threat. This second person is hidden and is known only to the PTSD sufferer and to those who have a close and extended contact with that person. This is the phenomenological depiction of PTSD, and it differs markedly from that of the symptom clusters delineated in the *DSM-5*.

While it is true, according to the DSM, that those with PTSD often re-experience the traumatic event in images, memories, and dreams; that they have sleep disturbance and are hyper aroused; that they consciously and unconsciously avoid anything that reminds them of their trauma; and that they have negative alterations in cognition and mood; their view of themselves and their perspective on the environment, the very notion of who they are is poorly described by the DSM-5 symptom clusters. The DSM clusters do not convey the felt experience of PTSD.

It is not at all unusual for the previously trusting and outgoing individual to become distrusting, withdrawn, and suspicious following a traumatic encounter. They become something they were not, and this thing is a negative version of their former self. An example here might be a young woman who was raped. Prior to the rape she was engaged in life and society and may have had an upbeat personality and enjoyed the company of others. After the rape she becomes moody, suspicious, and withdrawn. She has little desire to be around people for fear that, if she lets down her guard she might be attacked. She is often anxious and depressed. She may have a felt sense of having been sullied by her attacker and this negative self-view now becomes a central part of her identity. It is not at all uncommon for traumatized individuals to feel dehumanized and almost animal-like in their fear of the environment. The dramatic change in the person that one once was, is typical of those who have been traumatized.

A similar phenomenon is seen in veterans of war who may have entered the military with feelings of patriotism and high ideals. After exposure to gruesome images of war and after having participated in actions that are perceived as violations of their own moral code; and after having experienced extreme threats to their life, they are transformed. Often, they are no longer the patriotic, idealistic individual they once were. They may now see themselves as weary, suspicious, almost non-human beings that have been dramatically altered by their war experience. The DSM-5 does not capture the phenomenology, the felt sense of what it means to be traumatized.

In summary, trauma alters people and sometimes this alteration is permanent. Traumatized individuals often view their pre-trauma perspectives on life, relationships, the environment, fairness, ethics etc. as naively uninformed. They no longer see good as overcoming evil, justice as prevailing over injustice, etc. Their basic assumptions of themselves and their environments have been altered (McCann & Pearlman, 1990). Their distrust of others makes psychotherapeutic treatment of them, a challenging proposition.

Traditional Treatments for PTSD. The reputed "gold standards" for treating PTSD are Cognitive Behavioral Psychotherapy (CBT) and Prolonged Exposure (PE) to previously traumatizing stimuli (e.g., Preston, O'Neal, & Talaga, 2002). These are the "go to," treatments often advocated by the Veterans Health Administration (VHA or VA). What the VA fails to report is that most veterans find these approaches so threatening and anxiety provoking, that they avoid them and the therapists who espouse them. There is a good deal of controversy over the value of CBT in treating psychological trauma. Wompold (2015), for example, claims that the curative element in CBT and other therapies is the relationship and less so the specific technique. He refers to the relationship as the "common factor" in therapy.

A partial listing of the current "traditional" PTSD treatments are:

Acceptance and Commitment Therapy (ACT; Hayes et al., 2016). The goal of ACT is not to eliminate or negate negative thoughts and beliefs related to trauma or other disorders but rather to live with them, and to immerse oneself in, and explore them. The goal is to accept that trauma is a part of oneself and then move on to the learning of more adaptive ways of functioning. ACT often employs meditative techniques to teach the acceptance of the oneself and one's environment.

Dialectical Behavior Therapy (DBT; Linehan, 1993). The central components of DBT are distress tolerance, emotion regulation, and acceptance of change. In doing DBT the therapist partners with the client and helps the client to accept their dysfunctional behavior as an understandable response to an invalidating environment. At the same time the client is encouraged to see that their behavior is maladaptive, and that change is desirable. This is the dialectic, the synthesis of the opposites of understanding and accepting one's responses while moving toward adaptive change. DBT incorporates modules upon which the client works, including mindfulness (also emphasized in ACT), distress tolerance, emotion regulation, and interpersonal effectiveness. While DBT is associated with the treatment of borderline personality disorder, it is also used in treating PTSD.

Cognitive Processing Therapy (CPT; Resick, 2001). CPT, a manualized form of therapy, was initially developed for use with rape victims, but is also used in treating PTSD. Four elements of CPT are: educating clients about the nature of PTSD and the potential value of treatment; informing the client about the nature of their emotions and thoughts; assisting the client to challenge their dysfunctional thoughts; and helping the client see the change in their beliefs following therapeutic intervention. A typical 12 step structured protocol may begin with a psychoeducation component, followed by writing and reading about the traumatic event, the client's customary modes of thinking and acting, challenging these customary modes, and learning more adaptive modes of thinking and behaving.

Prolonged Exposure (PE; Foa, Hembree, & Rothbaum, 2007). One of the most common responses to distressing and anxiety laden experiences is avoidance of them (Motta, 2020). The central focus of PE is to change from the habitual tendency of avoiding uncomfortable thoughts, feelings, beliefs, and perceptions of their trauma to confronting them. Therapists often record sessions and encourage the client to listen these recording at home as a way of exposing the client to that which they have been avoiding. By confronting disturbing material, one eliminates the anxiety reduction that commonly follows the pushing away of this material from awareness. This anxiety reduction is what reinforces and maintains avoidance behavior. In other words, avoidance serves the short-term benefit of anxiety reduction but strengthens avoidance. Confronting and exposing oneself to this material weakens its negative impact and promotes the development of adaptive functioning. Available research shows that PE can be effective for those who stay with it, but the process of confronting one's trauma is aversive and therapy dropout is common (Motta, 2020). So, while it can be effective, PE is a difficult procedure to endure for many people and as a result they quit therapy.

The above list of traditional therapies is not exhaustive and there is no agreed upon compendium of traditional therapies for managing PTSD. In their book on *Effective Treatments for PTSD* (Foa, Keene, & Friedman, 2000), the following interventions are included: exposure therapy, systematic desensitization, CPT, stress inoculation training, cognitive therapy, assertiveness training, relaxation training, biofeedback, and others. One of the problems is selecting therapies specifically oriented toward treating PTSD is that many of them evoke such high levels of anxiety in the traumatized client that they are avoided. Many traumatized clients begin to associate their trauma therapists with anxiety producing material and end up avoiding the therapist and the therapy they are providing (Motta, 2020, p.6). For this reason, alternative forms of therapy, or non-traditional therapies are sought out. This seeking of non-traditional forms of treatment was revealed in a survey of those traumatized by the World Trade Center attack in 2001. Most sought out non-traditional treatments such as yoga, acupuncture, meditation, and relaxation exercises instead of various forms of CBT (van der Kolk, 2014).

Non-Traditional Treatment of PTSD. There is a wide array of alternatives to traditional treatments for PTSD (Benedek & Wynn, 2015; Motta, 2020). The material to follow will be a selection of these non-traditional treatments and with, one exception, i.e., MDMA (ecstasy), will not include mind altering, psychedelic drugs owing to a comparative scarcity of well controlled studies of them. MDMA, in contrast has been supported as a treatment of PTSD in many well controlled studies. Antidepressants and antianxiety agents have been used for comorbid symptoms of PTSD but do not appear to be effective in treating the disorder itself and for this reason will not be addressed in this chapter. The non-traditional treatments below meet the following criteria:

They have been shown to be effective in ameliorating PTSD.

They have amassed considerable empirical support and are therefore not "fringe" interventions.

They do not place a heavy emphasis on forced confronting to traumatic material.

Eye-Movement Desensitization and Reprocessing (EMDR; Shapiro, 1989). EMDR is included as a non-traditional treatment because it has not been widely embraced by the academic community despite its endorsement by the American Psychological Association (APA Presidential Task Force on Evidence-Based Practice, 2006). Although substantial empirical evidence shows that EMDR is effective in treating PTSD, the seemingly insufficient explanations as to why it works has led many academics to be skeptical of it and categorize it as a form of mesmerism.

The specific technique involves having the traumatized client consider specific imagery associated with their traumatic encounter, and particularly the negative cognitions associated with the event such as "I am weak and ineffective," I am powerless," "I should have acted more assertively," etc. While engaging in this imagery and while considering these thoughts, the therapist moves their index and middle finger, held together, across the client's visual field. The client visually tracks these approximately 20 bidirectional movements. When the movements are complete the therapist asks a non-directive question such as "What came up?" In this the therapist is inquiring as to what other images, beliefs, sensations etc. arose in response to the eye movement exercise. This non-directive question is unlike traditional therapies where the therapist guides the client to focus on specific maladaptive thoughts and beliefs. Whatever the client answers in response to the "what came up?" question is used as the next target for the EMDR procedure. This process continues through an approximate 90-minute session. The client is encouraged to practice self-management, relaxation procedures between sessions. As sessions progress, clients numerically rate the degree to which they continue to maintain negative cognitions, their degree of anxiety, and the degree to which they experience negative sensations.

One of the reputed benefits of EMDR is said to be the limited number of sessions (usually fewer than 10) required for treatment of PTSD and the resistance to relapse. While making eye movements is the most common approach to EMDR, moving light stimuli has also been used, as has alternating acoustic stimuli, alternating touch, and other procedures.

The question that has not been clearly addressed is why EMDR works in alleviating PTSD. Shapiro (1989) suggests an information processing explanation, whereby previously suppressed trauma memories which may have resided in the amygdala and other subcortical areas are brought into the cortex for processing. This transfer of information is brought about by the client consciously following the alternating stimuli across the visual field. The lack of definitive proof for this information transfer model has fomented a good deal of skepticism about EMDR. Despite this, many individual studies and meta-analyses have resulted in the American Psychological and Psychiatric Associations and many other professional organizations, including the World Health Organization, endorsing EMDR as an effective treatment for PTSD.

Yoga. Rape victims, military combatants, survivors of torture and natural disasters, and many other traumatized groups have found relief of their distress in the simple practice of yoga (Jackson 2014). Yoga has been practiced across the globe and has been in existence for over 5000 years. In Sanskrit the term means "union" or "connection," and implies the unification of physical, mental, and emotional states. PTSD is often linked to dissociation or a breakage of connection between body, mind, and emotion. Often PTSD involves intensely disruptive memories and images that the sufferer attempts to push out of awareness because they are so painful. There is thus a separation of one's thoughts from one's feelings and sensations. Yoga, with its focused attention to stretches and body postures, works to link or unite body and mind.

Most forms of yoga encompass breathing practices *(pranayama),* stretches (asanas), relaxation (savasana), and meditation. It could be argued that the focus on postures, breathing, etc. is a physical variant of meditation but meditation has been used in and of itself as an intervention for PTSD. "On a biochemical and physiological level, previous research has shown that yoga relaxes chronic muscle tension, restores natural diaphragmatic breathing, improves oxygen absorption and carbon dioxide elimination, increases alpha and theta brain waves, and regulates the thalamus at an optimum level." (Weintraub, 2012, p.14). In essence, yoga is a valid and empirically supported treatment for various types of psychological trauma (Motta, 2023).

Although empirical studies have provided support for the use of yoga with PTSD, it is often necessary to alter standard yoga practice when treating PTSD victims. In standard practice it is not unusual for the instructor to physically guide the yoga practitioner and provide specific suggestions and corrections regarding how they are conducting their asanas. Trauma victims have often felt themselves in situations where they are physically threatened and/or lack the ability to escape the fear inducing situation. For this reason, trauma victims may have an aversion for being touched and do not react well to having their movements limited or corrected. It is best for the yoga instructor who is working with trauma survivors to take a non-directive approach and accept the yoga participant's interpretation of how a given asana is done and to avoid physical contact with the practitioner. Again, touch and movement limitation may be uncomfortable triggers for traumatized individuals.

Despite the previously noted caveats, yoga is a valuable tool in treating trauma and is a form of intervention that is often sought out by trauma victims. Its emphasis on the body is endorsed by many therapists (e.g., van der Kolk, 2014) because it is recognized that "the body keeps the score" regarding the impact of trauma on human functioning. There are approximately 20 forms of yoga and in all there are 80,000 varied forms of asanas or stances (Emerson & Hooper, 2011).

Meditation. Meditation derives from the Latin *meditatum* and means to ponder. Meditation, like yoga, has a long history dating back about 5000 years (Dienstmann, 2018). The Hindus began the development of meditation as a way of getting closer to the nature of God. Since then, Islam, Christianity Judaism, Jainism, Sikhism, Taoism, Native American Sufism, and other traditions have all employed contemplative practices based on meditation.

Mindfulness meditation emphasizes a focus on the present moment and an elimination or reduction in mind-wandering and distracting, random thoughts that enter awareness. The dedicated practice of meditation can thus increase self-knowledge and eventuate in a reduction in the critical and negative evaluation of oneself and others. While empirical research shows that meditation can be of real benefit for PTSD sufferers, the nature of that disorder makes the practice of meditation particularly difficult. This is because those with PTSD are invested in past events which occupy their present awareness. They spend a good deal of time reliving and ruminating over past traumatic events. It takes a good deal of effort to master meditation but if one does, the practice can be liberating and enlightening. "We tend to be particularly unaware that we are thinking virtually all the time…Meditation means learning how to get out of this current, sit by the bank and listen to it, learn from it, and then use its energies to guide us rather than to tyrannize us (Kabat-Zinn, 1994, p.9).

The mechanics of meditation typically involve sitting on a straight-backed chair or meditation cushion (zafu) in an erect posture, as the latter fosters attention and awareness. The eyes are closed or looking downward but not focused. Attention is then paid to the process of breathing. Thoughts will invariably intrude and when they do, the content of the thought is noted and then one returns their attention to breathing. Being aware of this content and when thoughts intrude is a component of mindfulness. Once a facility is developed in focusing on breathing, one might focus on sensations of the body, sounds of traffic, degree of physical comfort, temperature of the room, etc. All thoughts, sensations, perceptions, emotions, and observations are accepted non-judgmentally. A typical session lasts about 20 minutes although this varies. With dedicated practice, a non-judgmental awareness develops so that the PTSD sufferer acquires a more positive view of themselves and others and learns to live in the present.

Many consider the dedicated practice of meditation to be difficult as it requires considerable self-discipline to sit daily and work on reducing distracting and intruding thoughts. Research shows that meditation is a learnable skill and that the ability to live in the present improves with practice and that this practice can reduce the symptoms of PTSD and improve non-judgmental self-acceptance. Meditation is a useful skill in managing PTSD, but it is not a skill that is easily attained.

Exercise. There is an abundance of high-quality empirical literature showing that exercise is beneficial in reducing negative emotional states such as anxiety, depression, and anger while enhancing self-esteem, concentration, well-being, and goal-directedness. Reviews of this research (e.g., Motta, 2018) also shows that exercise can also be of value in reducing PTSD. Why this is so is not well established and while early research focused on aerobic exercise of the type resulting from brisk walking, jogging, bicycling, swimming, etc., it is now clear that any form of exercise, even moderate levels, can reduce PTSD. It may be that because anxiety and depression are central components of PTSD and controlled research shows that exercise reduces these negative affective states, this may be why PTSD is positively impacted.

There are several theoretical views regarding why physical exercise impacts emotional states, but one provocative view is that of *bodymind* as espoused by Candace Pert (Pert, 1999). Pert's research strongly suggests that body and mind are not separate entities as is commonly accepted but rather represent a single entity composed of both physiological and mental states. If this is the case, then exercise which is beneficial to physical health has a corresponding benefit to psychological health. This mutual benefit is due to the unity of body and mind and thus the term *bodymind.* Pert is not restating the commonly held view of mind and body interaction but rather putting forth a new concept that challenges the conception of mind and body being separate systems. Her research shows both neurophysiological and neurochemical linkages among systems encompassing immunity, cognition, and emotion.

Among the other theoretical positions that attempt to explain the relationship between exercise and psychological states such as PTSD, are the following.

Thermogenic hypothesis. This hypothesis states that exercise elevates body temperature and such elevations have been associated with a calming of emotions. The body of available research has failed to support this position.

Endorphin and Endocannabinoid hypotheses. The position taken here is that when one exercises there is a release of *beta-endorphins* or endogenous opiates that produce beneficial effects like the "runners' high." A similar position is that exercise results in the release of endocannabinoids that are similar to tetrahydrocannabinol (THC) and this is what results in emotional benefits. The endorphin hypothesis has been popular for many years but certain inconsistencies in research finds have led to initial investigations of the competing endocannabinoid position.

Monoamine hypothesis. Like the endorphin and endocannabinoid hypotheses, the monoamine hypothesis proposes that exercise results in the release of neurotransmitters such as dopamine, serotonin, and norepinephrine and these are the cause of exercise benefits. While these elevations are seen in plasma and urine following exercise, it is unclear as to whether similar elevations are taking place in the brain.

Distraction and Self-efficacy hypotheses. Here the psychological benefits of exercise are said to be because when one exercises, they are distracted from their habitual concerns or that exercise improvements allow them to see themselves as more efficacious in managing their environments. While research tends to support both distraction and self-efficacy as resulting from exercise, it is less than clear that either result in long-term reductions in intractable states such as PTSD.

In summary, available empirical research (e.g., Manger & Motta, 2005) show that exercise results in significant reductions in PTSD and other negative emotional states such as anxiety and depression. The mechanism or theoretical model by which these benefits occur following exercise is for the most part, unknown. Nevertheless, both aerobic and anaerobic exercise are effective in reducing negative psychological states and improving health. Their positive impact in reducing PTSD and its symptoms shows that exercise is a valuable alternative to traditional psychotherapies.

Nature and Animal Assisted Therapies. Immersion in natural environment and interacting with animals have shown themselves to be valuable and empirically supported interventions for trauma-based disorders including PTSD. Their growing popularity may be due to several factors including available health services not being able to cope with the number of trauma cases that have resulted from the Covid epidemic and from our involvement in recent wars; the aversion to traditional therapies with their emphasis on confronting sensitive trauma issues; the avoidance of stigma associated with psychotherapy; the avoidance of medical interventions; and the expense and inconvenience of traditional therapy.

Nature assisted therapy (NAT) can take different forms including the discipline of plant care and propagation, wandering within natural environments, restoration and development of healing gardens, wilderness and outdoor therapy, adventure therapy, and others. In Japan it is common for stressed individuals to engage in supervised excursions into nature and this practice is referred to as *shirin yoku* (Japanese for "forest bathing"). "NAT is defined as an intervention with the aim to treat, hasten recovery, and/or rehabilitate patients with a disease or a condition of ill health, with the fundamental principle that the therapy involves plants, natural materials, and//or outdoor environments, without any therapeutic involvement of extra human mammals or other living creatures. (Annerstedt & Wahrborg, 2011, p. 372).

The most common types of NAT programs are sustained base camp expeditions often lasting 2 to 3 months. However, simply walking through parks and arboretums can have stress relieving effects. Clients in adventure programs engage in activities such as rope courses, group games, trust exercises, and expeditions into nature. Therapeutic goals can be anxiety reduction, building of social interaction skills, substance abuse reduction, and others (Bowen & Neill, 2013). Some of these adventure programs are designed for youngsters to develop self-confidence and social skills. Some are designed older adolescents and young adults. Other programs are for both adults and seniors and are intended to simply expose adults to the calming effects of being immersed in nature (Bowen & Nell, 2013).

Wilson (1984), an entomologist, was among the first to suggest that humans have an attraction to nature and is often credited with the use of the term *biophilia* to describe the in-born affiliation with nature. However, it was the social psychologist Eric Fromm who coined the term to describe the passionate love of life and living things. Natural environments present people with the sense of being away from the stresses of daily living and it is not uncommon for those going away on vacations and holidays to seek out natural environments, greenery, and water. The overall thrust of research (e.g., Poulsen et al., 2015) suggests that nature, in and of itself, can be beneficial to well-being, create stress reduction, bring about feelings of peace and tranquility, and be effective in managing PTSD.

In addition to natural environments, the presence of animals and animal assisted therapy (AAT) can have significant benefits in treating traumatized individuals (e.g. Parish-Plass, 2008) and PTSD. There are a variety of reasons for this including the fact that many animals are unconditionally accepting, are devoid of schemes and agendas, enjoy receiving and giving love and affection, require that the traumatized individual provide care and feeding and thereby reduce their self-absorption, and provide a non-threatening, stable presence. The range of problems that are improved by interacting with animals includes anxiety and depressive disorders, personality disorders, PTSD, ADD and ADHD, Alzheimer's and other dementias, autism spectrum disorders, reactions to abuse in its various forms. Dogs and cats are the most common house pets and are often seen as loving "family members." Their positive impact on well-being cannot be overstated.

Service dogs differ from pets and those used in therapy to assist in the therapeutic process (e.g., rabbits, horses, dogs, hamsters, cats, etc.) in that they are specifically trained to engage in behaviors that are oriented to help individual with specific difficulties. For example, a service dog may wake traumatized individuals during episodic nightmares; they may stand in the way of the individual to create barrier to anxiety provoking social encounters; provide physical and emotional connection; and reduce the need for medication owing to their stress reducing impact.

A study by O'Hare and Rodriguez (2018) systematically compared a group of traumatized veterans to another group of traumatized veterans who, like the first group, indicated a willingness to engage in a program involving service dogs. The second group had applied to be assigned a service dog and thus the variable of willingness to be with a service dog was controlled. Overall results revealed statistically significant reductions in PTSD for those who interacted with service dogs. These reductions were not seen in the control group. In comparison to controls those who did interact with dogs showed significantly improved willingness to engage in social interactions, had lower social isolation, and lower absenteeism from work due to health issues. The unanswered question in this study is whether veterans who were not positively oriented toward dogs would also have shown these benefits. Nevertheless, this well controlled study supported the beneficial effects of the presence of animals for those who are traumatized. Similar positive effects have been demonstrated with a wide variety of animals even those that are not typically associated with warm interactions with humans such as fish and amphibians. Data obtained from equine therapy programs provide empirical evidence for PTSD reductions in veterans who care for and are involved in horse riding programs. Overall, findings from a variety of studies provide substantial evidence for the health benefits of interacting with animals.

Acupuncture. The practice of acupuncture first arose approximately 2500 years ago as a way of uniting humans with nature and was based on the teachings of Taoism. Skeptics of acupuncture in treating PTSD find the procedure an easy target. Acupuncture is said to alter the flow of an energy or life force called *qi* (pronounced chi), and this alteration reportedly creates a balance between two opposing forces of yin and yang. There is also said to exist meridians or channels along which *qi* flows. Neither the flow of *qi,* nor meridians, nor the forces of yin and yang or any other underlying mechanisms of acupuncture have been demonstrated to the satisfaction of Western medicine. If there is a psychological or physical benefit, Western doubters attribute these benefits to the well-known placebo effect. However, the World Health Organization supports acupuncture for the treatment of physical and psychological distress owing to the existence of empirical studies showing that the impact of acupuncture exceeds that of placebos.

To some extent Western medicine's placebo critique of acupuncture is disingenuous. Meniscectomy is a surgical procedure to alleviate the pain of torn cartilage (the meniscus). Available evidence shows that arthroscopic meniscectomy, when compared to a sham procedure where surgical marks are made on the knee causing patients to believe they had actual surgery, but no actual surgery has taken place, reveals no difference in outcome between the two groups. Over the counter medication, rest, and exercise appear to be equally effective as surgery. This does not deter Western medicine from doing the surgical procedure on over 700,000 people a year for a cost of approximately $4 billion (Sihvonen et al., 2013). Whereas meniscectomy may not exceed the effect of placebo, it appears that acupuncture does.

The World Health Organization (WHO, 2002) reported a wide array of conditions "for which acupuncture has been proved" (p.33), including lower back pain, vomiting, neck and facial pain, headache, nausea, hypertension and hypotension, morning sickness, reaction chemotherapy and radiotherapy, and many others. It is of interest to note that acupuncture, when applied to those with high blood pressure, lowers that pressure. The reverse occurs in hypotension or low blood pressure. In those cases, acupuncture elevates blood pressure. This effect is said to occur because the *qi* is unblocked and allowed to flow along meridians. That explanation is likely to elicit skepticism and maybe even hypertension among many Western physicians.

One of the specific studies of acupuncture for PTSD (Hollifield, Sinclair-Lian, Warner, and Hammerschlag, 2007) was a randomized, controlled trial in which acupuncture was compared to CBT and a wait list control (WLC). Volunteers with PTSD and related problems were randomly assigned to the three groups. Sessions ran for two hours for a period of 12 weeks. Overall results showed statistically large reductions (effect size exceeding 1.0) for PTSD, anxiety and depression for the CBT and acupuncture groups in comparison to the WLC. The CBT and acupuncture groups were equivalent in their beneficial effects. This outcome is impressive as no actual psychotherapy was taking place in the acupuncture group and yet significant reductions in PTSD, anxiety, and depression occurred and was maintained in a follow-up assessment.

Studies such a Hollifield et al. (2007) provide substantial support for the use of acupuncture for PTSD, although it is likely that acupuncture is seldom sought out as a primary form of treatment. Acupuncture has established itself for many years as an effective intervention for pain and a variety of medical conditions and has only recently been viewed as a PTSD treatment. The fact that it can be effective with both physical and psychological conditions suggests a unity of these two entities and this falls in line with the *bodymind* concept of Candace Pert (1999) as mentioned above on the section on exercise as an intervention for PTSD.

Emotional Freedom Techniques. Emotional Freedom Techniques (EFT) are like acupuncture in that they take the position that various forms of physical and emotional difficulties arise from blockages or impedance of energy flow. While acupuncture primarily uses needles to rebalance this energy flow, EFT uses either tapping or rubbing of what are said to be meridians and meridian end points. EFT evolved from what was then called thought field therapy (TFT) and was originated by Roger Callahan (TFT; Callahan,1997). Callahan presented the case of Mary who had a severe water phobia, and this phobia was overcome through TFT and specifically by the activity of tapping below the eye. Continued follow-up over a period of 30 years revealed no return of the fear of water. After his death Callahan's wife, Joanne, coined the term Emotional Freedom Technique as an alternative to Thought Field Therapy.

Many techniques including EMDR, acupuncture, and perhaps even exercise have been branded as examples of charlatanism, voodoo, placebo effects and other pejoratives perhaps because explanations of how they work do not fit into Western materialistic, empirical interpretations. Most of the traditional treatments mentioned earlier such as CBT, ACT, DBT and others base their effects upon laboratory-based learning theory and cognitive science. In contrast EFT and acupuncture draw their validation from Eastern traditions involving concepts such as *qi*, meridians, and energy flow. Despite these differences in explaining therapeutic outcomes, empirical evidence does exist to support processes such as EFT and this evidence comes from randomized control group studies and metanalyses.

In 2016 the Substance Abuse and Mental Health Services Administration listed TFT as an empirically supported, evidence-based treatment for trauma related disorders, psychologically based stress disorders, and as enhancing overall resilience and ability to cope with stress. Similarly, in 2013 Dawson Church and David Feinstein initiated a series of studies that culminated in the position that the EFT method met, and in several cases, exceeded the criteria set by the Society of Clinical

Psychology (Division 12 of the American Psychological Association) for what is seen as empirically validated treatment.

The specifics of the technique involve series of steps. ***Step 1.****Identify the Problem.* For example: "my father's continued denigration of me when I was a child." "My sore leg." "My traumatic war experience." ***Step 2.*** Rate the intensity of the problem. Using the Subjective Units of Distress Scale (SUDS; Wolpe and Lazarus, 1966) the stated problem is rated from1 *(none or almost none)* to 10 (*maximum or most intense).****Step 3.*** Begin the setup phase. Here one acknowledges their problem yet does not engage in self-criticism or lack of self-acceptance. For example, the traumatized individual might state, "Even though I did not resist being demeaned by my sibling, I completely accept myself." ***Step 4.*** Start of the tapping process. While verbalizing the comment in step 3., one engages in tapping of various parts of the body approximately five to seven times. These body parts include the top of the head, beginning of the eyebrow, side of the eye, under the nose, and other body parts (see Motta, 2020; pp. 148 149). After completing the tapping sequence, one reassesses their distress rating by completing the subjective units of distress (SUDS) scale. The entire sequence is repeated until the SUDS rating is at a relatively low level of perhaps 1, 2, or 3.

Following a metanalysis by Sebastian and Nelms (2017), it was concluded that "the analysis of existing studies showed that a series of 4-10 EFT sessions is an efficacious treatment for PTSD with a variety of populations… (and) that it can be used both on a self-help basis and as a primary evidence-based treatment for PTSD." (p. 16). One of the real values of EFT is that it is a straightforward procedure that does not require a high level of training and can be self administered. And while these may be considered strengths to those who accept EFT as a treatment for PTSD, they might also be used as evidence to discredit the procedure as lacking in scientific rigor. Nevertheless, if one is looking for an empirically supported procedure that has amassed evidence for its efficacy, EFT is worthy of consideration.

MDMA (Ecstasy). MDMA or 3,4 methylenedioxymethamphetamine, also known Ecstasy, Adam, and Molly in the rave and party scene, is the only such drug that is nearing Food and Drug Administration (FDA) approval for the treatment of PTSD. MDMA differs from Ecstasy in that in the latter formulation it is often adulterated with other drugs. Pure MDMA had been used for many years as a chemical adjunct in treating trauma related disorders and this continued until 1985 when it was classified as a schedule 1 substance under the Federal Controlled Substances Act and once so scheduled, it was legally banned. It was banned because of safety concerns given the number of people who had overdosed on it in the party and rave scenes.

Now in its FDA Phase III trials, MDMA is in the final stages of showing both its effectiveness and safety in treating PTSD across a variety of traumatized groups. So far MDMA has been found to be more effective than placebo treatments, in randomized controlled clinical trials, even in cases of PTSD that have resisted other forms of treatment for decades. So far, the available data show MDMA to be effective in facilitating therapy for trauma related disorders in controlled studies. Although the drug has been fast tracked for FDA approval, several controlled studies are needed before MDMA receives the imprimatur of FDA approval. As such, its availability in treating PTSD is limited to those sites where government sanctioned research is taking place.

MDMA is technically not a hallucinogen as is LSD. The latter causes alterations in one's perceptions so that one might see images that are not actually there, and experience other radical alterations in the way reality is perceived. In contrast, MDMA is an empathogen that alters one's levels of empathy and acceptance of others and oneself. Its value in treating PTSD is that it allows one to accept and deal with their traumatic experiences rather than to avoid them. With MDMA one is better able to accept themselves and their responses that came about because of their trauma. Narcotics can produce tranquility and stupor and amphetamine-like substances produce mood alteration, energy, and behavioral activity. Empathogens produce feelings of peace and gentleness along with feelings of closeness and empathy and perhaps a new awareness of the value and importance of music. There are reported feelings of a loss of self-consciousness, feelings of joy, enhanced feelings of the importance of relationships, and an acceptance and joy in the appreciation of all things.

The typical treatment takes place in a welcoming room that often has a couch or bed, blankets, soothing music, beverages. and a male and female therapist. The therapists are trained to be non-directive and emotionally supportive. Medical supervision and oversight is also available on the premises. Treatment involves the use of MDMA administered over a period of days or weeks. After a period of approximately three, eight-hour sessions using MDMA, a period of an additional 8 to 16 weeks of non-drug therapy sessions follow. According to Holland (2001), what makes MDMA assisted therapy different from the usual non-drug treatment of PTSD "is that instead of feeling vulnerable and anxious during this experience, the patients remain relaxed, fearless, and show a stronger sense of self and purpose. Feelings of depression and anxiety are replaced with a sense of ease and safety.... " (P. 2).

It takes approximately 45 minutes for MDMA to start being felt. In the beginning there is some anxiety, a slight feeling of drunkenness, and a shift in consciousness. There is then an intense feeling of euphoria and an enhancement of sensations and feelings. There is an alteration in one's feeling for others. Whereas others may have previously been avoided, they are now welcomed and warmly accepted. There is a profound feeling of self-acceptance. After about three hours the impact of MDMA begins to wane but at this point the traumatized individual has encountered a self that may have been banned from awareness and pushed away from consciousness. This self that has been assiduously avoided, often for decades, is now seen, welcomed, and accepted. Some describe MDMA, not as a love drug but as a hug drug. While on MDMA one is inclined both literally and figuratively hug their inner self and the selves of others. Many traumatized individuals report MDMA therapy for PTSD to be life transforming.

As of this writing MDMA is about to be approved for the treatment of PTSD. It has not yet received official FDA approval but that appears to highly likely to occur. MDMA therapy might be resource demanding in that it requires multiple therapists, multiple sessions, and medical involvement. However, when one considers the costs of decades of therapy to treat thousands of veterans and others who have been severely traumatized, with little promise of improvement, the use of MDMA to treat PTSD is effective from both cost and outcome perspectives.

Other Alternative Therapies. There is a wide array of other therapies for treating PTSD that are found in the literature. These will not be covered fully either because a lack of a body of well controlled studies supporting their use, lack of metanalyses, or because they produce high levels of avoidance owing to their evoking elevations of anxiety and avoidance. A fuller description of each of these can be found in the literature (e.g., Motta, 2020. pp. 186-189).

Virtual Reality Exposure Therapy (VRET). This is computer-based form of trauma stimuli exposure often requiring the use of wearable electronic gear. Although it can be effective in treating PTSD, its anxiety producing imagery can evoke high levels of discomfort and subsequent avoidance of VRET.

Transcranial Magnetic Stimulation (TMS). TMS employs a magnetic field that induces firing in selected areas of the brain. Data is being gathered to date, but its overall effectiveness in treating PTSD has not been convincingly established.

Internet and Computer-Based Treatments. Computer based approaches going by names of apps such as Calm, VetChange, Interapy, DE-STRESS and many others have been implemented. High dropout rates have been reported and the evidence supporting these interventions is scant.

Neurofeedback. Some authors suggest that informational feedback on our brain's activity in the form of visual images and sounds can be helpful in altering dysfunctional brain activity due to PTSD. Wide acceptance of neurofeedback has not occurred perhaps because of the need for costly equipment and the lack of abundant empirical support for these procedures.

Propranolol Therapy. Propranolol is a beta blocker and shows promise in the treatment of PTSD. There are a handful of double-blind, placebo-controlled studies showing that the use of propranolol shortly after inducing of trauma memories helps to reduce their intensity and thereby the avoidance of those memories. Although promising, additional studies are needed to establish the utility of this medication in treating PTSD.

Stellate Ganglion Block (SGB). SGBs involve injection of an anesthetic into the sympathetic nerves around the neck. Although the procedure has been used to alleviate pain such as in severe headaches, refractory angina, and other medical concerns, it has also shown some evidence in being effective in reducing the psychological pain associated PTSD and particularly that due to war experiences. Like MDMA therapy, SGB therapy is not all that easy to initiate. Nevertheless, the Department of Defense has shown interest in pursuing further research in this form of treatment given the high cost and general ineffectiveness of other forms of PTSD treatment.

Summary. PTSD is a disabling disorder that can occur following extremely frightening and often life-threatening experiences. For some people, the consequences of PTSD can last a lifetime. While the DSM provides a series of symptoms that are characteristic of PTSD, it does not do well in describing the felt experience of this disorder. PTSD alters people both deeply and fundamentally. The disorder often produces changes in the way people see themselves. For example, the outgoing friendly extrovert can become an isolated, introverted, and suspicious individual. The person who previously trusted others and felt secure in their surroundings, is now suspicious, weary, and somber. PTSD alters people and most often those alterations are in the direction of negativism, doubt, suspiciousness, and distrust.

The various traditional therapies that have been used in treating PTSD often focus on altering the cognitions of the traumatized person. CBT and its variants are examples of traditional therapies. It is suggested that PTSD is not necessarily a cognitive or thinking problem but rather one of conditioned emotional reactions and avoidance of anxiety. As such a series of non-traditional therapies have been implemented and show considerable promise. The popularity of these alternative approaches such as yoga, meditation, exercise, acupuncture, and others may be that they do not elicit high levels of anxiety, they come with little stigma, they are cost effective, but mainly because they can be effective in reducing the pain of living with PTSD.

PTSD is a potentially disabling condition that has prompted a good deal of research on a variety of different treatment forms. It is a relatively new disorder as far as the DSM is concerned but it has obviously existed throughout history. It is fortunate that it has sparked so much research activity as this will eventually translate into a reduction of suffering for many who have lived with this disorder for most of their lives.

REFERENCES

American Psychiatric Association. (1980). *Diagnostic and statistical manual of mental disorders* (3rd ed.). Author.

American Psychiatric Association. (2013). *Diagnostic and statistical manual of mental disorders* (5th ed.). Author.

Annerstedt, M., & Wahrborg, P. (2011). Nature-assisted therapy: Systematic review of controlled and observational studies. *Scandinavian Journal of Public Health*, 39(4), 371–388. DOI: 10.1177/1403494810396400 PMID: 21273226

APA Presidential Task Force on Evidence-Based Practice. (2006). Evidence-based Practice in psychology. *The American Psychologist*, 61(4), 271–285. DOI: 10.1037/0003-066X.61.4.271 PMID: 16719673

Benedek, D. M., & Wynn, G. H. (2016). *Complementary and alternative medicine for PTSD*. DOI: 10.1093/med/9780190205959.001.0001

Bowen, D. J., & Neill, J. T. (2013). A meta-analysis of adventure therapy outcomes and moderators. *The Open Psychology Journal*, 6(1), 28–53. DOI: 10.2174/1874350120130802001

Breslau, N. (2009). The epidemiology of trauma. PTSD and other posttrauma disorders. *Trauma, Violence & Abuse*, 10(3), 198–210. DOI: 10.1177/1524838009334448 PMID: 19406860

Callahan, R. (1997). Thought field therapy: The case of Mary. *Traumatology*, 3(1), 30–37. DOI: 10.1177/153476569700300105

Church, D., & Feinstein, D. (2013). Energy psychology in the treatment of PTSD: Psychobiology and clinical principles. In T, Van Leeuwen & T. Van Brouwer (Eds.). *Psychology of trauma* (pp. 211-224). Hauppauge, N.Y: Nova Science

Dienstmann, G. (2018). Practical meditation: A simple step-by-step guide. New York, NY: DK.

Emerson, D., & Hopper, E. (2011). *Overcoming trauma through yoga: Reclaiming your body*. North Atlantic Books.

Foa, E. B., Hembree, E. A., & Rothbaum, B. O. (2007). *Prolonged exposure therapy for PTSD: Emotional process of traumatic experiences-Therapist guide*. Oxford University Press. DOI: 10.1093/med:psych/9780195308501.001.0001

Foa, E. B., Keane, T. M., & Friedman, M. J. (2000). *Effective treatments for PTSD*.

Hayes, S. C., Strosahl, K. D., & Wilson, G. (2016). *Acceptance and commitment therapy: The process and practice of mindful change*. Spiegel and Grau.

Holland, J. (2001). Medicine for the new millennium. In Holland, J. (Ed.), *Ecstasy: A complete guide-A comprehensive look at the risks and benefits of MDMA* (pp. 1–5). Park Street Press.

Hollifield, M., Sinclair-Lian, N., Warner, T. D., & Hammeschlag, R. (2007). Acupuncture for posttraumatic stress disorder: A randomized controlled pilot trial. *The Journal of Nervous and Mental Disease*, 195(6), 504–513. DOI: 10.1097/NMD.0b013e31803044f8 PMID: 17568299

Jackson, K. (2014). Treatment for veterans with PTSD – Outside the traditional toolbox. *Social Work Today*, 14, 18.

Kabat-Zinn, J. (1994). *Wherever you go, there you are: Mindfulness meditation in everyday life*. Hyperion.

Manger, T. A., & Motta, R. W. (2005). The impact of an exercise program on posttraumatic stress disorder, anxiety, and depression. *International Journal of Emergency Mental Health*, 7, 49–57. PMID: 15869081

McCann, I. L., & Pearlman, L. A. (1990). Vicarious traumatization: A framework for understanding the psychological effects of working with victims. *Journal of Traumatic Stress*, 3(1), 131–149. DOI: 10.1007/BF00975140

Motta, R.W. (2013, Winter). PTSD and secondary traumatization: A comprehensive review. *Mental Health News,* pp. 1, 6, 14, 16, 22, 26, 27, 30.

Motta, R. W. (2018). The role of exercise in reducing PTSD and negative emotional states. In Taukeni, S. G. (Ed.), *Psychology of health-Biopsychosocial approach.* InTech Open.

Motta, R. W. (2020). *Alternative therapies for PTSD: The science of mind-body treatments*. American Psychological Association. DOI: 10.1037/0000186-000

Motta, R. W. (2023). *Secondary trauma: Silent suffering and its treatment*. Springer. DOI: 10.1007/978-3-031-44308-4

O'Haire, M. E., & Rodriguez, K. E. (2018). Preliminary efficacy of service dogs as a complementary treatment for posttraumatic stress disorder in military members and veterans. *Journal of Consulting and Clinical Psychology*, 86(2), 179–188. DOI: 10.1037/ccp0000267 PMID: 29369663

Parish-Plass, N. (2008). Animal-assisted therapy with children suffering from insecure attachment due to abuse and neglect: A method to lower the risk of intergenerational transmission of abuse. *Clinical Child Psychology and Psychiatry*, 13(1), 7–30. DOI: 10.1177/1359104507086338 PMID: 18411863

Pert, C. (1999). *Molecules of emotion: The science behind mind-body medicine.* Scribner.

Poulsen, D. V., Stigsdotter, U. K., & Refshage, A. D. (2015). Whatever happened to the soldiers? Nature-assisted therapies for veterans diagnosed with post- traumatic stress disorder: A literature review. *Urban Forestry & Urban Greening*, 14(2), 438–445. DOI: 10.1016/j.ufug.2015.03.009

Preston, J. D., O'Neal, J. H., & Talaga, M. C. (2002). *Handbook of clinical psychopharmacology for therapists* (3rd ed.). New Harbinger.

Resick, P. A. (2001). Cognitive processing therapy: Generic version. University of Missouri: St. Lewis.

Sebastian, B., & Nelms, J. (2017). The effectiveness of emotional freedom techniques in the treatment of posttraumatic stress disorder: A meta- analysis. *Explore (New York, N.Y.)*, 13(1), 16–25. DOI: 10.1016/j.explore.2016.10.001 PMID: 27889444

Shapiro, F. (1989). Eye movement desensitization: A new treatment for post-traumatic stress disorder. *Journal of Behavior Therapy and Experimental Psychiatry*, 20(3), 211–217. DOI: 10.1016/0005-7916(89)90025-6 PMID: 2576656

Sihvonen, R., Paavola, M., Itala, A., Joukainen, A., Nurmi, H., & Jarvinen, T. L. N. (2013). Arthros.copic partial meniscectomy versus sham surgery for a degenerative meniscal tear. *The New England Journal of Medicine*, 369(26), 2515–2524. DOI: 10.1056/NEJMoa1305189 PMID: 24369076

van der Kolk, B. (2014). *The body keeps the score*. Viking.

Waters, L. M. (2018). *Factors influencing the vicarious effects of trauma in hotline volunteers.* (Unpublished doctoral dissertation). Hofstra University, New York.

Weintraub, A. (2012). *Yoga skills for therapists: Effective practices for mood management.* Norton.

Wilson, E. O. (1984). *Biophilia*. Harvard University Press. DOI: 10.4159/9780674045231

Wolpe, J., & Lazarus, A. A. (1966). *Behavior therapy techniques: A guide to the treatment of neuroses*. Pergamon Press.

Wompold, B. E. (2015). How important are common factors in psychotherapy? An update. *World Psychiatry; Official Journal of the World Psychiatric Association (WPA)*, 14(3), 270–277. DOI: 10.1002/wps.20238 PMID: 26407772

World Health Organization. (2002). *Acupuncture: Review and analysis of reports on controlled clinical trials*. Author.

Chapter 3
The Neurobiological Basis of Post-Traumatic Stress Disorder:
Insights Into the Underlying Pathophysiological Mechanisms

Bilal El-Mansoury
https://orcid.org/0000-0002-2583-7515
Chouaib Doukkali University, Morocco

Asmaa Haj-Khlifa
https://orcid.org/0000-0002-7809-839X
Cadi Ayyad University, Morocco

Jawad Laadraoui
https://orcid.org/0000-0002-9784-1265
University of Hassan II, Casablanca, Morocco

Hanane El Fatimi
Mohammed VI University of Health Sciences, Morocco

El Mehdi Dalil
Cadi Ayyad University, Morocco

Mohamed Hammani
Cadi Ayyad University, Morocco

Omar El Hiba
Chouaib Doukkali University, Morocco

Samira Boulbaroud
Université Sultan Moulay Slimane, Morocco

Abdelali Bitar
Chouaib Doukkali University, Morocco

Arumugam Jayakumar
University of Miami, USA

ABSTRACT

Post-traumatic stress disorder (PTSD) is a well-known mental health condition that affects millions of people worldwide. PTSD is characterized by a spectrum of psycho-

DOI: 10.4018/979-8-3693-2089-1.ch003

emotional and neurophysiological effects, such as re-experiencing the trauma in the form of vivid intrusive memories, flashbacks, or nightmares. These experiences often are followed by overwhelming fear and strong physical sensations. Neuroimaging studies in patients with PTSD as well as experimental studies show alterations in brain areas such as the amygdala, hippocampus and prefrontal cortex as well as in neurochemical stress response systems. Additionally, it is believed that the main neurochemical features of PTSD include abnormal regulation of catecholamines, monoamines, and opioid neurotransmitters among others, each of which is found in brain circuits that regulate/integrate stress and fear responses. This chapter will provide an overview on the recent pathophysiological mechanisms underlying the development of PTSD.

INTRODUCTION

Post-traumatic stress disorder (PTSD) is a mental health condition that develops after exposure to severely traumatic situations including interpersonal violence, dangerous accidents, combat, wars or natural disasters. PTSD symptoms include distressing and intrusive memories and nightmares of the trauma, impatience, hypervigilance, difficulty falling asleep, poor concentration, and emotional withdrawal. People who suffer from PTSD usually steer clear of situations, people, or objects that may trigger memories of the trauma (American Psychiatric Association & Association, 1994). In addition, significant medical comorbidities, such as persistent pain and inflammation, cardiometabolic diseases, and an increased risk of dementia, are also linked to PTSD (Lohr et al., 2015, 2015; Michopoulos et al., 2015). PTSD consists the most common psychopathological result of being exposed to stressful experiences. Depending on one's socioeconomic background and place of residence, the lifetime prevalence of PTSD can range from 1.3% to 12.2%, whereas the 1-year prevalence is between 0.2 and 3.8% (Marwit, 2003). Consequently, there is a very high overall illness burden (disability and early mortality) associated with PTSD (Yehuda et al., 2015).

When PTSD was first identified, it was believed to be a normal reaction at the extreme of a response continuum, the degree of which was mostly correlated with the severity of the trauma or stressor. Over time, it has been evident, therefore, that an individual's reaction to trauma is contingent upon both stressor attributes and individual traits (Sherin & Nemeroff, 2011). PTSD was almost exclusively understood in psychological terms, and the biological literature on the disorder only included a few scant psychophysiological observations. Understanding the neurobiological processes behind PTSD enhances research on the disease, even though it is still relevant from a psychiatric standpoint (Pitman et al., 2012). Recent neuroimaging studies in patients with PTSD as well as experimental studies have shown alterations in several brain structures including the cerebral cortex, cerebral white matter, amygdala, hippocampus, as well as in neurochemical stress response systems; imbalance in the functional aspects of hypothalamus-pituitary-adrenal axis and the hypothalamic-pituitary-thyroid axis (Pitman et al., 2001; Cooper et al., 2017 ; Daskalakis et al., 2013 ; Dominique, 2007; Schelling et al., 2004 ; Kim et al., 2019 ; Garfinkel et al., 2014; Karl et al., 2006 ; Dixon et al., 2017). Additionally, alteration in neurotransmission systems mainly catecholamines and monoamines as well neuropeptidergic systems have been reported. Moreover, several studies have shown impaired neurogenesis in PTSD (Peng et al., 2013 ; Ishikawa et al., 2019; Matsuoka, 2011 ; Terranova et al., 2019 ; Yoneda et al., 2008 ; Sun et al., 2020 ; Aliev et al., 2020). This chapter provides the pathophysiological mechanisms underpinning PTSD ranging from neuroimaging data to experimental studies.

NEUROCHEMICAL STRESS RESPONSE SYSTEMS

The Hypothalamic-Pituitary-Adrenal Axis

The hypothalamic-pituitary-adrenal (HPA) axis serves as the central regulator of the mammalian neuroendocrine stress response systems (Sherin & Nemeroff, 2011) through homeostatic mechanisms (Ursin & Olff, 1993). However, its dysfunction has been linked to several mental health disorders including PTSD. Indeed, recent studies have sustained this axis dysfunction in the pathogenesis of PTSD (Cooper et al., 2017), which makes it a focal point of investigation in patients with PTSD.

The HPA axis is made up of endocrine hypothalamic components, including the anterior pituitary and adrenal glands which act as an effector organs (Sherin & Nemeroff, 2011). Exposure to stress causes neurons in the hypothalamic paraventricular nucleus (PVN) to release corticotropin-releasing hormone (CRH) into the hypothalamo-hypophyseal portal circulation from nerve terminals in the median eminence, this process stimulates the anterior pituitary's production and release of adreno-corticotropin (ACTH) (Sherin & Nemeroff, 2011). ACTH in turn stimulates the release of glucocorticoids (GC) from the adrenal cortex, thereby orchestrating physiological behavior to manage stressors (Sherin & Nemeroff, 2011). Thus, the HPA axis function is regulated and restored in normal circumstances (Cooper et al., 2017). However, in PTSD, chronic exposure to repeated or severe stress leads to HPA axis dysfunction, leading to disrupted protective mechanisms that would normally stop the response to stressful stimuli (Cooper et al., 2017). This failure is manifested by lower cortisol levels and elevated catecholamine levels, which lead PTSD patients to exhibit a persistent response to an external challenge that is no longer actively present. Thus, patients continue to be hypervigilant, and exhibit autonomic reaction by intrusive memories of traumatic experiences (Fig. 1) (Daskalakis et al., 2013).

In addition to lower plasma or serum cortisol levels (Meewisse et al., 2007), PTSD patients exhibit reduced ACTH responses to CRH and that the cortisol response to stress is delayed in PTSD patients, with elevated (Rasmusson et al., 2001) or unchanged (Kellner et al., 2003) CRH-induced cortisol levels. In addition, it has been reported that PTSD patients can present hypocortisolism which could be associated with heightened negative feedback sensitivity of the HPA axis. Thus, hypocortisolism may make a person more susceptible to future PTSD and be a risk factor for maladaptive stress reactions (Sherin & Nemeroff, 2011).

It should be mentioned that GCs interfere with the retrieval of traumatic memories, an effect that may independently prevent or reduce symptoms of PTSD (Aerni et al., 2004). This hypothesis is supported in principle by the finding that exogenously administered hydrocortisone can prevent PTSD after exposure to psychological trauma (Dominique, 2007; Schelling et al., 2004). Furthermore, it has been demonstrated that the efficacy of exogenously injected hydrocortisone in simulating a normal diurnal cortisol rhythm for the treatment of PTSD (Aerni et al., 2004). In trauma or accident victims, both single-dose (Jovanovic et al., 2011; Zohar et al., 2011), and chronic cortisol treatment (Aerni et al., 2004) have been observed to enhance PTSD symptoms, suggesting that GC can attenuate symptoms even after the development of PTSD (Jacobson, 2014).

Furthermore, since GCs reduce sympathetic activity (Gustavson et al., 2008; Kvetnanský et al., 1995), low GC levels may allow excessive sympathetic arousal in PTSD, emulating an acute stress state (Yehuda, 2009; Yehuda & LeDoux, 2007). Interestingly, it has been reported that GCs obstruct memory retrieval (Dominique et al., 2009). As a result, inadequate GC secretion may permit the recurrence of the intrusive memories that are typical of PTSD (Yehuda, 2009). Moreover, processes controlling dendritic plasticity, neurogenesis, and neuronal survival may be adversely impacted by GCs (Radley et al., 2008). Changes in GC feedback mechanisms play a major role in the mechanisms leading to HPA axis dysfunction (Radley & Sawchenko, 2011). Indeed, the metabolic phenotype of PTSD may be caused partially by GC hypersensitivity, which may have an impact on oxidative stress, inflammation, insulin resistance, and energy deficiency (Somvanshi et al., 2019). Importantly, GCs hyposecretion is commonly associated with PTSD (Yehuda & Seckl, 2011).

Otherwise, it is believed that PTSD patients have suppressed HPA axis activity, which progressively leads to increased catecholamine levels, corticotropin-releasing factor (CRF), and reduced cortisol levels (T. D. Kim et al., 2020; Y.-K. Kim et al., 2019; Vasileva et al., 2019). Additionally, CRF-1-mediated signaling may also encourage increased corticotropins release, which are linked to other symptoms including "suicide" and "psychosis" under stress. CRF1 signaling may also have a role in the depression-related cognitive impairment that occurs following PTSD (Cacabelos et al., 2016). Moreover, adenylate cyclase-activating polypeptide (PACAP) in the pituitary may promote CRF secretion, which is further linked to stress incidence in PTSD patients, and thus PTSD comorbid symptoms may be effectively treated with new antagonists that target CRF-1 receptors (Bale & Vale, 2004; Holsboer & Ising, 2008).

It is worth mentioning that the HPA axis's negative feedback mechanism, which releases corticosteroids in response to stressful events, is mediated by the activation of the glucocorticoid receptor (GR) (Yehuda, 2009). Increased numbers and sensitivity of peripheral leukocyte GR to glucocorticoids have also been demonstrated in vitro, suggesting that alterations in GR sensitivity may occur throughout the body in PTSD (Yehuda, 2009; Yehuda & Seckl, 2011). Nonetheless, the mineralocorticoid receptor (MR) function seems to be normal (Jacobson, 2014). In PTSD patients, there is a report of increased GR expression and decreased overall methylation levels of GR promoter regions. For instance, individuals with PTSD who are military veterans have lower levels of methylation in the GR promoter than patients without PTSD, suggesting that pharmaceutical methods to alter methylation at the GR promoter may be useful (Yehuda, 2009). Thus, patients with PTSD have been found to have many GR-receptor gene polymorphisms (Castro-Vale et al., 2016; Yehuda, 2015).

Additionally, PTSD is linked also to immune response dysregulation, as evidenced by an increase in pro-inflammatory cytokines such as interleukins (IL-6 and IL-17) and a reduction of anti-inflammatory cytokines such as IL-4 (Mellon et al., 2018). Hence, some research indicates that PTSD symptoms may be exacerbated by disruption of the HPA axis and IL-6 (Furtado & Katzman, 2015). Of note, under stressful conditions, pro-inflammatory cytokines such as interferon γ (IFN-γ), tumor necrosis factor α (TNF-α), IL-6, and IL-12 are secreted less often and lymphocyte proliferation is inhibited by glucocorticoid secretions through the HPA axis (Y.-K. Kim et al., 2019).

Figure 1. The hypothalamic-pituitary-adrenal axis is the body's major response system for stress

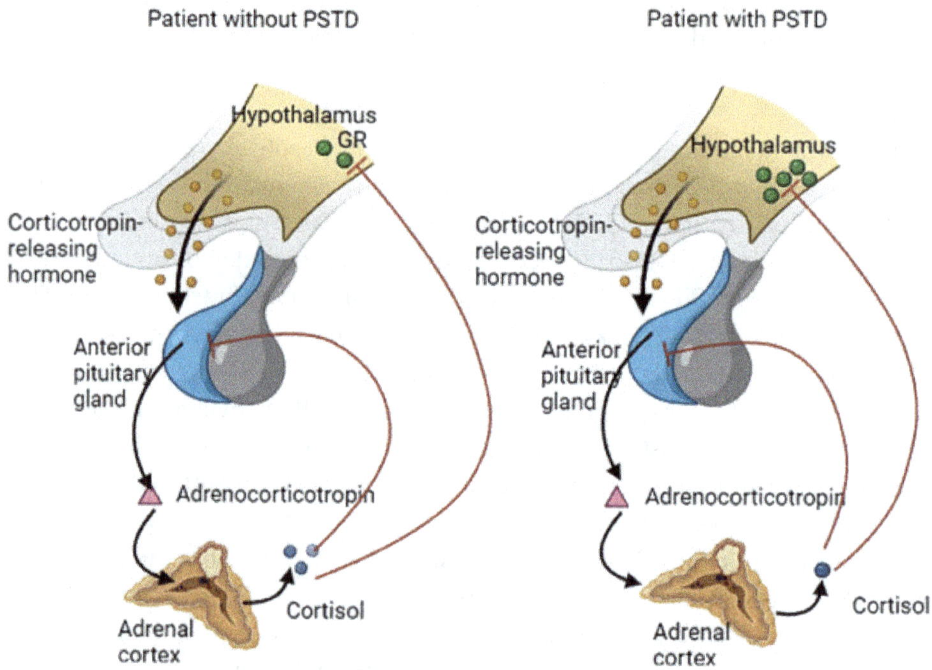

The Hypothalamic-Pituitary-Thyroid (HPT) Axis

Broadly speaking, the core endocrine features of PTSD involve the abnormal regulation of cortisol as aforementioned, and thyroid hormones (Sherin & Nemeroff, 2011), specifically through the hypothalamic-pituitary-thyroid (HPT) axis. It is well known that trauma events lead thyroid anomalies. Despite evidence linking traumatic stress to clinical hyperthyroidism, research on the HPT axis in PTSD has been limited. It has been shown that PTSD is associated with increased HPT axis activity (Bremner, Southwick, et al., 1999; Prange, 1999), revealing elevated levels of both total and free fractions of tri-iodothyronine (T3) and thyroxine (T4) (Sherin & Nemeroff, 2011).

It is worth mentioning that some studies on PTSD in Vietnam and World War II veterans have shown increased baseline levels of T3, T4, and T3 compared to T4, indicating improved peripheral deiodination of T4 to the more physiologically active T3 form of the hormone (Prange, 1999). In these individuals, isolated T3 levels were elevated whereas T4 levels were normal. Interestingly, in the standard thyrotropin-releasing hormone (TRH) stimulation test, an exaggerated thyrotropin-stimulating hormone (TSH) response has been reported in PTSD patients in contrast to the blunted TSH response observed in depression, although some depressed patients also exhibit an enhanced response (Newport & Nemeroff, 2000). Taken together, these studies suggest that over time the impact of trauma on T4 levels may abate. The authors suggest that elevated T3 may relate to subjective anxiety in these individuals with PTSD (Sherin & Nemeroff, 2011).

BRAIN NEURAL CIRCUITS AND MOLECULAR MECHANISMS DYSREGULATED IN PTSD

PTSD presents distinct symptoms, encompassing intrusive thoughts, heightened arousal, flashbacks, nightmares, sleep disturbances, altered memory and focus, and exaggerated startle reactions. These symptoms are believed to reflect changes in brain structure and function triggered by stress (Bremner, 2002; Pitman, Shin, & Rauch, 2001; Vermetten & Bremner, 2002), as the prefrontal cortex (PFC), which modulate memory functions (Bremner, 2003), and the amygdala (fig. 2; Bijanki et al., 2020).

Several neuroimaging studies have implicated a range of brain circuits, which encompass the hippocampus, amygdala, and PFC, in the behavioral and molecular anomalies in PTSD (fig. 2) (Garfinkel et al., 2014; Karl et al., 2006). These three brain regions are integral components of the neural circuit implicated in both fear and safety learning (Tovote et al., 2015).

In gaining a deeper comprehension of the neuropathology and diverse symptoms associated with PTSD, a crucial avenue lies in investigating the fundamental molecular changes influenced by this condition. While previous studies have unveiled various molecular mechanisms linked to PTSD (Liberzon & Abelson, 2016; Ressler et al., 2022), a deeper understanding of the these distinct molecular pathways in PTSD is imperative. A comprehensive exploration and categorization of different molecular mechanisms based on their involvement in fear acquisition and fear extinction, coupled with an analysis of their behavioral symptomatology, may facilitate the identification of more effective therapeutic targets for treating PTSD (Fig. 3).

Figure 2. The neural circuits involved in posttraumatic stress disorder (Iqbal et al., 2023)

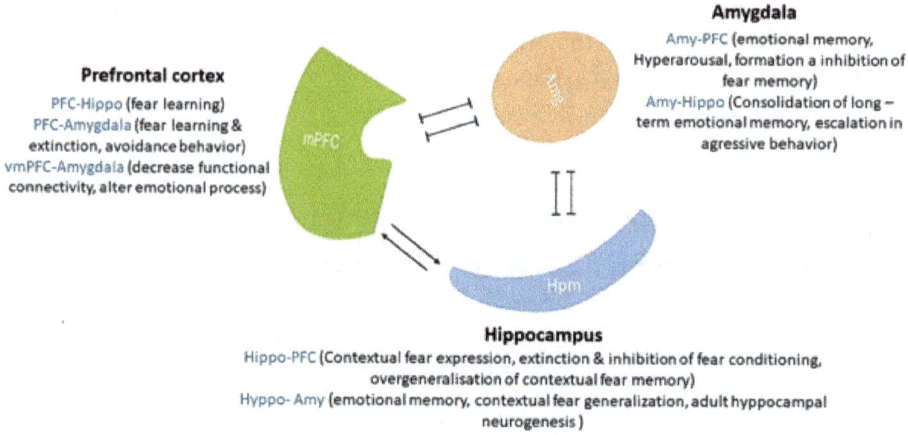

Figure 3. Molecular mechanisms affected by posttraumatic stress disorder (PTSD) (Iqbal et al., 2023)

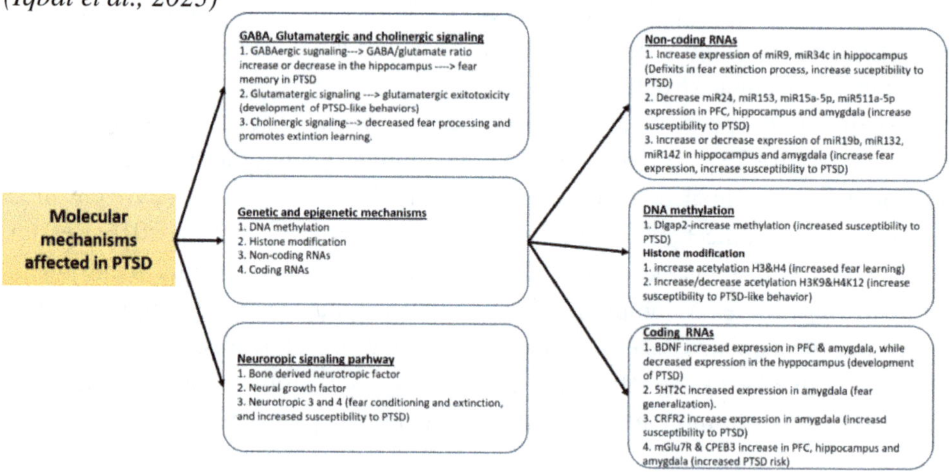

The Prefrontal Cortex Neural Circuit and PTSD

The prefrontal cortex (PFC), located in the frontal lobe region of the brain, plays crucial roles in decision-making and executive functions like working memory, regulating emotional behaviors, and attention (Dixon et al., 2017). Following PTSD, the PFC's communication with the hippocampus and amygdala significantly impacts the regulation of traumatic fear learning and its extinction (Gilmartin et al., 2014). Specifically, three subregions of the medial PFC (mPFC); the prelimbic cortex, the anterior cingulate cortex (ACC), and infralimbic cortex, show altered functions in PTSD (Gilmartin et al., 2014). These regions modulate emotional responses from other brain areas, with prelimbic and infralimbic cortices contributing to fear training and extinction processes respectively. The neuronal reserve within these regions influences the manifestation and preservation of fear behaviors and the retention of extinction memories (Do-Monte et al., 2015).

Individuals with PTSD who are undergoing traumatic symptoms exhibit diminished activity in the ventromedial PFC (vmPFC) (Hopper et al., 2007). The human vmPFC, similar to the infralimbic cortex in rodents, plays a crucial role in extinguishing fearful memories by activating safety signals and suppressing fear expression by interacting with the amygdala (Dunsmoor et al., 2019 ; Harrison et al., 2017). Similar alterations in connectivity are seen in PTSD, with decreased functional connectivity between specific brain regions in emotional tasks, both in women and men (Misaki et al., 2018). Structural changes are also noted in several brain areas of male PTSD patients, affecting fear-regulation circuits (Eckart et al., 2011).

The amygdala is under the normal homeostatic inhibitory control of the mPFC referred to as mPFC's "top-down" inhibitory regulation over the amygdala which maintains appropriate behavior patterns under stressful circumstances (Torrisi et al., 2019). However, in PTSD the hypoactive mPFC takes the brake off the amygdala, leading to amygdala hyperactivation which triggers hyperarousal and intrusion symptoms (fig 4). Importantly, alterations in connectivity between the vmPFC and the amygdala are linked to deficits in fear extinction in individuals with PTSD (Rauch et al., 2003; Stevens et al., 2013). This altered connectivity is implicated in disrupted emotional processing and compromised retention of fear extinction learning (Helpman et al., 2016).

Neuronal activity within the prelimbic cortex and infralimbic cortex proves essential for adapting fear learning in the face of stressful actions. The neural pathway from the prelimbic cortex to the basolateral amygdala (BLA) disturbs associative learning in females exposed to stress-inducing situations (Maeng & Shors, 2013). Stressful experiences, such as those induced by single prolonged stress, inhibit neural activity in the hippocampus, while simultaneously enhancing the functional connectivity between the vmPFC and BLA throughout emotional memory and learning processes. This inhibited neural activity and altered functional connectivity among the hippocampus, vmPFC and BLA contribute to in disruptions to the expression and retention of fear extinction memory (Knox et al., 2018).

Recent research suggested a negative correlation between the functional connectivity of two prefrontal regions, namely the left anterior middle frontal gyrus and the right orbitofrontal cortex, and the manifestation of anger symptoms in individuals with PTSD (Eshel et al., 2021). Additionally, in PTSD, the excitatory pathway originating from the posterior orbitofrontal cortex to amygdala inhibitory intercalated mass neurons plays a pivotal role in modulating autonomic function, primarily through the regulation of dopamine (DA) levels. Traumatic stress induces heightened release of DA, leading to the inhibition of intercalated mass neuron activity in the amygdala. This process disrupts the normally potent inhibitory mechanisms operating from the PFC to the amygdala, consequently intensifying autonomic drive (Zikopoulos et al., 2017).

During conditioned fear extinction procedures, there is a disruption in the functional connectivity between the insula, dorsal ACC, vmPFC, hippocampus, amygdala, and thalamus induced by the recall of extinction memory in individuals with PTSD. Irregular functional connectivity observed in fear- and anxiety-related disorders signifies deficits in cognitive and attention networks. Significantly, a positive correlation has been established between the parahippocampal cortex and trauma-related intrusive memories and avoidance behaviors in individuals diagnosed with PTSD (Steward et al., 2020). Moreover, an elevation in functional connectivity between the parahippocampus and the inferior frontal gyrus indicates the involvement of neural circuits extending from the PFC to the hippocampus during memory suppression in individuals experiencing PTSD.

Figure 4. Illustration of the inhibitory control failure exerted by the mPFC over the amygdala leading to hyperarousal and intrusion symptoms

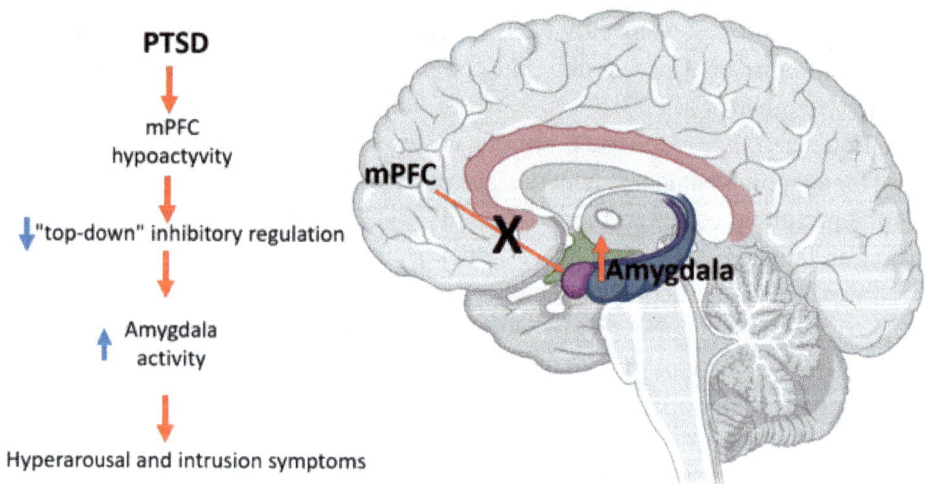

Amygdala Neural Circuits and PTSD

Animal studies investigating fear learning suggest that amygdala dysfunction; a central regulator of fear and stress (Simmons & Matthews, 2012), is a common characteristic across various anxiety disorders. Similarly, PTSD patients exhibit negative emotional processing (Shin et al., 2004; Williams et al., 2006), and some previous studies have indicated heightened amygdala activity among individuals with PTSD (Morey et al., 2009). While, contrasting findings exist, with certain studies reporting no discernible difference in amygdala activity between individuals with PTSD and control groups without the disorder (Clark et al., 2003; Ganzel et al., 2008).

Neuroimaging studies examining PTSD have consistently revealed heightened amygdala activation in response to personalized traumatic narratives (Shin et al., 2004), combat sounds and during fear conditioning in abuse survivors (Bremner et al., 2005). However, recent studies exploring amygdala activation levels suggest variability among individuals with PTSD. In a PET scanning study by Britton et al. (2005), involving 16 Vietnam veterans with PTSD, 15 veterans without PTSD (control group 1), and 14 healthy male subjects (control group 2), PTSD patients surprisingly did not show heightened amygdala activation when exposed to emotionally aversive stimuli, in contrast to the control groups. Interestingly, veterans without PTSD exhibited increased activation in the left amygdala in response to aversive stimuli (Britton et al., 2005). Moreover, Jacques et al. (2011) using fMRI indicated that, during the recollection of highly negative autobiographical memories, PTSD patients exhibited heightened amygdala activation, particularly in the right amygdala, in comparison to a control group (Jacques et al., 2011). This increased amygdala activation has been linked to the severity of PTSD symptoms (Shin et al., 2004). However, some studies have failed to detect amygdala activation during symptomatic conditions in PTSD, potentially due to limitations stemming from smaller sample sizes (Lanius et al., 2001).

Hippocampal Neural Circuits and PTSD

The hippocampus plays a pivotal role in regulating stress responses, declarative memory, and fear conditioning (Jovanovic et al., 2009; Milad et al., 2009). Consequently, it is one of the most extensively studied brain structures in relation to the effects of PTSD (Fuchs & Gould, 2000). Trauma and stress often lead to synaptic degeneration and neuronal atrophy in the hippocampus (Popoli et al., 2012). Several studies have consistently reported decreased hippocampal volume in individuals with PTSD (Kühn & Gallinat, 2013; Sussman et al., 2016). The scientific consortium "ENIGMA - Enhancing Neuroimaging Genetics through Meta-Analysis" conducted the most extensive neuroimaging study on PTSD, involving data from 1868 individuals across 16 cohorts. Their analysis confirmed a consistent association between PTSD and reduced hippocampal volume (Logue et al., 2018). In a comparative study by Apfel et al. (2011) examining individuals with chronic PTSD, acute PTSD, and acute depression symptoms, smaller average hippocampal volumes were observed in those with chronic PTSD. This raises questions about whether reduced hippocampal volume may impede recovery from PTSD or if it represents a reversible process post-withdrawal of PTSD symptoms (Apfel et al., 2011). This decreased hippocampal volume could be attributed to the fact that continuous exposure to stress and elevated glucocorticoid levels or increased sensitivity to glucocorticoids can cause hippocampal damage, leading to reduced dendrite numbers, loss of dendritic spines, and impaired neurogenesis (Conrad, 2008). However, the relationship between reduced hippocampal volume and PTSD remains uncertain, whether it signifies a risk factor for developing PTSD or if it is a consequence of the disorder itself (Heim & Nemeroff, 2009) and findings across studies are not always consistent with the decreased hippocampal volume (Golier et al., 2005; Pederson et al., 2004). For instance, in an MRI study conducted by Jatzko et al. (2006) comparing individuals with chronic PTSD from the 1988 air show plane crash in Germany to a healthy control group, voxel-based morphometry showed no difference in total hippocampal volume between patients and controls, including the left or right hippocampal regions (Jatzko et al., 2006). Moreover, Bonne et al. (2008) found no discrepancy in the volumes of the anterior hippocampus or subiculum (Bonne et al., 2008).

The Neural Circuitry of the Anterior Cingulate Gyrus Involved in PTSD

Certainly, two well-executed studies that compare the ACC in individuals with PTSD to those exposed to trauma without developing PTSD reveal reduced ACC activation in PTSD cases. In a PET study by Bremner et al. (1999) involving survivors of childhood sexual abuse, the PTSD group exhibited a lack of activation in the rostral ACC when exposed to traumatic versus neutral scripts, contrasting with those without PTSD (Bremner, Narayan, et al., 1999). Similarly, Hou et al. (2007) investigated individuals involved in a mining accident, finding decreased ACC activation in participants with severe acute PTSD compared to those without PTSD, especially in response to trauma-related versus neutral images. These findings suggest neurophysiological changes and memory deficits among individuals with severe acute PTSD (Hou et al., 2007).

However, there is a limited number of neuroimaging studies exploring energetic brain metabolism in PTSD. Shin et al. (2009) conducted a study among veterans with PTSD and their twins revealed significantly higher resting cerebral metabolic rate for glucose in the dorsal anterior cingulate/mid cingulate cortex. This increased activation in the dorsal ACC may represent a familial risk factor for PTSD (Shin et al., 2009). Additionally, PTSD symptoms have shown correlations with activation in the vmPFC in various studies (Hopper et al., 2007; Shin et al., 2005; Williams et al., 2006).

The Neural Circuitry of the Insula Involved in PTSD

Several studies have documented heightened activation in the insula in individuals with PTSD. Lindauer and colleagues utilized SPECT and script-driven imagery, revealed increased activation in the right insula in response to trauma-related scripts among individuals with PTSD compared to trauma-exposed control subjects (Lindauer et al., 2008). Moreover, in a study by Lanius and colleagues employing script-driven imagery during fMRI, activation patterns were compared in PTSD subjects with and without major depression (Lanius et al., 2007). They reported greater activation in the left insula during trauma in the PTSD-only group compared to the group with both PTSD and depression. Furthermore, combat veterans with PTSD also exhibited increased insula activation in response to trauma-related odors compared to veterans without PTSD (Vermetten et al., 2007).

In the other hand, studies using emotional stimuli unrelated to trauma have also reported increased insula activation. For instance, Bremner and colleagues, using PET, investigated regional cerebral blood flow associated with the retrieval of emotional and neutral word pairs in women with early childhood sexual abuse-related PTSD and non-traumatized women (Bremner et al., 2003). The PTSD group showed greater insula activation during the retrieval of negative words compared to the control group. Additionally, Simmons and colleagues found increased insula activation during the anticipation of negative versus positive images in women with intimate partner violence-related PTSD compared to healthy, trauma-unexposed control subjects (Simmons et al., 2008). Besides, Fonzo et al. (2010) observed increased insula activation while processing fearful (and angry) versus happy facial expressions in women with intimate partner violence-related PTSD relative to trauma-unexposed control subjects (Fonzo et al., 2010). Another study found increased insula recruitment in PTSD compared to both trauma-exposed and depressed control groups when retrieving neutral items encoded in emotional contexts versus neutral contexts (Whalley et al., 2009). Increased insula activation in PTSD has also been noted during an emotional counting Stroop task (Shin et al., 2001) and during the encoding of face–profession associations (Werner et al., 2009). Interestingly, several studies have established a positive correlation between insula activation and PTSD symptoms' severity (Bremner, Narayan, et al., 1999; Carrion et al., 2008; Hopper et al., 2007). Nevertheless, conflicting results exist, as some studies have reported no group differences or even decreased insula activation in individuals with PTSD (Shin et al., 1999 ; Bremner, Narayan, et al., 1999; Phan et al., 2006).

DYSREGULATION OF NEUROTRANSMITTERS AND NEUROPIPTIDES IN PTSD

Implication of Serotonin Dysfunction in PTSD

Serotonin (5-HT; 5-hydroxytryptamine), is a monoaminergic neurotransmitter found in the CNS and peripheral nervous system. Serotonergic neurons modulate a wide range of functions, including mood, perception, cognition, memory, aggression and reward processing (Cummings & Leiter, 2020; Paulus & Mintz, 2016; Pourhamzeh et al., 2022). Direct evidence confirms the contribution of altered serotonergic function in the pathophysiology of PTSD. This evidence is clearly illustrated both by the fact that animals suffering from inescapable shock exhibit a decrease in CNS serotonin levels, and by the fact that selective serotonin reuptake inhibitors (SSRIs) are highly effective pharmacological agents in the treatment of PTSD (Van Praag et al., 1990). Different serotonergic pathways regulate behaviors related to stress, anxiety and depression, with projections to different parts of the brain, or via different serotonin receptor subtypes (Van Praag et al., 1990). Preclinical studies have shown that chronic psychosocial stress decreases the density of 5-HT receptors in the limbic brain structures. In addition, fear conditioning in rodents has been shown to increase 5HT-2c receptors in the amygdala, while pharmacological antagonism of these receptors after conditioning decreases conditioned defensive behavior (Burghardt et al., 2007; Harada et al., 2008).

Learned helplessness is a psychological state showing that after exposure to stressful situations, individuals/animals give up learning to escape, even in a new, controllable environment (Song & Vilares, 2021). The learned helplessness paradigm is commonly used as a model for stress-induced behavioral disorders such as PTSD, and it has been associated with an *in vivo* reduction in serotonin release in the frontal cortex, probably reflecting a situation in which synthesis is unable to keep pace with demand (Petty et al., 1992, 1997). However, stress-induced learned helplessness has been restored by drugs that increase serotonin neurotransmission and by serotonin 5-HT1A receptor agonists. Learned helplessness in response to stress was also prevented by injection of serotonin into the frontal cortex of the brain (Bremner & Pearce, 2016). High levels of glucocorticoids, normally observed in chronic stress, also led to a decrease in hippocampal 5-HT1A receptor binding. Glucocorticoids modulate 5-HT1A receptor function as well, so this could represent, at least in part, the mechanism of stress-induced atrophy of the CA3 region of the hippocampus (Watanabe et al., 1993). Wu et al, (1999) reported that stress was associated with both reduced binding of 5-HT2A receptors in the amygdala and hypothalamus, and reduced binding of serotonin transporters in the frontal cortex (Wu et al., 1999). Furthermore, clinical studies on patients suffering from PTSD have shown an association between the symptoms observed in these patients, notably impulsivity, aggression, suicide and depression, and reduced serotonin function (Brown & Linnoila, 1990 ; Wu et al., 1999). Similarly, an increase in 5-HT2 receptor binding has been found in the frontal cortex of suicide victims, suggesting receptor upregulation (Arango et al., 1990; Mann et al., 1986). Furthermore, genetic studies also point in the direction of altered serotonin function in PTSD. Kuzelova et al, (2010) and Pietrzak et al, (2013) found that PTSD patients exhibited altered genotypic patterns for genes encoding the serotonin transporter and other serotonin receptors. Overall, there is ample evidence that serotonin dysfunction plays a role in PTSD (Kuzelova et al., 2010; Pietrzak et al., 2013).

Neuropeptide Y and PTSD

Neuropeptide Y (NPY) is a neuropeptide considered a key component of the stress response, with anxiolytic properties (Kuzelova et al., 2010; Pietrzak et al., 2013). The multiple effects of NPY are linked to its expression in many brain areas, including the hypothalamic arcuate nucleus (ARC), locus coeruleus (LC), nucleus solitarius is in the medulla oblongata (NTS) and septo-hippocampal nucleus (Kask et al., 2002). NPY is also present in numerous cortical interneurons, the hippocampus, amygdala, basal ganglia, nucleus accumbens (NAc) and thalamus (Holzer et al., 2012; Kask et al., 2002). Several preclinical and clinical studies strongly support a potential role for NPY dysfunction in the pathophysiology of PTSD. NPY and its receptors in limbic and brainstem areas are important in the regulation of stress and anxiety, extinction and retrieval of extinguished fear, learning and memory, as well as in the counter-regulation of corticotropin-releasing factor (CRF) and noradrenergic systems. Thus, reduced activation in the ventromedial PFC associated with impaired extinction recovery has been reported in subjects suffering from PTSD (Gøtzsche & Woldbye, 2016; Reichmann & Holzer, 2016; Tasan et al., 2016). Studies conducted in patients with PTSD show consistent alterations in peripheral or cerebrospinal fluid (CSF) levels of NPY. Other studies have shown reduced baseline plasma NPY levels in PTSD patients compared with normal subjects or non-PTSD subjects exposed to trauma (Rasmusson et al., 2000). Moreover, significantly higher plasma levels of NPY have been observed in individuals who have suffered from PTSD in the past but are currently recovered, suggesting a potential role for NPY in resilience (Schmeltzer et al., 2016; Yehuda et al., 2006). Reichmann and Holzer, (2016) reported that exposure to acute and chronic stress regulates NPY expression in the brain, on the basis of the modality of the stressor, the duration and the brain area examined (Reichmann & Holzer, 2016). In contrast to the effects of acute stress, chronic stress reduced plasma NPY levels and increased the noradrenergic response to a novel stressor. Exposure of rats to chronic stress resulted in a significant increase in prefrontal NPY expression, suggesting the sensitivity of this area to stress. Increased levels of prefrontal NPY could compromise the down-regulation of areas such as the amygdala, leading to impaired processing of conditioned fear and increased vulnerability to PTSD (Thorsell et al., 2000). However, injection of NPY into the amygdala showed anxiolytic effects and protects against the development of stress-induced gastric ulcers (Heilig et al., 1993; Penner et al., 1993). These studies confirm the role of NPY in the pathophysiology of PTSD, although further research is needed to elucidate its exact contributions in the development, diagnosis and treatment of PTSD.

Catecholamines in PTSD

Catecholamines have been identified as a group of monoaminergic neurotransmitters, comprising DA, noradrenaline and adrenaline. At the cerebral level, catecholamines are involved in traumatic memory. The sympathetic nervous system stimulates the release of catecholamines to mediate adaptive responses to acute stressors. In addition to this, they play an important role in modulating the mechanisms underlying different states of PTSD (Pan et al., 2018).

Dopaminergic System

Dopamine (DA) is a catecholamine produced in the substantia nigra pars compacta (SNpc) and ventral tegmental area (VTA) of the midbrain. DAergic neurons from the SN and VTA spread throughout many regions of the brain in which they release DA. DA plays a key role in functions such as reward processing, reinforcement, cognition, motivation, concentration, ability to experience pleasure and stress response (Baik, 2020; Sonnenschein et al., 2020). Studies of PTSD patients have revealed abnormalities in DAergic function. It is worth mentioning that DA release can be increased or inhibited depending on the intensity, duration and possibility to avoid the stressor. It has been reported that chronic stress leads to increased DA turnover in the PFC and NAc, with activation of several DAergic pathways, especially the mesofrontal pathway. However, uncontrollable stress stimulates DA release in the mPFC and blocks DA release in the NAc. Increased DA levels in PTSD may be due to desensitization of DA receptors and dysregulation of DA reuptake and degradation (Cabib et al., 2002; Deutch & Roth, 1991; Haaker et al., 2013; Hikind & Maroun, 2008). One of the hallmark symptoms of PTSD is the intrusive reliving of traumatic events (Brewin, 2015). Studies have shown that these intrusive symptoms are caused by the failure of top-down inhibitory control exerted by the mPFC over the amygdala. This alteration appears to be closely linked to disrupted fear extinction, contributing to exaggerated fear associated with the recurrence of traumatic memories in PTSD patients (Milad et al., 2009; Torrisi et al., 2019). In the PFC, DA plays a central role in regulating extinction memory consolidation. Fear extinction memory increases following D1 receptor activation in the nigrostriatal DAergic pathway and decreases with D1 receptor antagonism in the NAc or infralimbic cortex. D2 receptors in the mPFC, infralimbic cortex and basolateral amygdala (BLA) have been also found to be implicated in fear extinction learning in rat models of post-traumatic stress (Ney et al., 2021). Furthermore, Havelka Mestrovic et al, (2018) revealed a link between DAergic functioning and cognitive impairment in PTSD (Mestrovic et al., 2018).

Furthermore, clinical studies have demonstrated increased plasma and urinary DA in patients with PTSD such as veterans, adult female victims of childhood sexual abuse and in sexually abused children. Thus, a correlation has been established between increased urinary and plasma DA concentrations and symptom severity in PTSD patients (Glover et al., 2003; Hamner & Diamond, 1993). Overall, DA is a key element in the stress response, and PTSD is associated with long-term impairments in DAergic function. Therefore, functional modulation of DAergic networks is a promising approach to PTSD therapy.

Noradrenergic System

Noradrenaline (NA) also known as norepinephrine is a catecholamine produced primarily by noradrenergic neurons in the locus coeruleus (LC) and released in almost all brain areas. NA is involved in various behavioral and physiological processes such as attention, arousal, learning and memory, appetite, mood and reactivity to stress (Saboory et al., 2020). Clinical and basic neuroscience research has shown that the noradrenergic system is strongly involved in the pathophysiology of PTSD (Hendrickson & Raskind, 2016). It has been suggested that many PTSD symptoms, including irritability, reliving, hyperarousal and sleep disturbances, are in part related to impaired noradrenergic neuron function and reactivity to increased noradrenergic neuron sensitivity. Moreover, increased noradrenergic flux to neuroanatomical areas involved in memory formation and fear conditioning is thought to play a role in both the development and maintenance of PTSD symptoms (Bremner et al., 2010). A clinical study has revealed a significant increase in heart rate and systolic blood pressure in 11 veterans with PTSD compared to controls (Blanchard et al., 1982). In this vein, Blanchard et al. (1991) used auditory reminders of trauma as non-pharmacological in vivo probes of noradrenergic reactivity in combat veterans suffering from PTSD compared with non-mentally disturbed veterans. NA plasma samples were then collected before and after exposure to auditory stimuli reminiscent of combat. Results showed a 30% increase in plasma NA in the PTSD group, while no change was observed in the combat control group. Furthermore, exposure of PTSD patients to traumatic reminders has been associated with increased heart rate and blood pressure (Blanchard et al., 1991; Orr & Roth, 2000). The study carried out by Geracioti et al, (2001) revealed significantly higher levels of NA and its metabolites in the CSF of PTSD patients than in controls (Geracioti Jr et al., 2001). Therefore, CSF NA levels were correlated with the severity of PTSD symptoms. However, plasma levels of adrenaline and NA were found to be higher in PTSD patients than in controls after exposure to stress.

Assessment of urinary NA also revealed higher levels in PTSD patients than in controls (Bandelow et al., 2017; McFall et al., 1990). Southwick et al, (1991) suggested that the higher urinary excretion of NA in PTSD patients is due to noradrenergic hyperactivity in response to stressors. The neurochemical message of NA is translated, in part, by α2 adrenergic receptors. A decrease in the total number of platelets α2 adrenergic receptor binding sites has been reported in adults and children suffering from PTSD compared with controls. This reduction may be due to chronic elevation of circulating catecholamines, which in turn reduces the number of available receptor sites, and protects against agonist overstimulation (Southwick et al., 1999). A decrease in the activity of the second messenger, cyclic adenosine monophosphate (cAMP), and a decrease in platelet monoamine oxidase activity have also been noted in PTSD patients. These results are consistent with chronic increases in noradrenaline leading to compensatory changes in receptors and other parts of the pathways linked to noradrenergic function (Davidson et al., 1985; Lerer et al., 1990).

Adrenergic System

Adrenalin or epinephrine is a catecholamine naturally produced by the adrenal medulla in response to exhaustion or stress. Symptoms of PTSD occur when stress causes a sharp increase in the secretion of adrenaline in the bloodstream. High adrenaline levels trigger neurochemical and neurophysiological changes in the brain. These changes can persist for a long time, maintaining the person's sense of fear. The hippocampus is primarily responsible for memory processing. High levels of adrenalin released during stress can disrupt the normal functioning of the hippocampus, resulting in persistent and incorrect processing of memories of traumatic events and nightmares. However, if the stress subsides and adrenaline levels drop back to normal, the brain will be able to reverse the damage; bad memories will be processed and recognized correctly, and nightmares and other symptoms will disappear (Asalgoo et al., 2015). Delahanty et al, (2005) have shown that children with chronic PTSD excrete higher levels of cortisol and adrenaline than controls (Delahanty et al., 2005). In addition, elevated urinary cortisol and adrenaline levels after traumatic exposure are positively related to PTSD symptoms' severity in children after trauma. According to McFall and collegues (1990), increased plasma adrenaline was correlated with increased heart rate and blood pressure in veterans with PTSD during and after watching a combat movie, but not in response to a car accident movie. Besides, it has been found that patients hospitalized for chronic PTSD exhibited high levels of vanillylmandelic acid (VMA), a metabolite of adrenaline and NA (Dikanović et al., 2011; McFall et al., 1990). Adrenaline appears to enhance the persistence of traumatic memories, which may contribute to dysfunctional extinction of these memories. This is in line with what is observed in PTSD patients who exhibit deficits in the extinction of traumatic memories (Inslicht et al., 2013; Lissek et al., 2005).

NEUROGENESIS AND PTSD

The first evidence for adult mammalian neurogenesis was reported by Joseph Altman and colleagues in the 1960s who showed continual neuron production in the subventricular zone (SVZ) lining the anterior lateral ventricle (LV) wall (Altman, 1969) and the subgranular zone (SGZ) of the dentate gyrus (DG) of the hippocampus in rats (Altman & Das, 1965). Several studies have reported a link between hippocampal neurogenesis and the pathogenesis of PTSD (Ishikawa et al., 2019; Matsuoka, 2011).(Peng et al., 2013). (Terranova et al., 2019). (Yoneda et al., 2008). (Sun et al., 2020). (Aliev et al., 2020). Indeed, during development of PTSD, malfunctioned adult hippocampal neurogenesis contributes the cognitive and psychiatric episodes (Besnard & Sahay, 2016; Catlow et al., 2013; Malberg, 2004). A body line of evidence supports this link including atrophy of hippocampus in patients with PTSD (Bremner et al., 2007; Kitayama et al., 2005; Lindauer et al., 2006), suppressed hippocampal cell proliferation (Hendriksen et al., 2010; Kikuchi et al., 2008), and increased apoptosis in animal models of PTSD (X. Li et al., 2010; X. M. Li et al., 2010). Additionally, physical or psychosocial stress which consist the original cause of PTSD, might reduce the neurogenesis in the dentate gyrus (Peng et al., 2013).

Numerous studies have found that levels of adult hippocampal neurogenesis are highly sensitive to both aversive and enriching experiences and interventions (Aimone et al., 2014; Ernst & Frisén, 2015; Ming & Song, 2011; Opendak & Gould, 2015). Thus, it has been suggested that increased neurogenesis in the hippocampus may be important for the effective treatment of PTSD (Peng et al., 2013). Indeed, it has been suggested that neurogenesis enhancer not only enhanced the forgetting of traumatic memory but also improved PTSD (anxiety)-like behavior (Ishikawa et al., 2019). However, it is important to note that the possibility was not excluded that enhancement of hippocampal neurogenesis improved anxiety directly, but not indirectly through for- getting (Ishikawa et al., 2019).

In addition to the well-described rodent adult neurogenic regions, SVZ and SGZ, a novel adult neurogenic region was recently identified; the temporal germinal layer (TGL), within the white matter adjacent to the caudal edge of the lateral nucleus of the amygdala (LA) of rats (Takemura, 2005). TGL neurogenesis occurs within the fiber pathway connecting LA to other regions. An impaired TGL neurogenesis caused an increased amygdala excitation, and has led animals to hold a long-term fear memory (Takemura & Kato, 2007). This phenotype in an animal model reminds us of symptoms of human PTSD (Takemura & Kato, 2007). Because one of the underlying mechanisms for internal vulnerability factors to PTSD has been linked to anatomical/ functional abnormality in the amygdala, it is intriguing to speculate that an amygdala-relevant neurogenesis in humans might function as TGL neurogenesis in rodents (Takemura & Kato, 2007). Interestingly, postnatal neurogenesis in the human amygdala has been discovered recently (Roeder et al., 2022).

CLINICAL IMPLICATIONS

In healthcare, PTSD patients can benefit from several treatment plans which may include cognitive-behavioral therapy (CBT), eye movement desensitization and reprocessing (EMDR), and pharmacotherapy. CBT has been shown to be effective in reducing PTSD symptoms by helping individuals reframe their thoughts and develop coping strategies (Cusack et al., 2016). EMDR, another evidence-based therapy, uses guided eye movements to help individuals process and integrate traumatic memories, which helps in enhancing the patients (Shapiro, 2014). However, there is ongoing debate about the efficacy and ethical implications of exposure-based therapies like EMDR and prolonged exposure therapy, with some researchers questioning the methodological rigor of studies supporting these treatments (Cahill et al., 2009). Pharmacotherapy, particularly selective serotonin reuptake inhibitors (SSRIs), is often used to manage PTSD symptoms, with studies showing its efficacy in reducing anxiety and depressive symptoms (Hoskins et al., 2015). In the military, recognizing and addressing PTSD is vital for the mental health and operational readiness of service members. Programs such as the U.S. Department of Veterans Affairs' (VA) PTSD treatment programs have been established to provide comprehensive care, including therapy, medication, and support groups, which have been shown to improve outcomes for veterans (Seal et al., 2011). While some patients experience significant improvement, others may not respond as well or may experience adverse effects from medications (Bisson et al., 2013). This highlights the need for personalized treatment approaches and further research into the underlying mechanisms of PTSD and its treatment.

From the current study it appears that multiple mechanisms and pathways are involved in the development of PTSD. Therefore, understanding the neurobiological basis of PTSD has profound clinical implications, which can target disrupted several systems and pathways including impaired neurogenesis, dysregulated neurotransmitters, altered some brain areas connectivity (i.e., amygdala, PFC) and altered HPA-axis activity. It has been suggested that increased hippocampal neurogenesis may be important for the effective treatment of PTSD (Peng et al., 2013). Therefore, interventions that promote neurogenesis, such as certain antidepressants (e.g., SSRIs) and lifestyle modifications (e.g., exercise, diet), could be crucial in treating PTSD. Additionally, dysregulation of the HPA axis is common in PTSD which manifested by several changes including abnormal levels of cortisol and other stress hormones, thus medications that stabilize HPA axis function (e.g., glucocorticoid receptor antagonists) may help manage PTSD symptoms. Also, cortisol levels could be used to screen for PTSD risk and monitor treatment responses. Moreover, advanced imaging techniques (e.g., fMRI, PET scans) can aid in the diagnosis of PTSD by identifying specific brain changes. Imaging can track changes over the course of treatment, providing insights into the effectiveness of therapeutic interventions. On the other hand, PTSD is associated with imbalances in neurotransmitters such as serotonin, norepinephrine, and dopamine. Medications that modulate neurotransmitter levels (e.g., SSRIs, SNRIs, antipsychotics) are effective in managing PTSD symptoms. Importantly, combining pharmacotherapy with psychotherapy (e.g., cognitive-behavioral therapy, CBT) can be more effective due to their complementary effects on brain neurotransmitters and cognitive processes.

In a nutshell, by focusing on neurogenesis, the HPA axis, neuroimaging, and neurotransmitter dysregulation, clinicians can better address the complex and multifaceted nature of PTSD, ultimately enhancing patient outcomes. Therefore, the development of new therapies which target these specific brain systems known to be involved in PTSD is of great interest and should be addressed by further studies.

LIMITATIONS OF THE STUDY

Although this research is crucial to understand PTSD, it does not include all important aspects of PTSD including treatment options, prevention strategies, or the social and economic impacts of the disorder. Moreover, other relevant areas such as genetic factors, environmental influences, and psychological interventions are not thoroughly addressed. Additionally, the study does not discuss variability among individuals with PTSD. There may be a risk of overgeneralizing the findings without considering individual differences in PTSD presentation and response to stress. Moreover, existing research often focuses on specific populations, such as military personnel and first responders, potentially limiting the generalizability of findings to other groups, such as survivors of domestic violence or refugees. Future studies should aim to include more diverse populations to ensure broader applicability of the results (Kira et al., 2013). PTSD often co-occurs with other mental health conditions, such as depression and anxiety, and addressing the impact of such comorbidities on the pathophysiology of PTSD is also essential. While the current study aims to provide an overview of pathophysiological mechanisms, it may not delve into how these mechanisms translate into practical applications or interventions for PTSD patients.

CONCLUSION

Several neurobiological mechanisms are believed to underlie post-traumatic stress disorder including altered prefrontal cortex, amygdala and hippocampal circuits as well as neuroendocrine systems' dysfunctions, along with neurotransmissions abnormalities in addition to neurogenesis disruptions. A deeper understanding of these mechanisms will help to find suitable therapies, and thus treating the disorder and enhancing the patient's quality of life. Therefore, other studies investigating the molecular mechanisms underlying PTSD are urgently needed.

REFERENCES

Aerni, A., Traber, R., Hock, C., Roozendaal, B., Schelling, G., Papassotiropoulos, A., Nitsch, R. M., Schnyder, U., & de Quervain, D. J.-F. (2004). Low-dose cortisol for symptoms of posttraumatic stress disorder. *The American Journal of Psychiatry*, 161(8), 1488–1490. DOI: 10.1176/appi.ajp.161.8.1488 PMID: 15285979

Aimone, J. B., Li, Y., Lee, S. W., Clemenson, G. D., Deng, W., & Gage, F. H. (2014). Regulation and function of adult neurogenesis: From genes to cognition. *Physiological Reviews*, 94(4), 991–1026. DOI: 10.1152/physrev.00004.2014 PMID: 25287858

Aliev, G., Beeraka, N. M., Nikolenko, V. N., Svistunov, A. A., Rozhnova, T., Kostyuk, S., Cherkesov, I., Gavryushova, L. V., Chekhonatsky, A. A., Mikhaleva, L. M., Somasundaram, S. G., Avila-Rodriguez, M. F., & Kirkland, C. E. (2020). Neurophysiology and psychopathology underlying PTSD and recent insights into the PTSD therapies—A comprehensive review. *Journal of Clinical Medicine*, 9(9), 1–19. DOI: 10.3390/jcm9092951 PMID: 32932645

Altman, J. (1969). Autoradiographic and histological studies of postnatal neurogenesis. IV. Cell proliferation and migration in the anterior forebrain, with special reference to persisting neurogenesis in the olfactory bulb. *The Journal of Comparative Neurology*, 137(4), 433–457. DOI: 10.1002/cne.901370404 PMID: 5361244

Altman, J., & Das, G. D. (1965). Autoradiographic and histological evidence of postnatal hippocampal neurogenesis in rats. *The Journal of Comparative Neurology*, 124(3), 319–335. DOI: 10.1002/cne.901240303 PMID: 5861717

American Psychiatric Association. A. P., & Association, A. P. (1994). *Diagnostic and statistical manual of mental disorders: DSM-IV* (Vol. 4). American psychiatric association Washington, DC.

Apfel, B. A., Ross, J., Hlavin, J., Meyerhoff, D. J., Metzler, T. J., Marmar, C. R., Weiner, M. W., Schuff, N., & Neylan, T. C. (2011). Hippocampal volume differences in Gulf War veterans with current versus lifetime posttraumatic stress disorder symptoms. *Biological Psychiatry*, 69(6), 541–548. DOI: 10.1016/j.biopsych.2010.09.044 PMID: 21094937

Arango, V., Ernsberger, P., Marzuk, P. M., Chen, J.-S., Tierney, H., Stanley, M., Reis, D. J., & Mann, J. J. (1990). Autoradiographic demonstration of increased serotonin 5-HT2 and β-adrenergic receptor binding sites in the brain of suicide victims. *Archives of General Psychiatry*, 47(11), 1038–1047. DOI: 10.1001/archpsyc.1990.01810230054009 PMID: 2173513

Asalgoo, S., Jahromi, G. P., Meftahi, G. H., & Sahraei, H. (2015). Posttraumatic stress disorder (ptsd): Mechanisms and possible treatments. *Neurophysiology*, 47(6), 482–489. DOI: 10.1007/s11062-016-9559-9

Baik, J.-H. (2020). Stress and the dopaminergic reward system. *Experimental & Molecular Medicine*, 52(12), 1879–1890. DOI: 10.1038/s12276-020-00532-4 PMID: 33257725

Bale, T. L., & Vale, W. W. (2004). CRF and CRF receptors: Role in stress responsivity and other behaviors. *Annual Review of Pharmacology and Toxicology*, 44(1), 525–557. DOI: 10.1146/annurev.pharmtox.44.101802.121410 PMID: 14744257

Bandelow, B., Baldwin, D., Abelli, M., Bolea-Alamanac, B., Bourin, M., Chamberlain, S. R., Cinosi, E., Davies, S., Domschke, K., Fineberg, N., Grünblatt, E., Jarema, M., Kim, Y.-K., Maron, E., Masdrakis, V., Mikova, O., Nutt, D., Pallanti, S., Pini, S., & Riederer, P. (2017). Biological markers for anxiety disorders, OCD and PTSD: A consensus statement. Part II: Neurochemistry, neurophysiology and neurocognition. *The World Journal of Biological Psychiatry*, 18(3), 162–214. DOI: 10.1080/15622975.2016.1190867 PMID: 27419272

Besnard, A., & Sahay, A. (2016). Adult hippocampal neurogenesis, fear generalization, and stress. *Neuropsychopharmacology*, 41(1), 24–44. DOI: 10.1038/npp.2015.167 PMID: 26068726

Bijanki, K. R., Van Rooij, S. J. H., Ely, T. D., Stevens, J. S., Inman, C. S., Fasano, R. E., Carter, S. E., Winters, S. J., Baman, J. R., Drane, D. L., Jovanovic, T., & Willie, J. T. (2020). Case series: Unilateral amygdala ablation ameliorates post-traumatic stress disorder symptoms and biomarkers. *Neurosurgery*, 87(4), 796–802. DOI: 10.1093/neuros/nyaa051 PMID: 32259241

Bisson, J. I., Roberts, N. P., Andrew, M., Cooper, R., & Lewis, C. (2013). Psychological therapies for chronic post-traumatic stress disorder (PTSD) in adults. *Cochrane Database of Systematic Reviews*, 2015(8), 12. DOI: 10.1002/14651858.CD003388.pub4 PMID: 24338345

Blanchard, E. B., Kolb, L. C., Pallmeyer, T. P., & Gerardi, R. J. (1982). A psychophysiological study of post traumatic stress disorder in Vietnam veterans. *The Psychiatric Quarterly*, 54(4), 220–229. DOI: 10.1007/BF01064817 PMID: 7187510

Blanchard, E. B., Kolb, L. C., Prins, A., Gates, S., & McCOY, G. C. (1991). Changes in plasma norepinephrine to combat-related stimuli among Vietnam veterans with posttraumatic stress disorder. *The Journal of Nervous and Mental Disease*, 179(6), 371–373. DOI: 10.1097/00005053-199106000-00012 PMID: 2051153

Bonne, O., Vythilingam, M., Inagaki, M., Wood, S., Neumeister, A., Nugent, A. C., Snow, J., Luckenbaugh, D. A., Bain, E. E., Drevets, W. C., & Charney, D. S. (2008). Reduced posterior hippocampal volume in posttraumatic stress disorder. *The Journal of Clinical Psychiatry*, 69(7), 1087–1091. DOI: 10.4088/JCP.v69n0707 PMID: 18572983

Bremner, J. D. (2002). *Does stress damage the brain?: Understanding trauma-related disorders from a mind-body perspective*. WW Norton & Company.

Bremner, J. D. (2003). Functional neuroanatomical correlates of traumatic stress revisited 7 years later, this time with data. *Psychopharmacology Bulletin*, 37(2), 6–25. PMID: 14566211

Bremner, J. D., Charney, D. S., Stein, D. J., Hollander, E., & Rothbaum, B. O. (2010). *Neural circuits in fear and anxiety*.

Bremner, J. D., Elzinga, B., Schmahl, C., & Vermetten, E. (2007). Structural and functional plasticity of the human brain in posttraumatic stress disorder. *Progress in Brain Research*, 167, 171–186. DOI: 10.1016/S0079-6123(07)67012-5 PMID: 18037014

Bremner, J. D., Narayan, M., Staib, L. H., Southwick, S. M., McGlashan, T., & Charney, D. S. (1999). Neural correlates of memories of childhood sexual abuse in women with and without posttraumatic stress disorder. *The American Journal of Psychiatry*, 156(11), 1787–1795. DOI: 10.1176/ajp.156.11.1787 PMID: 10553744

Bremner, J. D., & Pearce, B. (2016). Neurotransmitter, neurohormonal, and neuropeptidal function in stress and PTSD. *Posttraumatic Stress Disorder*, 179–232.

Bremner, J. D., Southwick, S. M., & Charney, D. S. (1999). *The neurobiology of posttraumatic stress disorder: an integration of animal and human research*.

Bremner, J. D., Vythilingam, M., Vermetten, E., Southwick, S. M., McGlashan, T., Staib, L. H., Soufer, R., & Charney, D. S. (2003). Neural correlates of declarative memory for emotionally valenced words in women with posttraumatic stress disorder related to early childhood sexual abuse. *Biological Psychiatry*, 53(10), 879–889. DOI: 10.1016/S0006-3223(02)01891-7 PMID: 12742675

Brewin, C. R. (2015). Re-experiencing traumatic events in PTSD: New avenues in research on intrusive memories and flashbacks. *European Journal of Psychotraumatology*, 6(1), 27180. DOI: 10.3402/ejpt.v6.27180 PMID: 25994019

Britton, J. C., Phan, K. L., Taylor, S. F., Fig, L. M., & Liberzon, I. (2005). Corticolimbic blood flow in posttraumatic stress disorder during script-driven imagery. *Biological Psychiatry*, 57(8), 832–840. DOI: 10.1016/j.biopsych.2004.12.025 PMID: 15820703

Brown, G. L., & Linnoila, M. I. (1990). CSF serotonin metabolite (5-HIAA) studies in depression, impulsivity, and violence. *The Journal of Clinical Psychiatry*, 51, 31–41. PMID: 1691169

Burghardt, N. S., Bush, D. E. A., McEwen, B. S., & LeDoux, J. E. (2007). Acute selective serotonin reuptake inhibitors increase conditioned fear expression: Blockade with a 5-HT2C receptor antagonist. *Biological Psychiatry*, 62(10), 1111–1118. DOI: 10.1016/j.biopsych.2006.11.023 PMID: 17524369

Cabib, S., Ventura, R., & Puglisi-Allegra, S. (2002). Opposite imbalances between mesocortical and mesoaccumbens dopamine responses to stress by the same genotype depending on living conditions. *Behavioural Brain Research*, 129(1–2), 179–185. DOI: 10.1016/S0166-4328(01)00339-4 PMID: 11809509

Cacabelos, R., Torrellas, C., Fernandez-Novoa, L., & Aliev, G. (2016). Neuroimmune crosstalk in CNS disorders: The histamine connection. *Current Pharmaceutical Design*, 22(7), 819–848. DOI: 10.2174/1381612822666151209150954 PMID: 26648474

Cahill, S. P., Rothbaum, B. O., Resick, P. A., & Follette, V. M. (2009). *Cognitive-behavioral therapy for adults.*

Carrion, V. G., Garrett, A., Menon, V., Weems, C. F., & Reiss, A. L. (2008). Posttraumatic stress symptoms and brain function during a response-inhibition task: An fMRI study in youth. *Depression and Anxiety*, 25(6), 514–526. DOI: 10.1002/da.20346 PMID: 17598145

Castro-Vale, I., van Rossum, E. F. C., Machado, J. C., Mota-Cardoso, R., & Carvalho, D. (2016). Genetics of glucocorticoid regulation and posttraumatic stress disorder—What do we know? *Neuroscience and Biobehavioral Reviews*, 63, 143–157. DOI: 10.1016/j.neubiorev.2016.02.005 PMID: 26872620

Catlow, B. J., Song, S., Paredes, D. A., Kirstein, C. L., & Sanchez-Ramos, J. (2013). Effects of psilocybin on hippocampal neurogenesis and extinction of trace fear conditioning. *Experimental Brain Research*, 228(4), 481–491. DOI: 10.1007/s00221-013-3579-0 PMID: 23727882

Clark, C. R., McFarlane, A. C., Morris, P., Weber, D. L., Sonkkilla, C., Shaw, M., Marcina, J., Tochon-Danguy, H. J., & Egan, G. F. (2003). Cerebral function in posttraumatic stress disorder during verbal working memory updating: A positron emission tomography study. *Biological Psychiatry*, 53(6), 474–481. DOI: 10.1016/S0006-3223(02)01505-6 PMID: 12644352

Conrad, C. D. (2008). Chronic stress-induced hippocampal vulnerability: The glucocorticoid vulnerability hypothesis. *Reviews in the Neurosciences*, 19(6), 395–412. DOI: 10.1515/REVNEURO.2008.19.6.395 PMID: 19317179

Cooper, O., Bonert, V., Moser, F., Mirocha, J., & Melmed, S. (2017). Altered pituitary gland structure and function in posttraumatic stress disorder. *Journal of the Endocrine Society*, 1(6), 577–587. DOI: 10.1210/js.2017-00069 PMID: 29264511

Cummings, K. J., & Leiter, J. C. (2020). Take a deep breath and wake up: The protean role of serotonin preventing sudden death in infancy. *Experimental Neurology*, 326, 113165. DOI: 10.1016/j.expneurol.2019.113165 PMID: 31887304

Cusack, K., Jonas, D. E., Forneris, C. A., Wines, C., Sonis, J., Middleton, J. C., Feltner, C., Brownley, K. A., Olmsted, K. R., Greenblatt, A., Weil, A., & Gaynes, B. N. (2016). Psychological treatments for adults with posttraumatic stress disorder: A systematic review and meta-analysis. *Clinical Psychology Review*, 43, 128–141. DOI: 10.1016/j.cpr.2015.10.003 PMID: 26574151

Daskalakis, N. P., Lehrner, A., & Yehuda, R. (2013). Endocrine aspects of posttraumatic stress disorder and implications for diagnosis and treatment. *Endocrinology and Metabolism Clinics of North America*, 42(3), 503–513. DOI: 10.1016/j.ecl.2013.05.004 PMID: 24011883

Davidson, J., Swartz, M., Storck, M., Krishnan, R. R., & Hammett, E. (1985). A diagnostic and family study of posttraumatic stress disorder. *The American Journal of Psychiatry*, 142(1), 90–93. DOI: 10.1176/ajp.142.1.90 PMID: 3966591

Delahanty, D. L., Nugent, N. R., Christopher, N. C., & Walsh, M. (2005). Initial urinary epinephrine and cortisol levels predict acute PTSD symptoms in child trauma victims. *Psychoneuroendocrinology*, 30(2), 121–128. DOI: 10.1016/j.psyneuen.2004.06.004 PMID: 15471610

Deutch, A. Y., & Roth, R. H. (1991). The determinants of stress-induced activation of the prefrontal cortical dopamine system. *Progress in Brain Research*, 85, 367–403. DOI: 10.1016/S0079-6123(08)62691-6 PMID: 2094906

Dikanović, M., Demarin, V., Kadojić, D., Kadojić, M., Trkanjec, Z., Titlić, M., Bitunjac, M., & Soldo-Butković, S. (2011). Effect of elevated catecholamine levels on cerebral hemodynamics in patients with chronic post-traumatic stress disorder. *Collegium Antropologicum*, 35(2), 471–475. PMID: 21755720

Dixon, M. L., Thiruchselvam, R., Todd, R., & Christoff, K. (2017). Emotion and the prefrontal cortex: An integrative review. *Psychological Bulletin*, 143(10), 1033–1081. DOI: 10.1037/bul0000096 PMID: 28616997

Do-Monte, F. H., Manzano-Nieves, G., Quiñones-Laracuente, K., Ramos-Medina, L., & Quirk, G. J. (2015). Revisiting the role of infralimbic cortex in fear extinction with optogenetics. *The Journal of Neuroscience : The Official Journal of the Society for Neuroscience*, 35(8), 3607–3615. DOI: 10.1523/JNEUROSCI.3137-14.2015 PMID: 25716859

Dominique, J.-F. (2007). Glucocorticoid-induced reduction of traumatic memories: Implications for the treatment of PTSD. *Progress in Brain Research*, 167, 239–247. DOI: 10.1016/S0079-6123(07)67017-4 PMID: 18037019

Dominique, J.-F., Aerni, A., Schelling, G., & Roozendaal, B. (2009). Glucocorticoids and the regulation of memory in health and disease. *Frontiers in Neuroendocrinology*, 30(3), 358–370. DOI: 10.1016/j.yfrne.2009.03.002 PMID: 19341764

Dunsmoor, J. E., Kroes, M. C. W., Li, J., Daw, N. D., Simpson, H. B., & Phelps, E. A. (2019). Role of human ventromedial prefrontal cortex in learning and recall of enhanced extinction. *The Journal of Neuroscience : The Official Journal of the Society for Neuroscience*, 39(17), 3264–3276. DOI: 10.1523/JNEUROSCI.2713-18.2019 PMID: 30782974

Eckart, C., Stoppel, C., Kaufmann, J., Tempelmann, C., Hinrichs, H., Elbert, T., Heinze, H.-J., & Kolassa, I.-T. (2011). Structural alterations in lateral prefrontal, parietal and posterior midline regions of men with chronic posttraumatic stress disorder. *Journal of Psychiatry & Neuroscience*, 36(3), 176–186. DOI: 10.1503/jpn.100010 PMID: 21118656

Ernst, A., & Frisén, J. (2015). Adult neurogenesis in humans-common and unique traits in mammals. *PLoS Biology*, 13(1), e1002045. DOI: 10.1371/journal.pbio.1002045 PMID: 25621867

Eshel, N., Maron-Katz, A., Wu, W., Abu-Amara, D., Marmar, C. R., & Etkin, A. (2021). Neural correlates of anger expression in patients with PTSD. *Neuropsychopharmacology*, 46(9), 1635–1642. DOI: 10.1038/s41386-020-00942-y PMID: 33500557

Fonzo, G. A., Simmons, A. N., Thorp, S. R., Norman, S. B., Paulus, M. P., & Stein, M. B. (2010). Exaggerated and disconnected insular-amygdalar blood oxygenation level-dependent response to threat-related emotional faces in women with intimate-partner violence posttraumatic stress disorder. *Biological Psychiatry*, 68(5), 433–441. DOI: 10.1016/j.biopsych.2010.04.028 PMID: 20573339

Fuchs, E., & Gould, E. (2000). Mini-review: in vivo neurogenesis in the adult brain: regulation and functional implications. *The European Journal of Neuroscience*, 12(7), 2211–2214. DOI: 10.1046/j.1460-9568.2000.00130.x PMID: 10947799

Furtado, M., & Katzman, M. A. (2015). Examining the role of neuroinflammation in major depression. *Psychiatry Research*, 229(1–2), 27–36. DOI: 10.1016/j.psychres.2015.06.009 PMID: 26187338

Ganzel, B. L., Kim, P., Glover, G. H., & Temple, E. (2008). Resilience after 9/11: Multimodal neuroimaging evidence for stress-related change in the healthy adult brain. *NeuroImage*, 40(2), 788–795. DOI: 10.1016/j.neuroimage.2007.12.010 PMID: 18234524

Garfinkel, S. N., Abelson, J. L., King, A. P., Sripada, R. K., Wang, X., Gaines, L. M., & Liberzon, I. (2014). Impaired contextual modulation of memories in PTSD: An fMRI and psychophysiological study of extinction retention and fear renewal. *The Journal of Neuroscience : The Official Journal of the Society for Neuroscience*, 34(40), 13435–13443. DOI: 10.1523/JNEUROSCI.4287-13.2014 PMID: 25274821

Geracioti, T. D.Jr, Baker, D. G., Ekhator, N. N., West, S. A., Hill, K. K., Bruce, A. B., Schmidt, D., Rounds-Kugler, B., Yehuda, R., Keck, P. E.Jr, & Kasckow, J. W. (2001). CSF norepinephrine concentrations in posttraumatic stress disorder. *The American Journal of Psychiatry*, 158(8), 1227–1230. DOI: 10.1176/appi.ajp.158.8.1227 PMID: 11481155

Gilmartin, M. R., Balderston, N. L., & Helmstetter, F. J. (2014). Prefrontal cortical regulation of fear learning. *Trends in Neurosciences*, 37(8), 455–464. DOI: 10.1016/j.tins.2014.05.004 PMID: 24929864

Glover, D. A., Powers, M. B., Bergman, L., Smits, J. A. J., Telch, M. J., & Stuber, M. (2003). Urinary dopamine and turn bias in traumatized women with and without PTSD symptoms. *Behavioural Brain Research*, 144(1–2), 137–141. DOI: 10.1016/S0166-4328(03)00074-3 PMID: 12946604

Golier, J. A., Yehuda, R., De Santi, S., Segal, S., Dolan, S., & de Leon, M. J. (2005). Absence of hippocampal volume differences in survivors of the Nazi Holocaust with and without posttraumatic stress disorder. *Psychiatry Research: Neuroimaging*, 139(1), 53–64. DOI: 10.1016/j.pscychresns.2005.02.007 PMID: 15939577

Gøtzsche, C. R., & Woldbye, D. P. D. (2016). The role of NPY in learning and memory. *Neuropeptides*, 55, 79–89. DOI: 10.1016/j.npep.2015.09.010 PMID: 26454711

Gustavson, S. M., Sandoval, D. A., Ertl, A. C., Bao, S., Raj, S. R., & Davis, S. N. (2008). Stimulation of both type I and type II corticosteroid receptors blunts counterregulatory responses to subsequent hypoglycemia in healthy man. *American Journal of Physiology. Endocrinology and Metabolism*, 294(3), E506–E512. DOI: 10.1152/ajpendo.00589.2007 PMID: 18182467

Haaker, J., Gaburro, S., Sah, A., Gartmann, N., Lonsdorf, T. B., Meier, K., Singewald, N., Pape, H.-C., Morellini, F., & Kalisch, R. (2013). Single dose of L-dopa makes extinction memories context-independent and prevents the return of fear. *Proceedings of the National Academy of Sciences of the United States of America*, 110(26), E2428–E2436. DOI: 10.1073/pnas.1303061110 PMID: 23754384

Hamner, M. B., & Diamond, B. I. (1993). Elevated plasma dopamine in posttraumatic stress disorder: A preliminary report. *Biological Psychiatry*, 33(4), 304–306. DOI: 10.1016/0006-3223(93)90302-T PMID: 8471687

Harada, K., Yamaji, T., & Matsuoka, N. (2008). Activation of the serotonin 5-HT2C receptor is involved in the enhanced anxiety in rats after single-prolonged stress. *Pharmacology, Biochemistry, and Behavior*, 89(1), 11–16. DOI: 10.1016/j.pbb.2007.10.016 PMID: 18067955

Harrison, B. J., Fullana, M. A., Via, E., Soriano-Mas, C., Vervliet, B., Martínez-Zalacaín, I., Pujol, J., Davey, C. G., Kircher, T., Straube, B., & Cardoner, N. (2017). Human ventromedial prefrontal cortex and the positive affective processing of safety signals. *NeuroImage*, 152, 12–18. DOI: 10.1016/j.neuroimage.2017.02.080 PMID: 28254509

Heilig, M., McLeod, S., Brot, M., Heinrichs, S. C., Menzaghi, F., Koob, G. F., & Britton, K. T. (1993). Anxiolytic-like action of neuropeptide Y: Mediation by Y1 receptors in amygdala, and dissociation from food intake effects. *Neuropsychopharmacology*, 8(4), 357–363. DOI: 10.1038/npp.1993.35 PMID: 8099792

Heim, C., & Nemeroff, C. B. (2009). Neurobiology of posttraumatic stress disorder. *CNS Spectrums*, 14(1, Suppl 1), 13–24. PMID: 19169190

Helpman, L., Marin, M.-F., Papini, S., Zhu, X. I., Sullivan, G. M., Schneier, F., Neria, M., Shvil, E., Aragon, M. J. M., & Markowitz, J. C. (2016). Neural changes in extinction recall following prolonged exposure treatment for PTSD: A longitudinal fMRI study. *NeuroImage. Clinical*, 12, 715–723. DOI: 10.1016/j.nicl.2016.10.007 PMID: 27761402

Hendrickson, R. C., & Raskind, M. A. (2016). Noradrenergic dysregulation in the pathophysiology of PTSD. *Experimental Neurology*, 284, 181–195. DOI: 10.1016/j.expneurol.2016.05.014 PMID: 27222130

Hendriksen, H., Prins, J., Olivier, B., & Oosting, R. S. (2010). Environmental enrichment induces behavioral recovery and enhanced hippocampal cell proliferation in an antidepressant-resistant animal model for PTSD. *PLoS One*, 5(8), e11943. DOI: 10.1371/journal.pone.0011943 PMID: 20700523

Hikind, N., & Maroun, M. (2008). Microinfusion of the D1 receptor antagonist, SCH23390 into the IL but not the BLA impairs consolidation of extinction of auditory fear conditioning. *Neurobiology of Learning and Memory*, 90(1), 217–222. DOI: 10.1016/j.nlm.2008.03.003 PMID: 18442937

Holsboer, F., & Ising, M. (2008). Central CRH system in depression and anxiety—Evidence from clinical studies with CRH1 receptor antagonists. *European Journal of Pharmacology*, 583(2–3), 350–357. DOI: 10.1016/j.ejphar.2007.12.032 PMID: 18272149

Holzer, P., Reichmann, F., & Farzi, A. (2012). Neuropeptide Y, peptide YY and pancreatic polypeptide in the gut–brain axis. *Neuropeptides*, 46(6), 261–274. DOI: 10.1016/j.npep.2012.08.005 PMID: 22979996

Hopper, J. W., Frewen, P. A., van der Kolk, B. A., & Lanius, R. A. (2007). Neural correlates of reexperiencing, avoidance, and dissociation in PTSD: Symptom dimensions and emotion dysregulation in responses to script-driven trauma imagery. *Journal of Traumatic Stress*, 20(5), 713–725. DOI: 10.1002/jts.20284 PMID: 17955540

Hoskins, M., Pearce, J., Bethell, A., Dankova, L., Barbui, C., Tol, W. A., Van Ommeren, M., De Jong, J., Seedat, S., Chen, H., & Bisson, J. I. (2015). Pharmacotherapy for post-traumatic stress disorder: Systematic review and meta-analysis. *The British Journal of Psychiatry*, 206(2), 93–100. DOI: 10.1192/bjp.bp.114.148551 PMID: 25644881

Hou, C., Liu, J., Wang, K., Li, L., Liang, M., He, Z., Liu, Y., Zhang, Y., Li, W., & Jiang, T. (2007). Brain responses to symptom provocation and trauma-related short-term memory recall in coal mining accident survivors with acute severe PTSD. *Brain Research*, 1144, 165–174. DOI: 10.1016/j.brainres.2007.01.089 PMID: 17331476

Inslicht, S. S., Metzler, T. J., Garcia, N. M., Pineles, S. L., Milad, M. R., Orr, S. P., Marmar, C. R., & Neylan, T. C. (2013). Sex differences in fear conditioning in posttraumatic stress disorder. *Journal of Psychiatric Research*, 47(1), 64–71. DOI: 10.1016/j.jpsychires.2012.08.027 PMID: 23107307

Iqbal, J., Huang, G.-D., Xue, Y.-X., Yang, M., & Jia, X.-J. (2023). The neural circuits and molecular mechanisms underlying fear dysregulation in posttraumatic stress disorder. *Frontiers in Neuroscience*, 17, 17. DOI: 10.3389/fnins.2023.1281401 PMID: 38116070

Ishikawa, R., Uchida, C., Kitaoka, S., Furuyashiki, T., & Kida, S. (2019). Improvement of PTSD-like behavior by the forgetting effect of hippocampal neurogenesis enhancer memantine in a social defeat stress paradigm. *Molecular Brain*, 12(1), 4–9. DOI: 10.1186/s13041-019-0488-6 PMID: 31370877

Jacobson, L. (2014). Hypothalamic-pituitary-adrenocortical axis: Neuropsychiatric aspects. *Comprehensive Physiology*, 4(2), 715–738. DOI: 10.1002/cphy.c130036 PMID: 24715565

Jacques, P. L. S., Botzung, A., Miles, A., & Rubin, D. C. (2011). Functional neuroimaging of emotionally intense autobiographical memories in post-traumatic stress disorder. *Journal of Psychiatric Research*, 45(5), 630–637. DOI: 10.1016/j.jpsychires.2010.10.011 PMID: 21109253

Jatzko, A., Rothenhöfer, S., Schmitt, A., Gaser, C., Demirakca, T., Weber-Fahr, W., Wessa, M., Magnotta, V., & Braus, D. F. (2006). Hippocampal volume in chronic posttraumatic stress disorder (PTSD): MRI study using two different evaluation methods. *Journal of Affective Disorders*, 94(1–3), 121–126. DOI: 10.1016/j.jad.2006.03.010 PMID: 16701903

Jovanovic, T., Norrholm, S. D., Fennell, J. E., Keyes, M., Fiallos, A. M., Myers, K. M., Davis, M., & Duncan, E. J. (2009). Posttraumatic stress disorder may be associated with impaired fear inhibition: Relation to symptom severity. *Psychiatry Research*, 167(1–2), 151–160. DOI: 10.1016/j.psychres.2007.12.014 PMID: 19345420

Jovanovic, T., Phifer, J. E., Sicking, K., Weiss, T., Norrholm, S. D., Bradley, B., & Ressler, K. J. (2011). Cortisol suppression by dexamethasone reduces exaggerated fear responses in posttraumatic stress disorder. *Psychoneuroendocrinology*, 36(10), 1540–1552. DOI: 10.1016/j.psyneuen.2011.04.008 PMID: 21601366

Karl, A., Schaefer, M., Malta, L. S., Dörfel, D., Rohleder, N., & Werner, A. (2006). A meta-analysis of structural brain abnormalities in PTSD. *Neuroscience and Biobehavioral Reviews*, 30(7), 1004–1031. DOI: 10.1016/j.neubiorev.2006.03.004 PMID: 16730374

Kask, A., Harro, J., von Hörsten, S., Redrobe, J. P., Dumont, Y., & Quirion, R. (2002). The neurocircuitry and receptor subtypes mediating anxiolytic-like effects of neuropeptide Y. *Neuroscience and Biobehavioral Reviews*, 26(3), 259–283. DOI: 10.1016/S0149-7634(01)00066-5 PMID: 12034130

Kellner, M., Yassouridis, A., Hübner, R., Baker, D. G., & Wiedemann, K. (2003). Endocrine and cardiovascular responses to corticotropin-releasing hormone in patients with posttraumatic stress disorder: A role for atrial natriuretic peptide? *Neuropsychobiology*, 47(2), 102–108. DOI: 10.1159/000070018 PMID: 12707494

Kikuchi, A., Shimizu, K., Nibuya, M., Hiramoto, T., Kanda, Y., Tanaka, T., Watanabe, Y., Takahashi, Y., & Nomura, S. (2008). Relationship between post-traumatic stress disorder-like behavior and reduction of hippocampal 5-bromo-2′-deoxyuridine-positive cells after inescapable shock in rats. *Psychiatry and Clinical Neurosciences*, 62(6), 713–720. DOI: 10.1111/j.1440-1819.2008.01875.x PMID: 19068009

Kim, T. D., Lee, S., & Yoon, S. (2020). Inflammation in post-traumatic stress disorder (PTSD): A review of potential correlates of PTSD with a neurological perspective. *Antioxidants*, 9(2), 107. DOI: 10.3390/antiox9020107 PMID: 31991875

Kim, Y.-K., Amidfar, M., & Won, E. (2019). A review on inflammatory cytokine-induced alterations of the brain as potential neural biomarkers in post-traumatic stress disorder. *Progress in Neuro-Psychopharmacology & Biological Psychiatry*, 91, 103–112. DOI: 10.1016/j.pnpbp.2018.06.008 PMID: 29932946

Kira, I. A., Ashby, J. S., Lewandowski, L., Alawneh, A. W. N., Mohanesh, J., & Odenat, L. (2013). Advances in continuous traumatic stress theory: Traumatogenic dynamics and consequences of intergroup conflict: The Palestinian adolescents case. *Psychology (Irvine, Calif.)*, 4(04), 396–409. DOI: 10.4236/psych.2013.44057

Kitayama, N., Vaccarino, V., Kutner, M., Weiss, P., & Bremner, J. D. (2005). Magnetic resonance imaging (MRI) measurement of hippocampal volume in posttraumatic stress disorder: A meta-analysis. *Journal of Affective Disorders*, 88(1), 79–86. DOI: 10.1016/j.jad.2005.05.014 PMID: 16033700

Knox, D., Stanfield, B. R., Staib, J. M., David, N. P., DePietro, T., Chamness, M., Schneider, E. K., Keller, S. M., & Lawless, C. (2018). Using c-Jun to identify fear extinction learning-specific patterns of neural activity that are affected by single prolonged stress. *Behavioural Brain Research*, 341, 189–197. DOI: 10.1016/j.bbr.2017.12.037 PMID: 29292158

Kühn, S., & Gallinat, J. (2013). Gray matter correlates of posttraumatic stress disorder: A quantitative meta-analysis. *Biological Psychiatry*, 73(1), 70–74. DOI: 10.1016/j.biopsych.2012.06.029 PMID: 22840760

Kuzelova, H., Ptacek, R., & Macek, M. (2010). The serotonin transporter gene (5-HTT) variant and psychiatric disorders: Review of current literature. *Neuroendocrinology Letters*, 31(1), 4–10. PMID: 20150867

Kvetnanský, R., Pacák, K., Fukuhara, K., Viskupic, E., Hiremagalur, B., Nankova, B., Goldstein, D. S., Sabban, E. L., & Kopin, I. J. (1995). Sympathoadrenal system in stress. Interaction with the hypothalamic-pituitary-adrenocortical system. *Annals of the New York Academy of Sciences*, 771(1), 131–158. DOI: 10.1111/j.1749-6632.1995.tb44676.x PMID: 8597393

Lanius, R. A., Frewen, P. A., Girotti, M., Neufeld, R. W. J., Stevens, T. K., & Densmore, M. (2007). Neural correlates of trauma script-imagery in posttraumatic stress disorder with and without comorbid major depression: A functional MRI investigation. *Psychiatry Research: Neuroimaging*, 155(1), 45–56. DOI: 10.1016/j.pscychresns.2006.11.006 PMID: 17412567

Lanius, R. A., Williamson, P. C., Densmore, M., Boksman, K., Gupta, M. A., Neufeld, R. W., Gati, J. S., & Menon, R. S. (2001). Neural correlates of traumatic memories in posttraumatic stress disorder: A functional MRI investigation. *The American Journal of Psychiatry*, 158(11), 1920–1922. DOI: 10.1176/appi.ajp.158.11.1920 PMID: 11691703

Lerer, B., Bleich, A., Bennett, E. R., Ebstein, R. P., & Balkin, J. (1990). Platelet adenylate cyclase and phospholipase C activity in posttraumatic stress disorder. *Biological Psychiatry*, 27(7), 735–740. DOI: 10.1016/0006-3223(90)90588-S PMID: 2328269

Li, X., Han, F., Liu, D., & Shi, Y. (2010). Changes of Bax, Bcl-2 and apoptosis in hippocampus in the rat model of post-traumatic stress disorder. *Neurological Research*, 32(6), 579–586. DOI: 10.1179/016164110X12556180206194 PMID: 20092675

Li, X. M., Han, F., Liu, D. J., & Shi, Y. X. (2010). Single-prolonged stress induced mitochondrial-dependent apoptosis in hippocampus in the rat model of post-traumatic stress disorder. *Journal of Chemical Neuroanatomy*, 40(3), 248–255. DOI: 10.1016/j.jchemneu.2010.07.001 PMID: 20624456

Liberzon, I., & Abelson, J. L. (2016). Context processing and the neurobiology of post-traumatic stress disorder. *Neuron*, 92(1), 14–30. DOI: 10.1016/j.neuron.2016.09.039 PMID: 27710783

Lindauer, R. J. L., Booij, J., Habraken, J. B. A., van Meijel, E. P. M., Uylings, H. B. M., Olff, M., Carlier, I. V. E., den Heeten, G. J., van Eck-Smit, B. L. F., & Gersons, B. P. R. (2008). Effects of psychotherapy on regional cerebral blood flow during trauma imagery in patients with post-traumatic stress disorder: A randomized clinical trial. *Psychological Medicine*, 38(4), 543–554. DOI: 10.1017/S0033291707001432 PMID: 17803835

Lindauer, R. J. L., Olff, M., Van Meijel, E. L. S. P. M., Carlier, I. V. E., & Gersons, B. P. R. (2006). Cortisol, learning, memory, and attention in relation to smaller hippocampal volume in police officers with posttraumatic stress disorder. *Biological Psychiatry*, 59(2), 171–177. DOI: 10.1016/j.biopsych.2005.06.033 PMID: 16154543

Lissek, S., Powers, A. S., McClure, E. B., Phelps, E. A., Woldehawariat, G., Grillon, C., & Pine, D. S. (2005). Classical fear conditioning in the anxiety disorders: A meta-analysis. *Behaviour Research and Therapy*, 43(11), 1391–1424. DOI: 10.1016/j.brat.2004.10.007 PMID: 15885654

Logue, M. W., van Rooij, S. J. H., Dennis, E. L., Davis, S. L., Hayes, J. P., Stevens, J. S., Densmore, M., Haswell, C. C., Ipser, J., Koch, S. B. J., Korgaonkar, M., Lebois, L. A. M., Peverill, M., Baker, J. T., Boedhoe, P. S. W., Frijling, J. L., Gruber, S. A., Harpaz-Rotem, I., Jahanshad, N., & Morey, R. A. (2018). Smaller hippocampal volume in posttraumatic stress disorder: a multisite ENIGMA-PGC study: subcortical volumetry results from posttraumatic stress disorder consortia. *Biological Psychiatry*, 83(3), 244–253. DOI: 10.1016/j.biopsych.2017.09.006 PMID: 29217296

Lohr, J. B., Palmer, B. W., Eidt, C. A., Aailaboyina, S., Mausbach, B. T., Wolkowitz, O. M., Thorp, S. R., & Jeste, D. V. (2015). Is post-traumatic stress disorder associated with premature senescence? A review of the literature. *The American Journal of Geriatric Psychiatry*, 23(7), 709–725. DOI: 10.1016/j.jagp.2015.04.001 PMID: 25959921

Maeng, L. Y., & Shors, T. J. (2013). The stressed female brain: Neuronal activity in the prelimbic but not infralimbic region of the medial prefrontal cortex suppresses learning after acute stress. *Frontiers in Neural Circuits*, 7, 198. DOI: 10.3389/fncir.2013.00198 PMID: 24391548

Malberg, J. E. (2004). Implications of adult hippocampal neurogenesis in antidepressant action. *Journal of Psychiatry & Neuroscience*, 29(3), 196–205. PMID: 15173896

Mann, J. J., Stanley, M., McBride, P. A., & McEwen, B. S. (1986). Increased serotonin2 and β-adrenergic receptor binding in the frontal cortices of suicide victims. *Archives of General Psychiatry*, 43(10), 954–959. DOI: 10.1001/archpsyc.1986.01800100048007 PMID: 3019268

Marwit, S. J. (2003). Post-Traumatic Stress Disorder. *Encyclopedia of Death and Dying, Table 1*, 364–366. DOI: 10.1056/NEJMra1612499

Matsuoka, Y. (2011). Clearance of fear memory from the hippocampus through neurogenesis by omega-3 fatty acids: A novel preventive strategy for posttraumatic stress disorder? *BioPsychoSocial Medicine*, 5(February), 3. Advance online publication. DOI: 10.1186/1751-0759-5-3 PMID: 21303552

McFall, M. E., Murburg, M. M., Ko, G. N., & Veith, R. C. (1990). Autonomic responses to stress in Vietnam combat veterans with posttraumatic stress disorder. *Biological Psychiatry*, 27(10), 1165–1175. DOI: 10.1016/0006-3223(90)90053-5 PMID: 2340325

Meewisse, M.-L., Reitsma, J. B., De Vries, G.-J., Gersons, B. P. R., & Olff, M. (2007). Cortisol and post-traumatic stress disorder in adults: Systematic review and meta-analysis. *The British Journal of Psychiatry*, 191(5), 387–392. DOI: 10.1192/bjp.bp.106.024877 PMID: 17978317

Mellon, S. H., Gautam, A., Hammamieh, R., Jett, M., & Wolkowitz, O. M. (2018). Metabolism, metabolomics, and inflammation in posttraumatic stress disorder. *Biological Psychiatry*, 83(10), 866–875. DOI: 10.1016/j.biopsych.2018.02.007 PMID: 29628193

Mestrovic, A. H., Tudor, L., Perkovic, M. N., Erjavec, G. N., Petrovic, Z. K., Strac, D. S., Konjevod, M., & Pivac, N. (2018). Significant association between catechol-O-methyltransferase (COMT) Val158/108Met polymorphism and cognitive function in veterans with PTSD. *Neuroscience Letters*, 666, 38–43. DOI: 10.1016/j.neulet.2017.12.033 PMID: 29248614

Michopoulos, V., Rothbaum, A. O., Jovanovic, T., Almli, L. M., Bradley, B., Rothbaum, B. O., Gillespie, C. F., & Ressler, K. J. (2015). Association of CRP genetic variation and CRP level with elevated PTSD symptoms and physiological responses in a civilian population with high levels of trauma. *The American Journal of Psychiatry*, 172(4), 353–362. DOI: 10.1176/appi.ajp.2014.14020263 PMID: 25827033

Milad, M. R., Pitman, R. K., Ellis, C. B., Gold, A. L., Shin, L. M., Lasko, N. B., Zeidan, M. A., Handwerger, K., Orr, S. P., & Rauch, S. L. (2009). Neurobiological basis of failure to recall extinction memory in posttraumatic stress disorder. *Biological Psychiatry*, 66(12), 1075–1082. DOI: 10.1016/j.biopsych.2009.06.026 PMID: 19748076

Ming, G., & Song, H. (2011). Adult neurogenesis in the mammalian brain: Significant answers and significant questions. *Neuron*, 70(4), 687–702. DOI: 10.1016/j.neuron.2011.05.001 PMID: 21609825

Morey, R. A., Dolcos, F., Petty, C. M., Cooper, D. A., Hayes, J. P., LaBar, K. S., & McCarthy, G. (2009). The role of trauma-related distractors on neural systems for working memory and emotion processing in posttraumatic stress disorder. *Journal of Psychiatric Research*, 43(8), 809–817. DOI: 10.1016/j.jpsychires.2008.10.014 PMID: 19091328

Newport, D. J., & Nemeroff, C. B. (2000). Neurobiology of posttraumatic stress disorder. *Current Opinion in Neurobiology*, 10(2), 211–218. DOI: 10.1016/S0959-4388(00)00080-5 PMID: 10753802

Ney, L. J., Akhurst, J., Bruno, R., Laing, P. A. F., Matthews, A., & Felmingham, K. L. (2021). Dopamine, endocannabinoids and their interaction in fear extinction and negative affect in PTSD. *Progress in Neuro-Psychopharmacology & Biological Psychiatry*, 105, 110118. DOI: 10.1016/j.pnpbp.2020.110118 PMID: 32991952

Opendak, M., & Gould, E. (2015). Adult neurogenesis: A substrate for experience-dependent change. *Trends in Cognitive Sciences*, 19(3), 151–161. DOI: 10.1016/j.tics.2015.01.001 PMID: 25715908

Orr, S. P., & Roth, W. T. (2000). Psychophysiological assessment: Clinical applications for PTSD. *Journal of Affective Disorders*, 61(3), 225–240. DOI: 10.1016/S0165-0327(00)00340-2 PMID: 11163424

Pan, X., Kaminga, A. C., Wen, S. W., & Liu, A. (2018). Catecholamines in post-traumatic stress disorder: A systematic review and meta-analysis. *Frontiers in Molecular Neuroscience*, 11, 450. DOI: 10.3389/fnmol.2018.00450 PMID: 30564100

Paulus, E. V., & Mintz, E. M. (2016). Circadian rhythms of clock gene expression in the cerebellum of serotonin-deficient Pet-1 knockout mice. *Brain Research*, 1630, 10–17. DOI: 10.1016/j.brainres.2015.10.044 PMID: 26529643

Pederson, C. L., Maurer, S. H., Kaminski, P. L., Zander, K. A., Peters, C. M., Stokes-Crowe, L. A., & Osborn, R. E. (2004). Hippocampal volume and memory performance in a community-based sample of women with posttraumatic stress disorder secondary to child abuse. *Journal of Traumatic Stress*, 17(1), 37–40. DOI: 10.1023/B:JOTS.0000014674.84517.46 PMID: 15027791

Peng, Z., Zhang, R., Wang, H., Chen, Y., Xue, F., Wang, L., Yang, F., Chen, Y., Liu, L., Kuang, F., & Tan, Q. (2013). Ziprasidone ameliorates anxiety-like behaviors in a rat model of PTSD and up-regulates neurogenesis in the hippocampus and hippocampus-derived neural stem cells. *Behavioural Brain Research*, 244, 1–8. DOI: 10.1016/j.bbr.2013.01.032 PMID: 23384713

Penner, S. B., Smyth, D. D., & Glavin, G. B. (1993). Effects of neuropeptide Y and [Leu31, Pro34] neuropeptide Y on experimental gastric lesion formation and gastric secretion in the rat. *The Journal of Pharmacology and Experimental Therapeutics*, 266(1), 339–343. PMID: 8101219

Petty, F., Kramer, G., & Wilson, L. (1992). Prevention of learned helplessness: In vivo correlation with cortical serotonin. *Pharmacology, Biochemistry, and Behavior*, 43(2), 361–367. DOI: 10.1016/0091-3057(92)90163-A PMID: 1438477

Petty, F., Kramer, G. L., & Wu, J. (1997). Serotonergic modulation of learned helplessness. *Annals of the New York Academy of Sciences*, 821(1), 538–541. DOI: 10.1111/j.1749-6632.1997.tb48324.x PMID: 9238247

Phan, K. L., Britton, J. C., Taylor, S. F., Fig, L. M., & Liberzon, I. (2006). Corticolimbic blood flow during nontraumatic emotional processing in posttraumatic stress disorder. *Archives of General Psychiatry*, 63(2), 184–192. DOI: 10.1001/archpsyc.63.2.184 PMID: 16461862

Pietrzak, R. H., Galea, S., Southwick, S. M., & Gelernter, J. (2013). Examining the relation between the serotonin transporter 5-HTTPLR genotype x trauma exposure interaction on a contemporary phenotypic model of posttraumatic stress symptomatology: A pilot study. *Journal of Affective Disorders*, 148(1), 123–128. DOI: 10.1016/j.jad.2012.11.003 PMID: 23183127

Pitman, R. K., Rasmusson, A. M., Koenen, K. C., Shin, L. M., Orr, S. P., Gilbertson, M. W., Milad, M. R., & Liberzon, I. (2012). Biological studies of post-traumatic stress disorder. *Nature Reviews. Neuroscience*, 13(11), 769–787. DOI: 10.1038/nrn3339 PMID: 23047775

Pitman, R. K., Shin, L. M., Ph, D., & Rauch, S. L. (2001). *Posttraumatic Stress Disorder With Neuroimaging rig ht a du. 62*(suppl 17).

Pitman, R. K., Shin, L. M., & Rauch, S. L. (2001). Investigating the pathogenesis of posttraumatic stress disorder with neuroimaging. *The Journal of Clinical Psychiatry*, 62(Suppl 17), 47–54. PMID: 11495097

Popoli, M., Yan, Z., McEwen, B. S., & Sanacora, G. (2012). The stressed synapse: The impact of stress and glucocorticoids on glutamate transmission. *Nature Reviews. Neuroscience*, 13(1), 22–37. DOI: 10.1038/nrn3138 PMID: 22127301

Pourhamzeh, M., Moravej, F. G., Arabi, M., Shahriari, E., Mehrabi, S., Ward, R., Ahadi, R., & Joghataei, M. T. (2022). The roles of serotonin in neuropsychiatric disorders. *Cellular and Molecular Neurobiology*, 42(6), 1671–1692. DOI: 10.1007/s10571-021-01064-9 PMID: 33651238

Prange, A. J. (1999). Thyroid axis sustaining hypothesis of posttraumatic stress disorder. *Psychosomatic Medicine*, 61(2), 139–140. DOI: 10.1097/00006842-199903000-00002 PMID: 10204963

Radley, J. J., & Sawchenko, P. E. (2011). A common substrate for prefrontal and hippocampal inhibition of the neuroendocrine stress response. *The Journal of Neuroscience : The Official Journal of the Society for Neuroscience*, 31(26), 9683–9695. DOI: 10.1523/JNEUROSCI.6040-10.2011 PMID: 21715634

Radley, J. J., Williams, B., & Sawchenko, P. E. (2008). Noradrenergic innervation of the dorsal medial prefrontal cortex modulates hypothalamo-pituitary-adrenal responses to acute emotional stress. *The Journal of Neuroscience : The Official Journal of the Society for Neuroscience*, 28(22), 5806–5816. DOI: 10.1523/JNEUROSCI.0552-08.2008 PMID: 18509042

Rasmusson, A. M., Hauger, R. L., Morgan, C. A.III, Bremner, J. D., Charney, D. S., & Southwick, S. M. (2000). Low baseline and yohimbine-stimulated plasma neuropeptide Y (NPY) levels in combat-related PTSD. *Biological Psychiatry*, 47(6), 526–539. DOI: 10.1016/S0006-3223(99)00185-7 PMID: 10715359

Rasmusson, A. M., Lipschitz, D. S., Wang, S., Hu, S., Vojvoda, D., Bremner, J. D., Southwick, S. M., & Charney, D. S. (2001). Increased pituitary and adrenal reactivity in premenopausal women with posttraumatic stress disorder. *Biological Psychiatry*, 50(12), 965–977. DOI: 10.1016/S0006-3223(01)01264-1 PMID: 11750893

Rauch, S. L., Shin, L. M., Segal, E., Pitman, R. K., Carson, M. A., McMullin, K., Whalen, P. J., & Makris, N. (2003). Selectively reduced regional cortical volumes in post-traumatic stress disorder. *Neuroreport*, 14(7), 913–916. PMID: 12802174

Reichmann, F., & Holzer, P. (2016). Neuropeptide Y: A stressful review. *Neuropeptides*, 55, 99–109. DOI: 10.1016/j.npep.2015.09.008 PMID: 26441327

Ressler, K. J., Berretta, S., Bolshakov, V. Y., Rosso, I. M., Meloni, E. G., Rauch, S. L., & Carlezon, W. A.Jr. (2022). Post-traumatic stress disorder: Clinical and translational neuroscience from cells to circuits. *Nature Reviews. Neurology*, 18(5), 273–288. DOI: 10.1038/s41582-022-00635-8 PMID: 35352034

Roeder, S. S., Burkardt, P., Rost, F., Rode, J., Brusch, L., Coras, R., Englund, E., Håkansson, K., Possnert, G., Salehpour, M., Primetzhofer, D., Csiba, L., Molnár, S., Méhes, G., Tonchev, A. B., Schwab, S., Bergmann, O., & Huttner, H. B. (2022). Evidence for postnatal neurogenesis in the human amygdala. *Communications Biology*, 5(1), 1–8. DOI: 10.1038/s42003-022-03299-8 PMID: 35440676

Saboory, E., Ghasemi, M., & Mehranfard, N. (2020). Norepinephrine, neurodevelopment and behavior. *Neurochemistry International*, 135, 104706. DOI: 10.1016/j.neuint.2020.104706 PMID: 32092327

Schelling, G., Kilger, E., Roozendaal, B., Dominique, J.-F., Briegel, J., Dagge, A., Rothenhäusler, H.-B., Krauseneck, T., Nollert, G., & Kapfhammer, H.-P. (2004). Stress doses of hydrocortisone, traumatic memories, and symptoms of posttraumatic stress disorder in patients after cardiac surgery: A randomized study. *Biological Psychiatry*, 55(6), 627–633. DOI: 10.1016/j.biopsych.2003.09.014 PMID: 15013832

Schmeltzer, S. N., Herman, J. P., & Sah, R. (2016). Neuropeptide Y (NPY) and posttraumatic stress disorder (PTSD): A translational update. *Experimental Neurology*, 284, 196–210. DOI: 10.1016/j.expneurol.2016.06.020 PMID: 27377319

Seal, K. H., Cohen, G., Waldrop, A., Cohen, B. E., Maguen, S., & Ren, L. (2011). Substance use disorders in Iraq and Afghanistan veterans in VA healthcare, 2001–2010: Implications for screening, diagnosis and treatment. *Drug and Alcohol Dependence*, 116(1–3), 93–101. DOI: 10.1016/j.drugalcdep.2010.11.027 PMID: 21277712

Shapiro, F. (2014). The role of eye movement desensitization and reprocessing (EMDR) therapy in medicine: Addressing the psychological and physical symptoms stemming from adverse life experiences. *The Permanente Journal*, 18(1), 71–77. DOI: 10.7812/TPP/13-098 PMID: 24626074

Sherin, J. E., & Nemeroff, C. B. (2011). Post-traumatic stress disorder: The neurobiological impact of psychological trauma. *Dialogues in Clinical Neuroscience*, 13(3), 263–278. DOI: 10.31887/DCNS.2011.13.2/jsherin PMID: 22034143

Shin, L. M., Lasko, N. B., Macklin, M. L., Karpf, R. D., Milad, M. R., Orr, S. P., Goetz, J. M., Fischman, A. J., Rauch, S. L., & Pitman, R. K. (2009). Resting metabolic activity in the cingulate cortex and vulnerability to posttraumatic stress disorder. *Archives of General Psychiatry*, 66(10), 1099–1107. DOI: 10.1001/archgenpsychiatry.2009.138 PMID: 19805700

Shin, L. M., McNally, R. J., Kosslyn, S. M., Thompson, W. L., Rauch, S. L., Alpert, N. M., Metzger, L. J., Lasko, N. B., Orr, S. P., & Pitman, R. K. (1999). Regional cerebral blood flow during script-driven imagery in childhood sexual abuse-related PTSD: A PET investigation. *The American Journal of Psychiatry*, 156(4), 575–584. DOI: 10.1176/ajp.156.4.575 PMID: 10200737

Shin, L. M., Orr, S. P., Carson, M. A., Rauch, S. L., Macklin, M. L., Lasko, N. B., Peters, P. M., Metzger, L. J., Dougherty, D. D., Cannistraro, P. A., Alpert, N. M., Fischman, A. J., & Pitman, R. K. (2004). Regional cerebral blood flow in the amygdala and medial prefrontalcortex during traumatic imagery in male and female vietnam veterans with ptsd. *Archives of General Psychiatry*, 61(2), 168–176. DOI: 10.1001/archpsyc.61.2.168 PMID: 14757593

Shin, L. M., Whalen, P. J., Pitman, R. K., Bush, G., Macklin, M. L., Lasko, N. B., Orr, S. P., McInerney, S. C., & Rauch, S. L. (2001). An fMRI study of anterior cingulate function in posttraumatic stress disorder. *Biological Psychiatry*, 50(12), 932–942. DOI: 10.1016/S0006-3223(01)01215-X PMID: 11750889

Shin, L. M., Wright, C. I., Cannistraro, P. A., Wedig, M. M., McMullin, K., Martis, B., Macklin, M. L., Lasko, N. B., Cavanagh, S. R., Krangel, T. S., Orr, S. P., Pitman, R. K., Whalen, P. J., & Rauch, S. L. (2005). A functional magnetic resonance imaging study of amygdala and medial prefrontal cortex responses to overtly presented fearful faces in posttraumatic stress disorder. *Archives of General Psychiatry*, 62(3), 273–281. DOI: 10.1001/archpsyc.62.3.273 PMID: 15753240

Simmons, A. N., & Matthews, S. C. (2012). Neural circuitry of PTSD with or without mild traumatic brain injury: A meta-analysis. *Neuropharmacology*, 62(2), 598–606. DOI: 10.1016/j.neuropharm.2011.03.016 PMID: 21420986

Simmons, A. N., Paulus, M. P., Thorp, S. R., Matthews, S. C., Norman, S. B., & Stein, M. B. (2008). Functional activation and neural networks in women with posttraumatic stress disorder related to intimate partner violence. *Biological Psychiatry*, 64(8), 681–690. DOI: 10.1016/j.biopsych.2008.05.027 PMID: 18639236

Somvanshi, P. R., Mellon, S. H., Flory, J. D., Abu-Amara, D., Wolkowitz, O. M., Yehuda, R., Jett, M., Hood, L., Marmar, C., & Doyle, F. J. (2019). Mechanistic inferences on metabolic dysfunction in PTSD from an integrated model and multiomic analysis: Role of glucocorticoid receptor sensitivity. *American Journal of Physiology. Endocrinology and Metabolism*. Advance online publication. DOI: 10.1152/ajpendo.00065.2019

Song, X., & Vilares, I. (2021). Assessing the relationship between the human learned helplessness depression model and anhedonia. *PLoS One*, 16(3), e0249056. DOI: 10.1371/journal.pone.0249056 PMID: 33784324

Sonnenschein, S. F., Gomes, F. V., & Grace, A. A. (2020). Dysregulation of midbrain dopamine system and the pathophysiology of schizophrenia. *Frontiers in Psychiatry*, 11, 613. DOI: 10.3389/fpsyt.2020.00613 PMID: 32719622

Southwick, S. M., Bremner, J. D., Rasmusson, A., Morgan, C. A.III, Arnsten, A., & Charney, D. S. (1999). Role of norepinephrine in the pathophysiology and treatment of posttraumatic stress disorder. *Biological Psychiatry*, 46(9), 1192–1204. DOI: 10.1016/S0006-3223(99)00219-X PMID: 10560025

Stevens, J. S., Jovanovic, T., Fani, N., Ely, T. D., Glover, E. M., Bradley, B., & Ressler, K. J. (2013). Disrupted amygdala-prefrontal functional connectivity in civilian women with posttraumatic stress disorder. *Journal of Psychiatric Research*, 47(10), 1469–1478. DOI: 10.1016/j.jpsychires.2013.05.031 PMID: 23827769

Steward, T., Das, P., Malhi, G. S., Bryant, R. A., & Felmingham, K. L. (2020). Dysfunctional coupling of the parahippocampal cortex and inferior frontal gyrus during memory suppression in posttraumatic stress disorder. *European Neuropsychopharmacology*, 41, 146–151. DOI: 10.1016/j.euroneuro.2020.09.634 PMID: 32967787

Sun, L., Cui, K., Xing, F., & Liu, X. (2020). Akt dependent adult hippocampal neurogenesis regulates the behavioral improvement of treadmill running to mice model of post-traumatic stress disorder. *Behavioural Brain Research, 379*(October 2019), 112375. DOI: 10.1016/j.bbr.2019.112375

Sussman, D., Pang, E. W., Jetly, R., Dunkley, B. T., & Taylor, M. J. (2016). Neuroanatomical features in soldiers with post-traumatic stress disorder. *BMC Neuroscience*, 17(1), 1–11. DOI: 10.1186/s12868-016-0247-x PMID: 27029195

Takemura, N. U. (2005). Evidence for neurogenesis within the white matter beneath the temporal neocortex of the adult rat brain. *Neuroscience*, 134(1), 121–132. DOI: 10.1016/j.neuroscience.2005.04.033 PMID: 15964698

Takemura, N. U., & Kato, N. (2007). Adult neurogenesis and systemic adaptation: Animal experiments and clinical perspectives for PTSD. *Progress in Brain Research*, 167(07), 99–109. DOI: 10.1016/S0079-6123(07)67007-1 PMID: 18037009

Tasan, R. O., Verma, D., Wood, J., Lach, G., Hörmer, B., de Lima, T. C. M., Herzog, H., & Sperk, G. (2016). The role of Neuropeptide Y in fear conditioning and extinction. *Neuropeptides*, 55, 111–126. DOI: 10.1016/j.npep.2015.09.007 PMID: 26444585

Terranova, J. I., Ogawa, S. K., & Kitamura, T. (2019). Adult hippocampal neurogenesis for systems consolidation of memory. *Behavioural Brain Research*, 372(June), 112035. DOI: 10.1016/j.bbr.2019.112035 PMID: 31201874

Thorsell, A., Michalkiewicz, M., Dumont, Y., Quirion, R., Caberlotto, L., Rimondini, R., Mathe, A. A., & Heilig, M. (2000). Behavioral insensitivity to restraint stress, absent fear suppression of behavior and impaired spatial learning in transgenic rats with hippocampal neuropeptide Y overexpression. *Proceedings of the National Academy of Sciences of the United States of America*, 97(23), 12852–12857. DOI: 10.1073/pnas.220232997 PMID: 11058155

Torrisi, S. A., Leggio, G. M., Drago, F., & Salomone, S. (2019). Therapeutic challenges of post-traumatic stress disorder: Focus on the dopaminergic system. *Frontiers in Pharmacology*, 10, 404. DOI: 10.3389/fphar.2019.00404 PMID: 31057408

Tovote, P., Fadok, J. P., & Lüthi, A. (2015). Neuronal circuits for fear and anxiety. *Nature Reviews. Neuroscience*, 16(6), 317–331. DOI: 10.1038/nrn3945 PMID: 25991441

Ursin, H., & Olff, M. (1993). Psychobiology of coping and defence strategies. *Neuropsychobiology*, 28(1–2), 66–71. DOI: 10.1159/000119002 PMID: 8255412

Van Praag, H. M., Asnis, G. M., Kahn, R. S., Brown, S. L., Korn, M., Friedman, J. M., & Wetzler, S. (1990). Nosological tunnel vision in biological psychiatry. A plea for a functional psychopathology. *Annals of the New York Academy of Sciences*, 600(1), 501–510. DOI: 10.1111/j.1749-6632.1990.tb16905.x PMID: 2252329

Vasileva, L. V., Ivanovska, M. V., Murdjeva, M. A., Saracheva, K. E., & Georgiev, M. I. (2019). Immunoregulatory natural compounds in stress-induced depression: An alternative or an adjunct to conventional antidepressant therapy? *Food and Chemical Toxicology*, 127, 81–88. DOI: 10.1016/j.fct.2019.03.004 PMID: 30858105

Vermetten, E., & Bremner, J. D. (2002). Circuits and systems in stress. I. Preclinical studies. *Depression and Anxiety*, 15(3), 126–147. DOI: 10.1002/da.10016 PMID: 12001181

Vermetten, E., Schmahl, C., Southwick, S. M., & Bremner, J. D. (2007). A positron tomographic emission study of olfactory induced emotional recall in veterans with and without combat-related posttraumatic stress disorder. *Psychopharmacology Bulletin*, 40(1), 8. PMID: 17285093

Watanabe, Y., Sakai, R. R., McEwen, B. S., & Mendelson, S. (1993). Stress and antidepressant effects on hippocampal and cortical 5-HT1A and 5-HT2 receptors and transport sites for serotonin. *Brain Research*, 615(1), 87–94. DOI: 10.1016/0006-8993(93)91117-B PMID: 8364729

Werner, N. S., Meindl, T., Engel, R. R., Rosner, R., Riedel, M., Reiser, M., & Fast, K. (2009). Hippocampal function during associative learning in patients with post-traumatic stress disorder. *Journal of Psychiatric Research*, 43(3), 309–318. DOI: 10.1016/j.jpsychires.2008.03.011 PMID: 18490028

Whalley, M. G., Rugg, M. D., Smith, A. P. R., Dolan, R. J., & Brewin, C. R. (2009). Incidental retrieval of emotional contexts in post-traumatic stress disorder and depression: An fMRI study. *Brain and Cognition*, 69(1), 98–107. DOI: 10.1016/j.bandc.2008.05.008 PMID: 18614265

Williams, L. M., Kemp, A. H., Felmingham, K., Barton, M., Olivieri, G., Peduto, A., Gordon, E., & Bryant, R. A. (2006). Trauma modulates amygdala and medial prefrontal responses to consciously attended fear. *NeuroImage*, 29(2), 347–357. DOI: 10.1016/j.neuroimage.2005.03.047 PMID: 16216534

Wu, J., Kramer, G. L., Kram, M., Steciuk, M., Crawford, I. L., & Petty, F. (1999). Serotonin and learned helplessness: A regional study of 5-HT1A, 5-HT2A receptors and the serotonin transport site in rat brain. *Journal of Psychiatric Research*, 33(1), 17–22. DOI: 10.1016/S0022-3956(98)00041-7 PMID: 10094235

Yehuda, R. (2009). Status of glucocorticoid alterations in post-traumatic stress disorder. *Annals of the New York Academy of Sciences*, 1179(1), 56–69. DOI: 10.1111/j.1749-6632.2009.04979.x PMID: 19906232

Yehuda, R. (2015). Is the glucocorticoid receptor a therapeutic target for the treatment of PTSD. *Psychoneuroendocrinology*, 61, 2. DOI: 10.1016/j.psyneuen.2015.07.391

Yehuda, R., Brand, S., & Yang, R.-K. (2006). Plasma neuropeptide Y concentrations in combat exposed veterans: Relationship to trauma exposure, recovery from PTSD, and coping. *Biological Psychiatry*, 59(7), 660–663. DOI: 10.1016/j.biopsych.2005.08.027 PMID: 16325152

Yehuda, R., Hoge, C. W., McFarlane, A. C., Vermetten, E., Lanius, R. A., Nievergelt, C. M., Hobfoll, S. E., Koenen, K. C., Neylan, T. C., & Hyman, S. E. (2015). Post-traumatic stress disorder. *Nature Reviews. Disease Primers*, 1(October), 1–22. DOI: 10.1038/nrdp.2015.57 PMID: 27189040

Yehuda, R., & LeDoux, J. (2007). Response variation following trauma: A translational neuroscience approach to understanding PTSD. *Neuron*, 56(1), 19–32. DOI: 10.1016/j.neuron.2007.09.006 PMID: 17920012

Yehuda, R., & Seckl, J. (2011). Minireview: stress-related psychiatric disorders with low cortisol levels: a metabolic hypothesis. *Endocrinology*, 152(12), 4496–4503. DOI: 10.1210/en.2011-1218 PMID: 21971152

Yoneda, Y., Tamaki, K., & Kakuda, T. (2008). Disturbance of adult neurogenesis by PTSD. *The International Journal of Neuropsychopharmacology*, 11, 50.

Zikopoulos, B., Höistad, M., John, Y., & Barbas, H. (2017). Posterior orbitofrontal and anterior cingulate pathways to the amygdala target inhibitory and excitatory systems with opposite functions. *The Journal of Neuroscience : The Official Journal of the Society for Neuroscience*, 37(20), 5051–5064. DOI: 10.1523/JNEUROSCI.3940-16.2017 PMID: 28411274

Zohar, J., Yahalom, H., Kozlovsky, N., Cwikel-Hamzany, S., Matar, M. A., Kaplan, Z., Yehuda, R., & Cohen, H. (2011). High dose hydrocortisone immediately after trauma may alter the trajectory of PTSD: Interplay between clinical and animal studies. *European Neuropsychopharmacology*, 21(11), 796–809. DOI: 10.1016/j.euroneuro.2011.06.001 PMID: 21741804

Chapter 4
Decoding PTSD and Paving the Way for Healing

Rati Kailash Prasad Tripathi
Assam University, India

ABSTRACT

Post-Traumatic Stress Disorder (PTSD) stands as a complex and pervasive mental health challenge, woven into the fabric of individual and collective experiences. The chapter sheds light into the heart of PTSD, seeking to understand its multifaceted origins, and intricacies of its development focussing on psychological, neurological, and sociological influences playing roles in shaping PTSD trajectory. It covers holistic understanding of PTSD, from the profound impact of trauma on brain's architecture to cultural and environmental factors amplifying its effects, laying the groundwork for subtle analysis of disorder. It stresses on importance of tailored-treatment approaches that address the unique needs of individuals. Traditional therapies like cognitive-behavioral and exposure therapies are scrutinized alongside pharmacological interventions and innovative modalities like technology-assisted, art, and nature-based interventions, including mind-body practices like yoga and meditation. Impact of community on PTSD treatment, emerging trends and research frontiers are also highlighted.

1. INTRODUCTION

Post-Traumatic Stress Disorder (PTSD) stands as a profound testament to the enduring impact of trauma on the human psyche. It transcends the boundaries of mere psychological affliction, weaving its intricate threads into the very fabric of

DOI: 10.4018/979-8-3693-2089-1.ch004

an individual's identity. Defined by a constellation of symptoms that range from intrusive memories and hypervigilance to emotional numbness, PTSD is a complex and often debilitating condition that can manifest in the wake of exposure to deeply distressing events (Asmundson & Taylor, 2009).

The echoes of trauma reverberate through time, and those grappling with PTSD find themselves navigating a landscape marked by the shadows of past experiences. While traditionally associated with the aftermath of combat, PTSD extends its reach to encompass a spectrum of traumatic incidents, from natural disasters and accidents to interpersonal violence. It is a universal response to the extraordinary challenges that life may present, emphasizing the inherent vulnerability of the human mind when confronted with the extreme (Asmundson & Taylor, 2009).

The present chapter sheds light on the complexities inherent in the development of PTSD. It delves into the development of PTSD, acknowledging the multifaceted nature of its origins. It explores the myriad of pathophysiological factors associated with it and subsequently examines a diverse array of treatment approaches that extend beyond the conventional, inviting a holistic perspective towards recovery. It illuminates the intricate association of personal history, neurological responses, and societal influences that converge to shape an individual's mental landscape in the aftermath of trauma. From acute, singular incidents to the insidious effects of chronic stressors, understanding the multifaceted dimensions of PTSD development becomes essential for comprehensive treatment strategies. In addition, the chapter also explores diverse manifestations of PTSD, ranging from classic symptoms such as flashbacks and hypervigilance to the less-explored realm of developmental trauma. This section sheds light on the varied ways PTSD manifests across the lifespan, emphasizing the importance of tailored treatment approaches that address the unique needs of individuals. Further, traditional therapies such as cognitive-behavioural and exposure therapies are scrutinized alongside pharmacological interventions. The spotlight extends to innovative modalities like technology-assisted therapies, art, and nature-based interventions, as well as mind-body practices such as yoga and meditation. The emphasis is on embracing a diverse arsenal of treatment options, recognizing that the path to recovery is as varied as the individuals seeking it. In addition, the importance of social support is highlighted. This section explores the impact of community on the treatment of PTSD and addresses the persistent stigma surrounding PTSD, suggesting that a comprehensive approach to treatment extends beyond individual therapy to encompass the broader support systems that contribute to resilience. Finally, it also gives a glimpse of emerging trends and research frontiers which are still under development phase for the intervention of PTSD.

2. ORIGIN OF PTSD

Post-Traumatic Stress Disorder (PTSD) has a complex origin rooted in the understanding of the ways by which the individuals respond to and cope with traumatic experiences. The recognition and understanding of this mental health condition have evolved over time, and its origin can be traced through historical, medical, and psychological perspectives (Veith, 1965; van der Kolk et al., 1996; Green, 1982) (Figure 1).

Figure 1. Origin of PTSD

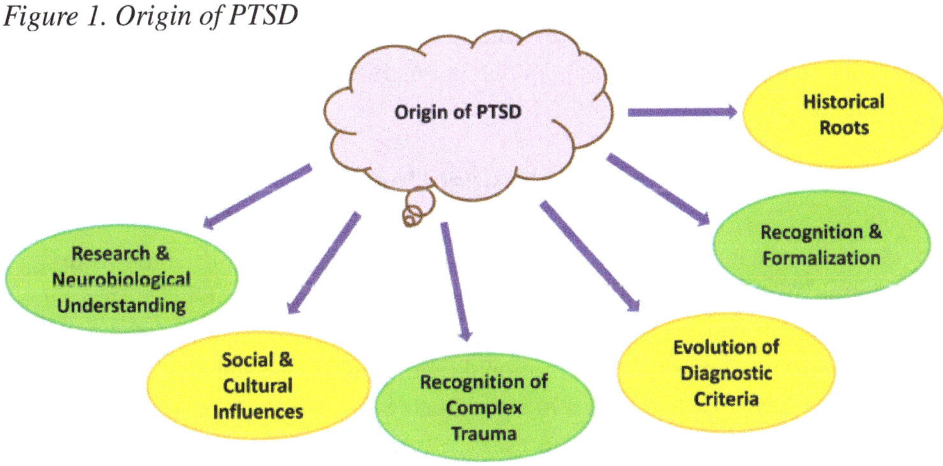

2.1. Historical Roots

The concept of psychological distress following exposure to traumatic events is not a recent development. Throughout history, accounts of soldiers experiencing lingering psychological effects after war can be found. Various terms, such as "shell shock" during World War I and "combat fatigue" during World War II, were used to describe these symptoms. However, it was in the aftermath of the Vietnam War that the modern understanding of PTSD began to take shape (Rivers, 1918; Blank, 1985; Kulka et al., 1990).

2.2. Recognition and Formalization

The formal recognition of PTSD as a distinct psychological disorder gained traction with the inclusion of "Post-Vietnam Syndrome" in the third edition of the Diagnostic and Statistical Manual of Mental Disorders (DSM-III) in 1980 (American

Psychiatric Association, 1980). This marked a shift from viewing the symptoms as a transient reaction to stress to recognizing them as a persistent and diagnosable condition (Kulka et al., 1990; Herman, 1992).

2.3. Evolution of Diagnostic Criteria

The diagnostic criteria for PTSD have undergone refinements over subsequent editions of the DSM. Initially, the focus was largely on trauma related to combat experiences, but the criteria have broadened to encompass a range of traumatic events, including natural disasters, accidents, and interpersonal violence (Regier et al., 2013). The DSM-5, published in 2013, further refined the criteria to better capture the diverse ways in which PTSD can manifest (American Psychiatric Association, 2013).

2.4. Research and Neurobiological Understanding

Advances in neurobiological research have contributed significantly to understanding the origins of PTSD. Studies have revealed alterations in brain structures, particularly the amygdala, hippocampus, and prefrontal cortex, associated with the processing of fear, memory, and emotional regulation. These changes help explain the persistent nature of symptoms in individuals with PTSD (Bremner, 2006).

2.5. Recognition of Complex Trauma

The understanding of trauma has expanded beyond isolated incidents to include complex and cumulative forms of trauma, such as developmental trauma and chronic interpersonal stress. This recognition acknowledges that the origins of PTSD are not confined to single, acute events but can encompass a broader spectrum of experiences over time (Cruz et al., 2022).

2.6. Social and Cultural Influences

Societal attitudes and cultural factors play a role in shaping the experience and expression of trauma. The acknowledgment of PTSD has grown alongside increased awareness of mental health issues in society. Cultural factors influence the way trauma is perceived, and societal responses impact the stigma associated with seeking help for mental health conditions (Ford et al., 2015).

Thus, the origin of PTSD is multifaceted, encompassing historical, diagnostic, neurobiological, and societal dimensions. Today, ongoing research continues to refine our understanding of the origins of PTSD, leading to improved diagnostic criteria and more effective treatment approaches.

3. PATHOPHYSIOLOGY OF PTSD

The pathophysiology of PTSD is a complex interplay of neurobiological, hormonal, and psychological factors that collectively shape the persistent and often debilitating symptoms observed in individuals who have experienced trauma. Understanding the pathophysiological mechanisms (Figure 2) underlying PTSD is crucial for developing targeted interventions and advancing our comprehension of this complex mental health condition (Mann & Marwaha, 2023; Sherin & Nemeroff, 2011).

Figure 2. Pathophysiological factors associated with PTSD

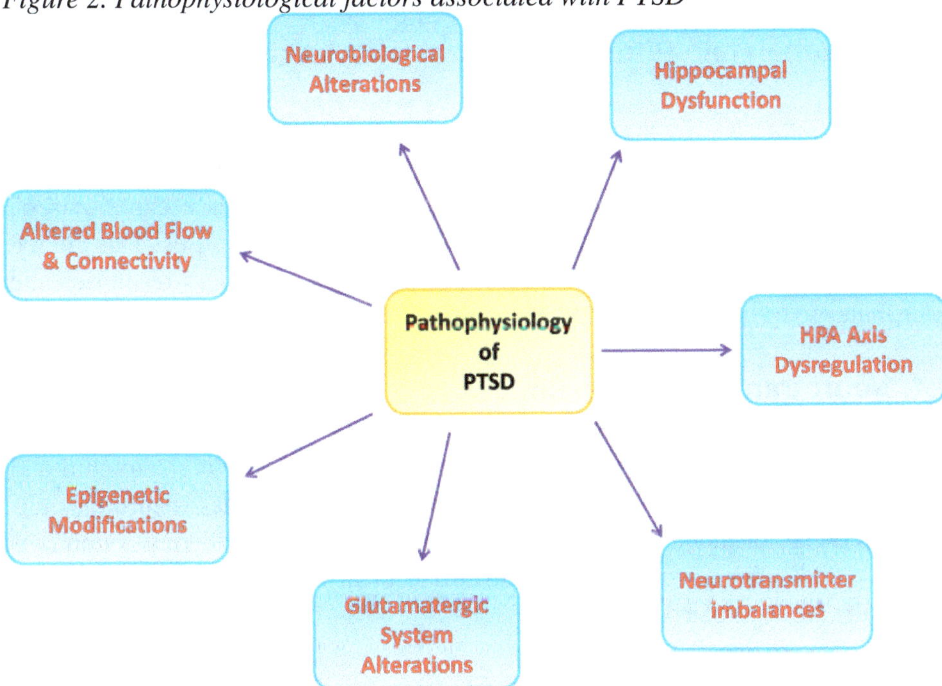

3.1. Neurobiological Alterations

Changes in brain structures associated with the processing of stress, fear, and emotions are central to the pathophysiology of PTSD. The amygdala, a key region involved in emotional responses, is often hyperactive in individuals with PTSD, leading to heightened fear responses and emotional reactivity. Conversely, the prefrontal cortex, responsible for cognitive control and emotional regulation, may exhibit reduced activity, contributing to difficulties in emotional modulation (Bremner, 2006; Ressler, 2011; Sherin & Nemeroff, 2011).

3.2. Hippocampal Dysfunction

The hippocampus, a brain region crucial for memory formation and contextual understanding, is adversely affected in PTSD. Chronic stress and exposure to trauma can lead to a reduction in hippocampal volume. This shrinkage is thought to contribute to memory disturbances observed in PTSD, particularly the intrusive recollections and flashbacks associated with traumatic events (Sherin & Nemeroff, 2011; Acheson et al., 2012).

3.3. Hypothalamic-Pituitary-Adrenal (HPA) Axis Dysregulation

The HPA axis, a key component of the body's stress response system, is dysregulated in individuals with PTSD. This dysregulation can result in abnormal cortisol levels. While acute stress typically leads to increased cortisol release, chronic stress, as seen in PTSD, may be associated with blunted cortisol responses. This altered HPA axis functioning is linked to difficulties in regulating stress responses and contributes to the persistence of PTSD symptoms (Herman et al., 2016).

3.4. Neurotransmitter Imbalances

Disruptions in neurotransmitter systems, particularly involving serotonin and norepinephrine, play a role in the pathophysiology of PTSD. These neurotransmitters are crucial for mood regulation, and imbalances may contribute to symptoms such as mood swings, irritability, and disturbances in sleep and arousal (Sherin & Nemeroff, 2011; Skolariki et al., 2023).

3.5. Glutamatergic System Alterations

Dysfunction in the glutamatergic system, which plays a vital role in synaptic plasticity and learning, is implicated in the pathophysiology of PTSD. Abnormalities in glutamate transmission may contribute to difficulties in memory consolidation and the encoding of safety cues, perpetuating the heightened fear responses characteristic of PTSD (Sherin & Nemeroff, 2011; Averill et al., 2017).

3.6. Epigenetic Modifications

Emerging research suggests that exposure to trauma can induce epigenetic modifications - changes in gene expression without alterations to the underlying DNA sequence. These modifications may influence stress response systems and contribute to the heritability of vulnerability to PTSD (Jiang et al., 2019; Nie et al., 2022).

3.7. Altered Blood Flow and Connectivity

Functional neuroimaging studies have revealed altered patterns of blood flow and connectivity in the brains of individuals with PTSD. These changes highlight disruptions in neural circuits involved in emotional regulation, memory processing, and threat perception (Francati et al., 2007).

Overall, understanding the pathophysiology of PTSD as a dynamic interplay of these neurobiological factors offers valuable insights into potential targets for therapeutic interventions. Targeted treatments aimed at restoring neurobiological balance and addressing the intricate mechanisms involved in the persistence of PTSD symptoms are central to advancing our ability to effectively alleviate the impact of trauma on individuals' lives.

4. FACTORS CONTRIBUTING TO EMERGENCE AND MANIFESTATION OF PTSD

Figure 3. Factors contributing to emergence and manifestation of PTSD

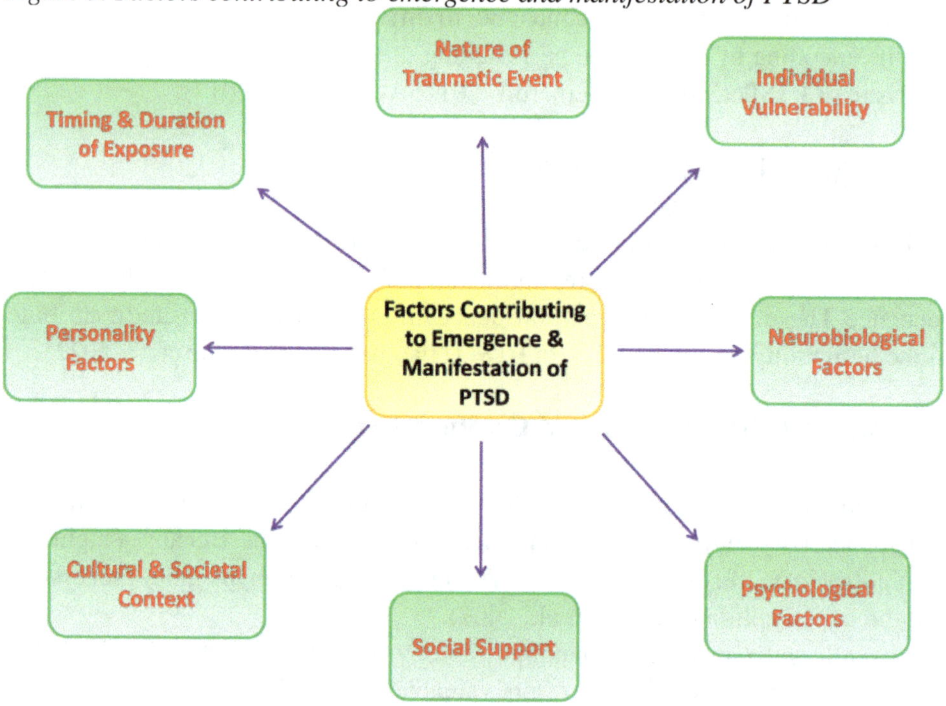

The genesis of PTSD is a complex interplay of various factors that converge to shape the trajectory of an individual's psychological response to trauma. Understanding these factors is crucial for unravelling the intricacies of PTSD development and implementing effective interventions. The key dimensions that contribute to the emergence and manifestation of PTSD (Figure 3) has been explored and are discussed below (Bomyea et al., 2012).

4.1. Nature of the Traumatic Event

The type, intensity, and duration of the traumatic incident play a pivotal role in PTSD development. Events involving physical harm, threat to life, or severe emotional distress are more likely to lead to the development of PTSD. Combat experiences, natural disasters, and incidents of violence often carry a higher risk (Sareen, 2014).

4.2. Individual Vulnerability

Not all individuals exposed to trauma develop PTSD, indicating the influence of pre-existing vulnerabilities. Factors such as genetic predispositions, family history of mental health disorders, and personal resilience play a significant role. Understanding an individual's inherent vulnerability can provide insights into their susceptibility to PTSD (Sareen, 2014).

4.3. Neurobiological Factors

PTSD is intricately linked to neurobiological changes in response to trauma. The brain's stress response systems, particularly the amygdala and hippocampus, undergo alterations, impacting memory, emotional regulation, and the perception of threat. Examining these neurobiological mechanisms offers a deeper understanding of PTSD's physiological underpinnings (Sherin & Nemeroff, 2011; Ressler, 2010; Acheson et al., 2012).

4.4. Psychological Factors

Pre-existing mental health conditions, coping mechanisms, and cognitive processes influence how individuals process and respond to trauma. Those with a history of anxiety, depression, or prior traumatic experiences may be more susceptible. Additionally, the way individuals interpret and make meaning of the traumatic event can impact the development and severity of PTSD (Green, 1982).

4.5. Social Support

The presence or absence of a robust support system can significantly shape the aftermath of trauma. Strong social support acts as a protective factor, buffering against the development of PTSD. Conversely, isolation or a lack of understanding from others may contribute to the exacerbation of symptoms (Ford et al., 2015).

4.6. Cultural and Societal Context

Cultural norms, societal attitudes toward trauma, and the availability of resources can influence how individuals and communities experience and cope with traumatic events. Variations in cultural expectations and coping strategies underscore the importance of considering these contextual factors in understanding PTSD development (Ford et al., 2015).

In their social-interpersonal model of PTSD, Maercker and Horn (2013) proposed three tiers of factors influencing the onset and persistence of PTSD. On the intrapersonal level, emotional reactions like shame, guilt, anger, and revenge play a central role. The interpersonal level highlights the significance of processes such as disclosure and social support as key determinants of PTSD. Meanwhile, on the cultural and societal level, more distal contextual factors, including the collective experience of trauma, societal acknowledgment of injustice, and cultural value orientations, may contribute to the prevalence of PTSD and other common mental disorders (Maercker & Horn, 2013).

Empirical evidence supports this assumption. In a study by Mueller and team, two interpersonal variables, *viz.* disclosure intentions and social acknowledgment as a victim, were assessed among survivors of crimes in Germany and China. The study revealed that both variables were predictors of PTSD symptomatology in both cultural groups. However, cultural differences were observed. Chinese crime victims experienced significantly more social acknowledgment and significantly less general disapproval from family, friends, acquaintances, and local authorities. In contrast, German crime victims reported more expressive disclosure attitudes (such as the urge to talk and emotional reactions while disclosing), while Chinese participants expressed more reluctance to discuss the trauma. The urge to talk about the traumatic experience emerged as a stronger predictor of PTSD among Chinese participants than among Germans. Conversely, reluctance to talk was a significant predictor of PTSD in the German sample but not among Chinese participants (Muller et al. 2009).

Evidence suggests that relational disturbances, the third DSO symptom, vary depending on culture. Nickerson et al. (2016) used two items - a sense of alienation from others and a reluctance to become overly intimate - to quantify relationship disruptions in a sample of refugees in Switzerland, the majority of whom had experienced torture. More people reported experiencing feelings of alienation than avoiding close relationships. The studies concluded that whereas the latter would suggest a more active approach that could result in interpersonal dysfunction, the former might reflect an interior experience. The writers further argue that "in collectivist societies, the experience of avoiding becoming too close to others may be particularly subject to cultural influence and may have a different meaning" (Nickerson et al., 2016).

In a recent study by Hansford and Jobson (2021), cultural variations were identified in terms of the efficacy of social support in moderating the connection between trauma exposure and PTSD. The researchers explored the impact of independent *versus* interdependent self-construal, diverse forms of social support, and PTSD symptoms among trauma survivors from European Australian and Asian Australian backgrounds. Their findings indicated that emotional support, involving expressions of empathy and understanding, played a moderating role in the relationship between lifetime trauma exposure and PTSD symptoms for both groups. However, concerning other types of social support such as appraisal support (providing advice or assistance in understanding, defining, or coping with the stressor), belonging support (engagement without the need for disclosing the stressor), and tangible support (material aid and assistance), the study revealed a moderating effect of interdependence. When perceived social support was low, higher levels of interdependence were associated with a more pronounced relationship between lifetime trauma exposure and PTSD symptoms. The authors concluded that, within individuals valuing interdependence, social support exerts a more favourable impact on mental health compared to those with independent values. Simultaneously, the absence of social support has a more detrimental effect among individuals with interdependent values than among those with independent values (Hansford & Jobson, 2021).

Research indicates the efficacy of PTSD treatments across diverse cultural groups (Barbui et al., 2020). In a systematic review and meta-analysis by Karatzias et al. focusing on the effectiveness of treatments for complex PTSD, cognitive-behavioural therapy (CBT), exposure therapy, and eye movement desensitization and reprocessing (EMDR) demonstrated moderate to large effects on negative self-concept and disturbed relationships. However, evidence regarding the impact of treatments on affect dysregulation was found to be lacking. Additionally, the study noted that the advantages of trauma-specific interventions were somewhat diminished when compared to non-specific treatments, suggesting that a considerable portion of the effectiveness stemmed from non-specific factors (Karatzias et al., 2019).

4.7. Timing and Duration of Exposure

The duration and chronicity of exposure to trauma impact the likelihood of developing PTSD. Prolonged exposure or repeated traumatic events may increase the risk, as seen in situations such as ongoing abuse or military deployments with multiple deployments (Sareen, 2014; van der Kolk, 2000a).

4.8. Personality Factors

Individual differences in personality traits, such as resilience, coping styles, and temperament, contribute to the diverse responses observed in the aftermath of trauma. Personality factors can either mitigate or exacerbate the development of PTSD symptoms (Mattson et al., 2018).

The above-mentioned factors clearly indicate that PTSD is not a uniform consequence of trauma but a nuanced outcome shaped by a complex interplay of individual, biological, social, and contextual elements. A comprehensive understanding of these factors provides a foundation for tailoring interventions that address the unique needs of individuals grappling with the aftermath of trauma.

5. MANIFESTATIONS OF PTSD

The manifestations of PTSD are diverse and profound, encapsulating a range of symptoms that impact an individual's thoughts, emotions, and behaviours. These manifestations often arise in response to exposure to traumatic events and can persist, affecting various aspects of daily life. Understanding the multifaceted nature of these manifestations is crucial for identifying and addressing the challenges faced by individuals grappling with PTSD (D'Souza, 1995; Davidson et al., 1991; van der Kolk, 2000a; van der Kolk, 2000b) (Figure 4).

5.1. Re-Experiencing Symptoms

Individuals with PTSD often re-experience the trauma through intrusive memories, distressing dreams, or flashbacks. These symptoms vividly transport the person back to the traumatic event, creating a sense of reliving the experience. Intrusive thoughts can be triggered by reminders in the environment, leading to emotional distress.

Figure 4. Manifestations of PTSD

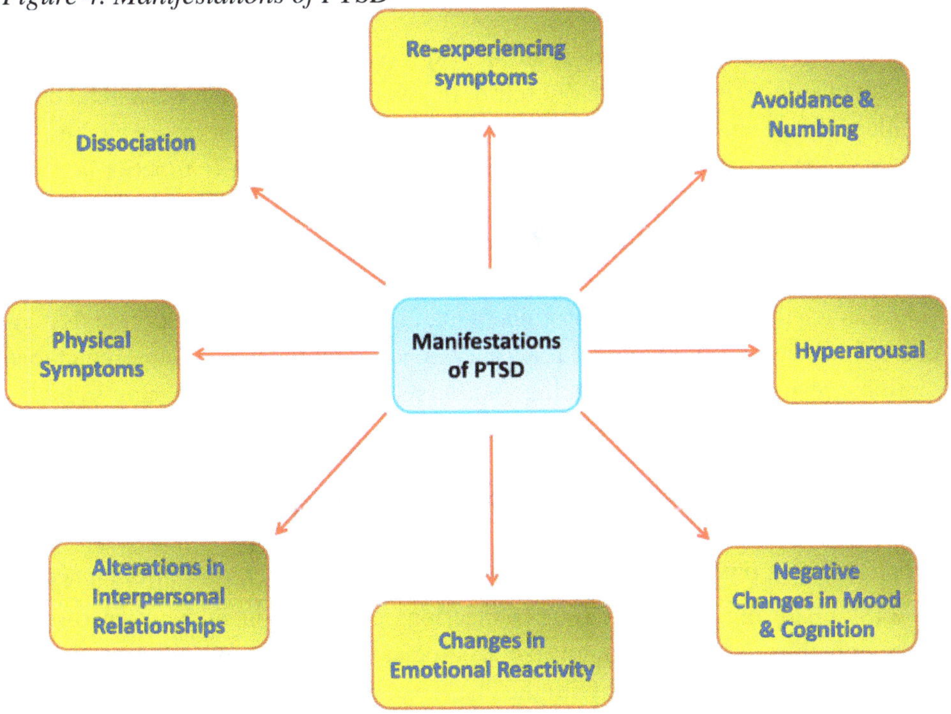

5.2. Avoidance and Numbing

A hallmark of PTSD is the avoidance of reminders associated with the trauma, including places, people, or activities that evoke distressing memories. This avoidance extends to discussing the traumatic event, and individuals may also experience emotional numbness, detachment, or a sense of estrangement from others.

5.3. Hyperarousal

Individuals with PTSD often exhibit heightened arousal and vigilance in response to perceived threats. This state of hyperarousal can manifest as irritability, difficulty concentrating, exaggerated startle responses, and sleep disturbances. Hypervigilance is a common feature, as individuals remain on constant alert for potential danger.

5.4. Negative Changes in Mood and Cognition

PTSD can significantly impact an individual's mood and cognitive processes. Persistent negative beliefs about oneself or the world, distorted blame, and feelings of guilt or shame are common. Additionally, individuals may experience challenges in memory and concentration, contributing to difficulties in daily functioning.

5.5. Changes in Emotional Reactivity

Emotional dysregulation is a prominent manifestation of PTSD. Individuals may experience heightened emotional reactivity, marked by intense and unpredictable emotional responses. This can include outbursts of anger, overwhelming sadness, or a general sense of emotional numbness.

5.6. Alterations in Interpersonal Relationships

The effects of PTSD often extend to interpersonal relationships. Individuals may struggle with forming or maintaining connections, experiencing difficulties trusting others, or feeling detached from loved ones. Social withdrawal and isolation may be common as a means of coping with the challenges posed by PTSD.

5.7. Physical Symptoms

The impact of PTSD is not confined to the psychological realm; it can also manifest in physical symptoms. Chronic pain, gastrointestinal issues, and cardiovascular problems are among the physical manifestations that can accompany PTSD, highlighting the intricate mind-body connection.

5.8. Dissociation

Some individuals with PTSD may experience dissociative symptoms, where they feel disconnected from themselves or their surroundings. This can include a sense of being in a daze, amnesia regarding aspects of the traumatic event, or feeling as though the world is unreal.

Thus, the manifestations of PTSD are not one-size-fits-all, and individuals may experience a unique combination and intensity of symptoms. These manifestations often create a complex and challenging landscape for those affected, underscoring the importance of personalized and comprehensive approaches to assessment, diagnosis, and treatment.

6. PTSD IN CHILDREN AND ADULTS

The manifestation of PTSD symptoms in children is anticipated to differ from adolescents and adults based on not only their developmental stage and varying levels of cognitive and emotional maturity but also upon the traumatic event itself, its severity and duration of exposure and the child's demographic variable like gender, age and ethnicity. Prevalence of PTSD diagnosis is elevated among females, middle school students, and Hispanics. PTSD is more likely to occur following interpersonal traumas, including sexual and physical assaults, as compared to exposure to natural or technological disasters.

Fundamental symptoms used for diagnosing PTSD in children aged 7 and older closely resemble those employed for adults. Nevertheless, consensus diminishes, particularly below the age of 5 years, where there is less alignment on the diagnostic criteria. Symptoms of trauma impact in younger children may include regression to immature behaviours (like increased anxiety and clinginess, and difficulty settling to sleep), aggression (like irritability, temper tantrums, or destructive behaviour), repetitive re-enactment in play or drawings, with nightmares occurring less frequently. La Greca and team conducted a review on the prevalence of PTSD in children who experienced natural or man-made disasters, revealing that 5–10% of these children meet the diagnostic criteria for PTSD. In alternative traumatic situations, such as fires, sexual assaults, and wars, surveys indicate that the prevalence of PTSD in children varies widely, ranging from 25 to 75% (La Greca et al., 2012).

It is crucial to recognize the symptomatology of children, adolescents and adults in relation to their functioning. Children might not voluntarily communicate their psychological responses to trauma unless prompted with specific inquiries. Cognitive immaturity can limit their chances to discuss the event, and even when given the opportunity, the limited cognitive and expressive language skills of children can hinder the smooth articulation of their thoughts and feelings. Despite parents and teachers often being unreliable reporters of children's symptoms, it is almost always necessary to directly inquire about the children's experiences.

Numerous assessment instruments have been created for appraising the responses and symptoms of children and adults who have experienced traumatic events. These assessment tools can be broadly categorized into two groups (a) subjective instruments and (b) structured and semi-structured interview tools.

6.1. Subjective Instruments

Subjective instruments consist of self-rating or other-rating scales, typically provided by parents or caregivers, and are regarded as effective instruments for screening PTSD in children and adolescents. These scales can offer insights into the current stress response of the patient to some extent and are convenient for widespread use in populations exposed to trauma. Subjective instruments include (a) Impact of Event Scale-Revised (IES-R); (b) The Children's Revised Impact of Event Scale (CRIES-13); (c) Child PTSD Symptom Scale (CPSS); and (d) The UCLA PTSD Reaction Index for DSM-IV, revision 1 (UCLA CPTSD-R).

6.1.1. Impact of Event Scale-Revised (IES-R)

A self-report instrument used to gauge ongoing subjective discomfort in reaction to a particular traumatic experience is the Impact of Event Scale-Revised (IES-R) (Creamer et al. 2003). This measure, which was created initially for adults, is helpful for tracking symptoms of PTSD as well as to monitor the outcomes of programs for those older than seven years (Motlagh, 2010).

IES-R is the revised version of The Impact of Event Scale. It consists of 22 items that measure three main PTSD symptom clusters: hyperarousal (6 items related to difficulty concentrating, anger and irritability, psychophysiological arousal upon exposure to reminders, and hypervigilance), avoidance (8 items related to avoiding feelings, situations, and ideas), and intrusion (8 items related to intrusive thoughts, nightmares, and imagery associated with the traumatic event). No particular training is needed to administer the IES-R questionnaire, which takes around 10 minutes to complete and scores on the degree of distress rather than the frequency of symptoms. Additionally, it demonstrated strong validity, reliability, and change sensitivity.

6.1.2. The Children's Revised Impact of Event Scale (CRIES-13)

CRIES-13 is a short, kid-friendly test that is intended to evaluate kids who may be at risk for PTSD. It has strong validity and reliability as well as a stable components structure. It has been used to assess a sizable number of children who are considered to be at-risk after experiencing various forms of trauma. Based on the DSM criteria, CRIES identified a three-factor solution that corresponded to the intrusion (4 items), avoidance (4 items), and arousal (5 items) subscales of the PTSD symptoms across three symptom clusters. Greater ratings are indicative of children's increased susceptibility to PTSD (Perrin et al., 2005). Smith et al. stated that the scores were associated with the children's degree of anxiety, despair, and traumatic exposure in addition to the suffering that mothers and teachers reported (Smith et al., 2001).

6.1.3. Child PTSD Symptom Scale (CPSS)

According to DSM–IV 4th ed. (APA, 1994), the CPSS is a self-report measure of PTSD severity among children aged 8 to 18 years. Children appear to understand it well, and administering it takes them only a little while. With each item assessed on a 4-point Likert-type scale (0 = not at all, 1 = once a week or less, 2 = two–four times a week, and 3 = five or more times per week), the CPSS measures the frequency of the 17 PTSD symptoms (DSM–IV). Seven dichotomously scored items are used to measure the impact of symptoms on daily function. These items cover topics including academics and family relationships (Nixon et al., 2013).

6.1.4. The UCLA PTSD Reaction Index for DSM-IV, revision 1 (UCLA CPTSD-RI)

The UCLA Trauma Psychiatry Program created the UCLA PTSD Reaction Index in 1985 as a screening tool based on DSM diagnostic criteria to evaluate post-traumatic stress reactions in children and adolescents. The UCLA PTSD-RI is a self-report tool extensively used worldwide to measure childhood PTSD (Steinberg et al., 2004). It demonstrates satisfactory, reliability and validity. There are two components to the 33-item scale: The DSM-IV criteria A (the objective and subjective experiences and memories of the traumatic event) was met by (1) a section of 13 questions (scored dichotomously); (2) a section of 20 questions, with each item scored from 0 (never or rarely) to 4 (most or all of the time), directly corresponds to the DSM-IV criteria B (intrusion), C (sense of "numbness" and avoidance), and D (arousal) for PTSD.

6.2. Structured and Semi-structured Interview Tools

Contrastingly, structured and semi-structured diagnostic interview schedules require precise implementation procedures and should be administered by professionals or rigorously trained surveyors for an objective evaluation of the subject's symptoms. Due to their enhanced diagnostic reliability, these tools have become pivotal assets in assessing treatment effectiveness, epidemiological patterns of psychopathology, and the continuity and validity of psychiatric syndromes observed in children and adults. While the content of most of these interview schedules is typically symptom-based, their formats may vary. These include (a) The schedule for affective disorders and schizophrenia for school-age children present and lifetime version (K SADS PL); and (b) Mini international neuropsychiatric interview for children and adolescents (MINI-KID) (Li et al., 2020).

6.2.1. The schedule for affective disorders and schizophrenia for school-age children present and lifetime version (K-SADS-PL)

DSM-IV compatible, K-SADS-PL is a semi-structured diagnostic interview schedule used by professionals in child and adolescent psychiatry to determine the lifetime and present status of mental illness in children and adolescents. It is designed to interview kids as well as parents. If the symptoms of the severe current episode have subsided, score sheet margin notations are necessary (Ambrosini, 2000).

6.2.2. Mini international neuropsychiatric interview for children and adolescents (MINI-KID)

The MINI-KID is a structured clinical diagnostic interview that is intended to evaluate children and adolescents aged 6 to 17 years without mental retardation for the presence of psychiatric illnesses based on DSM-IV and ICD-10 criteria. It is a quick, yet reliable and valid diagnostic tool that can be applied in psychiatric therapeutic settings (Adamowska et al., 2014). A skilled surveyor can readily conduct MINI-KID, making it a convenient tool for large-scale epidemiological research. The surveyors must take into account elements related to their own experience, the familiarity of the instruments, and the objective conditions while choosing the right evaluation tool and creating an evaluation strategy. Surveyors ought to start by thinking about the goal and target of the evaluation. The type and severity of trauma, the assessment of risk and protective factors, the evaluation of children's social functions, the features of children and adolescents' psychological development at different ages, and evaluations of parents' mental health should all be taken into account when choosing and organizing assessment tools. It should be noted, however, that cultural variations could lessen their initial impact.

Promptly establishing "child-friendly" spaces and activities aimed at normalizing the lives of children providing them with a sense of safety plays a significant role. It is crucial to concentrate efforts on interventions that bolster the resilience and resources of the population. Effective strategies should focus on enhancing the psychological adaptation of children and adolescents in the aftermath of the disaster.

7. PTSD AND GENDER DIFFERENCES

Research on gender differences in PTSD prevalence indicates that females are diagnosed with PTSD approximately twice or thrice as males (Hu et al., 2017; Christiansen & Hansen, 2015). A report demonstrated that children and adolescents living through disaster do experience long-term PTSD symptoms (63.1%). A significant gender difference in the mean score on CPTSD-RI was observed; female students had higher scores than male. However, there is no association between age and severity of PTSD symptoms (Agustini & Matsuo, 2012).

Further, during the acute phase also, women typically exhibit higher scores than men on subjective responses such as threat perception, peritraumatic dissociation, and known PTSD predictors. Women employs distinct strategies in handling stressful situations, evolving differentially to support varied behaviours. For example, women may engage in tend-and-befriend responses instead of the commonly assumed fight-or-flight reaction. Emotion-focused, defensive, and palliative coping mechanisms are more prevalent among women, whereas problem-focused coping is more commonly observed in men. Women tend to seek greater social support, with the lack of it being a consistently identified predictor of negative trauma outcomes. Literatures report that there seems to be a greater sensitivity of hypothalamus-pituitary-axis in women compared to men, while men exhibit a heightened physiological hyper-arousal system. PTSD consistently correlates with amygdala hyperactivity, reduced ventromedial prefrontal cortex (vmPFC) activity, and diminished communication (functional connectivity) between the vmPFC and amygdala. This reduced control of the amygdala by the lower PFC offers an explanation for the exaggerated fear response observed in PTSD (Olff, 2017). A study by Frijling (2017) demonstrated sex-specific routes for the effects of single oxytocin administration on the potential to diminish anxiety (fear learning) and fear expression by the amygdala: increased inhibitory control of the vmPFC over the centromedial nucleus in men and fewer excitatory dorsal anterior cingulate cortex projections to the basolateral nucleus in women. Their findings indicate that oxytocin administration could potentially enhance treatment response in PTSD, although the routes in men and women differ (Frijling, 2017). Further, women derive greater benefits from psychotherapy than men in terms of reducing PTSD symptoms (Olff, 2017).

8. HOLISTIC HEALING: TREATMENT APPROACHES BEYOND THE CONVENTIONAL

8.1. Traditional Therapies

Traditional therapies for PTSD encompass evidence-based approaches that have been widely utilized and studied for their efficacy in alleviating symptoms and promoting recovery. These therapies typically involve structured interventions that target various aspects of the individual's experience, aiming to address the cognitive, emotional, and behavioural manifestations of PTSD. Here are some of the traditional therapies commonly employed for individuals with PTSD (Foa et al.,

2003; Bradley et al., 2005; Turner et al., 2005; Hembree & Foa, 2000; Davidson & Parker, 2001) (Figure 5).

Figure 5. Treatment approaches of PTSD

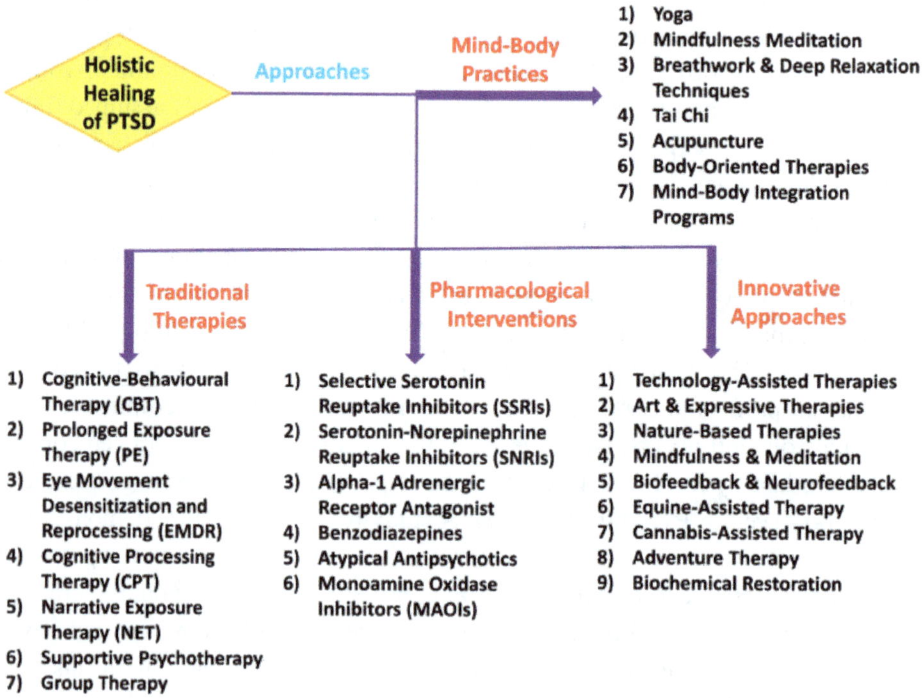

8.1.1. Cognitive-Behavioural Therapy (CBT)

CBT is a well-established and widely used therapeutic approach for PTSD. It focuses on identifying and challenging negative thought patterns and beliefs associated with the traumatic event. Cognitive restructuring helps individuals develop healthier thought processes, while exposure therapy encourages gradual confrontation with trauma-related memories or situations in a controlled and supportive environment (Foa et al., 2003).

8.1.2. Prolonged Exposure Therapy (PE)

PE is a specific form of CBT designed to reduce avoidance behaviours commonly associated with PTSD. Through repeated and controlled exposure to memories and reminders of the traumatic event, individuals learn to confront and process their emotions, gradually reducing the anxiety and distress associated with these memories. This approach aims to promote desensitization and emotional processing (Bradley et al., 2005).

8.1.3. Eye Movement Desensitization and Reprocessing (EMDR)

EMDR is a therapeutic approach that incorporates elements of cognitive-behavioural therapy with bilateral stimulation, typically through guided eye movements. During EMDR sessions, individuals focus on distressing memories while engaging in specific eye movements. The goal is to facilitate the processing of traumatic memories, ultimately reducing their emotional charge and alleviating symptoms (Davidson & Parker, 2001).

8.1.4. Cognitive Processing Therapy (CPT)

CPT is a cognitive-behavioural approach that targets maladaptive beliefs and thoughts related to the traumatic event. Through structured writing exercises and discussions, individuals work to challenge and reframe distorted cognitions. The emphasis is on understanding the impact of trauma on beliefs about oneself, others, and the world (Monson et al., 2006).

8.1.5. Narrative Exposure Therapy (NET)

NET is an evidence-based therapy that focuses on constructing a detailed narrative of the individual's life, including traumatic experiences. Through the therapeutic retelling of their life story, individuals can gain a sense of coherence and integration, promoting the processing and integration of traumatic memories (Lely et al., 2019).

8.1.6. Supportive Psychotherapy

Supportive psychotherapy involves creating a safe and empathetic space for individuals to express their thoughts and emotions related to the trauma. While it may not be as structured as CBT or EMDR, supportive therapy provides a valuable foundation for individuals to explore and process their experiences, fostering a therapeutic alliance and promoting emotional expression (Turner et al., 2005).

8.1.7. Group Therapy

Group therapy brings individuals with PTSD together, providing a supportive community where they can share their experiences and coping strategies. Group settings offer a sense of validation, normalization, and connection, reducing feelings of isolation commonly experienced by those with PTSD (Hembree & Foa, 2000).

These traditional therapies for PTSD are typically implemented by trained mental health professionals and are often tailored to the specific needs and preferences of the individual.

8.2. Pharmacological Interventions

Pharmacotherapy plays a significant role in the comprehensive treatment of PTSD. While medications do not provide a cure, they can help alleviate specific symptoms associated with PTSD, improving overall well-being. Here is an overview of common pharmacological interventions used in the management of PTSD (Ehret, 2019) (Figure 5 and Table 1).

Table 1. Pharmacological interventions in the management of PTSD

Class	Drug	Daily Dose (mg)	Specific Side-effects	General Side-effects	Contraindications
SSRIs	Sertraline	50-150	Sedation	Gastrointestinal, Nausea, Loose motions, Interferes with ejaculation or orgasm; Mild side-effects, viz. nervous restlessness, insomnia, anorexia, dyskinesia and headache, epistaxis and ecchymosis, serotonin syndrome	Inhibit drug metabolizing isoenzymes CYP2D6 and CYP3A4; elevate plasma levels of TCAs (tricyclic antidepressants), haloperidol, clozapine, terfenadine, astemizole, warfarin, β blockers, some BZDs and carbamazepine; Precipitation of serotonin syndrome with MAOIs, tramadol and pethidine
	Fluoxetine	20-40	Sedation, seizure precipitation, agitation, dermatological reactions		
	Paroxetine	20-50	Sedation, anti-muscarinic effects, GI side effects, sexual distress, agitation, discontinuation reaction with other SSRIs		

continued on following page

Table 1. Continued

Class	Drug	Daily Dose (mg)	Specific Side-effects	General Side-effects	Contraindications
SNRIs	Venlafaxine	75-150	Cardiac arrhythmia	Depress BP, nausea, sweating, anxiety, dizziness, impotence, withdrawal reactions on discontinuation	MAOIs, TCAs, Triptans, Anticoagulants, Antihistamines, Alcohol, Theophylline, Ketoconazole
	Duloxetine	30-80	Difficulty sleeping, headache, dizziness, blurred vision, dry mouth	Gastrointestinal, Sexual problems, Agitation, Insomnia, Rise in BP	
Alpha-1 adrenergic receptor antagonist	Prazosin	1-20	Postural hypotension, palpitation	Dizziness, headache, drowsiness, weakness, nausea, bloating, constipation	Not recommended for congestive heart failure due to mechanical obstruction; when giving first dose monitor for excessive hypotension or give at bedtime
BZDs	Diazepam	5-10	Accumulation, prolonged anxiolytic effect, rebound insomnia, withdrawal phenomenon	Dizziness, vertigo, ataxia, disorientation, amnesia, prolongation of reaction time, impairment of psychomotor skills, hangover, weakness, blurring of vision, dry mouth, urinary incontinence, sleep apnoea, psychomotor side effects restlessness, malaise, loss of appetite, bad dreams are prominent; Agitation, panic reaction, tremors and delirium are occasional; convulsions are rare	Alcohol and other CNS depressants leads to excessive impairment; sodium valproate provokes psychotic symptoms; ketoconazole and erythromycin increases BZDs metabolism; cimetidine, isoniazid and oral contraceptives retard BZD metabolism
	Clonazepam	0.5-5	Sedation, dullness, lack of concentration, irritability, temper and other behavioural abnormalities in children, motor disturbances, ataxia, salvation, increased respiratory secretions		

continued on following page

Table 1. Continued

Class	Drug	Daily Dose (mg)	Specific Side-effects	General Side-effects	Contraindications
Atypical antipsychotics	Risperidone	2-8	Disproportionate increase in prolactin levels, agitation, increase in new-onset diabetes	Extrapyramidal effects, sedation, hypotension, weight gain, increased risk of stroke in elderly	Potentiates all CND depressants; block actions of levodopa and direct DA agonists; antihypertensive action of clonidine and methyldopa is reduced
	Olanzapine	2.5-20	Little rise in prolactin levels, high risk of impairing glucose tolerance or worsening diabetes, elevates serum triglycerides,		
MAOIs	Phenelzine	15-90	Restlessness, confusion, hallucinations, hypertensive crisis, photophobia, serotonin syndrome, allergic reactions	Headache, weakness, diarrhoea, nausea, sweating, chest pain, neck stiffness	Patients exhibiting hypersensitivity to the drug or who have pheochromocytoma, congestive heart failure, severe renal impairment or renal pathology, abnormal LFTs, or a history of liver disease; antidepressants, appetite suppressants, drugs for attention deficit disorder, street drugs

(Tripathi, 2013)

8.2.1. Selective Serotonin Reuptake Inhibitors (SSRIs)

SSRIs are a class of antidepressant medications frequently prescribed for PTSD. Medications such as sertraline, fluoxetine, and paroxetine are among the SSRIs commonly used (Figure 6). These medications work by increasing the availability of serotonin, a neurotransmitter that plays a role in mood regulation. SSRIs are considered a first-line pharmacological treatment for PTSD and may help reduce symptoms such as anxiety, intrusive thoughts, and irritability.

8.2.2. Serotonin-Norepinephrine Reuptake Inhibitors (SNRIs)

SNRIs, such as venlafaxine and duloxetine, are another class of antidepressants used in the treatment of PTSD (Figure 6). They increase the levels of both serotonin and norepinephrine, addressing symptoms related to mood, arousal, and emotional regulation. SNRIs may be particularly helpful for individuals who do not respond adequately to SSRIs.

8.2.3. Alpha-1 Adrenergic Receptor Antagonist

Prazosin is an alpha-1 adrenergic receptor antagonist primarily used to address nightmares and sleep disturbances associated with PTSD (Figure 6). By blocking the effects of norepinephrine, prazosin can reduce the intensity and frequency of traumatic nightmares, promoting improved sleep quality. It is often prescribed in addition to other medications or psychotherapeutic interventions.

Figure 6. Examples of SSRIs, SNRIs, and Alpha-1 adrenergic receptor antagonists used in PTSD treatment

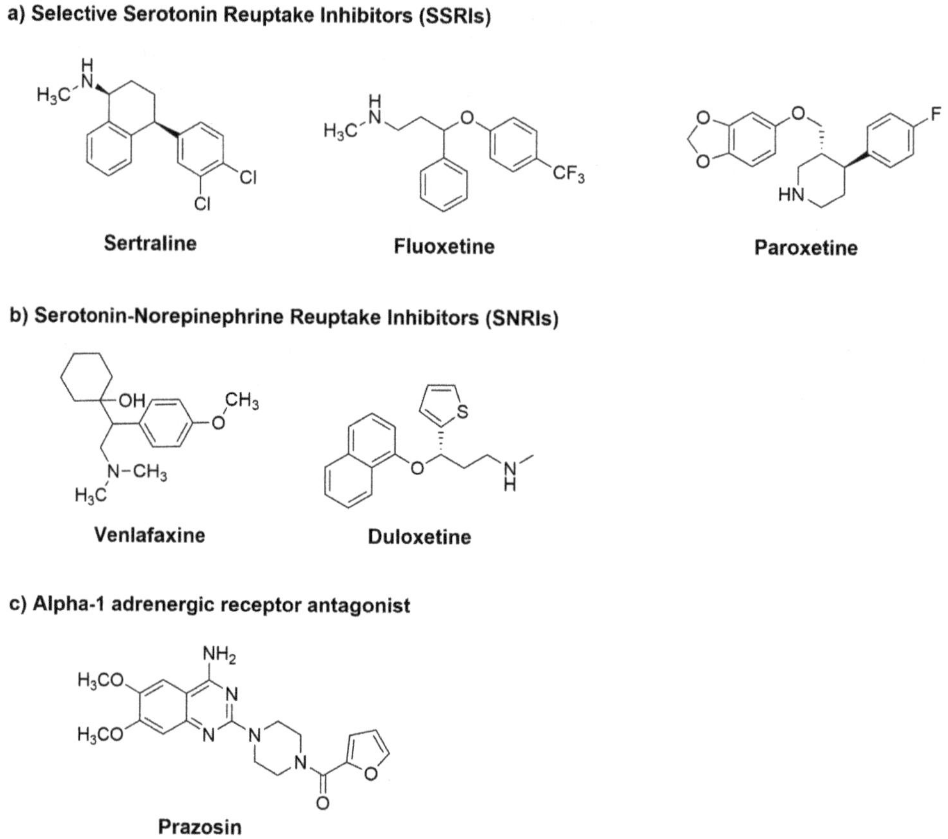

8.2.4. Benzodiazepines (Cautionary Use)

Benzodiazepines (BZDs), such as diazepam and clonazepam, may be prescribed to manage symptoms of anxiety and insomnia in individuals with PTSD (Figure 7). However, their use is generally approached with caution due to the risk of dependence and potential for worsening symptoms over the long term. Benzodiazepines are typically reserved for short-term use or situations where other treatments are ineffective or contraindicated.

8.2.5. Atypical Antipsychotics

In some cases, atypical antipsychotic medications, such as risperidone or olanzapine (Figure 7), may be prescribed to address symptoms such as severe irritability, aggression, or disorganized thinking. These medications are often used as adjunctive treatments when other interventions have not provided sufficient relief.

Figure 7. Examples of SSRIs, SNRIs, and Alpha-1 adrenergic receptor antagonists used in PTSD treatment

a) Benzodiazepines

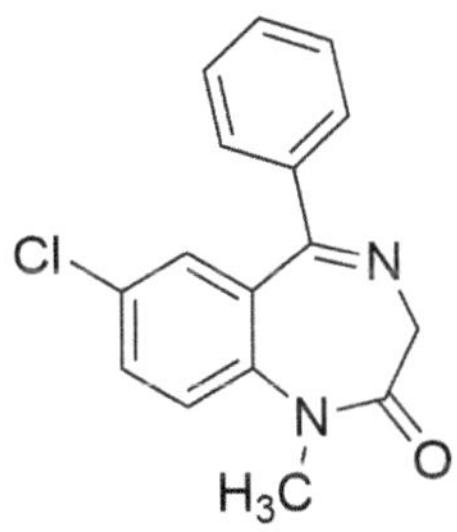

Diazepam

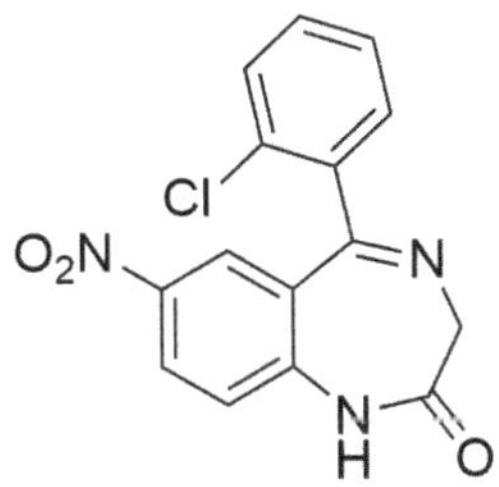

Clonazepam

b) Atypical Antipsycotics

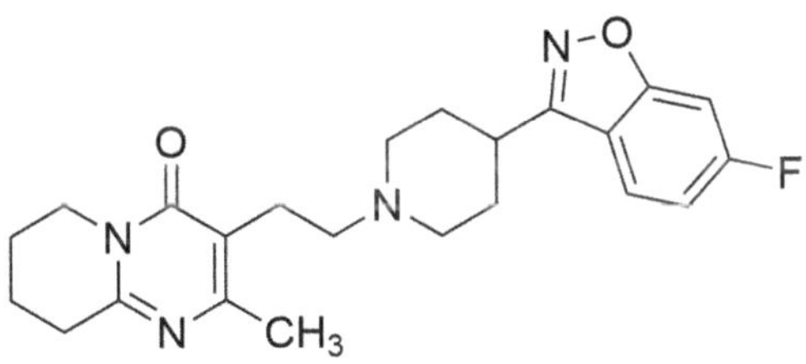

Resperidone

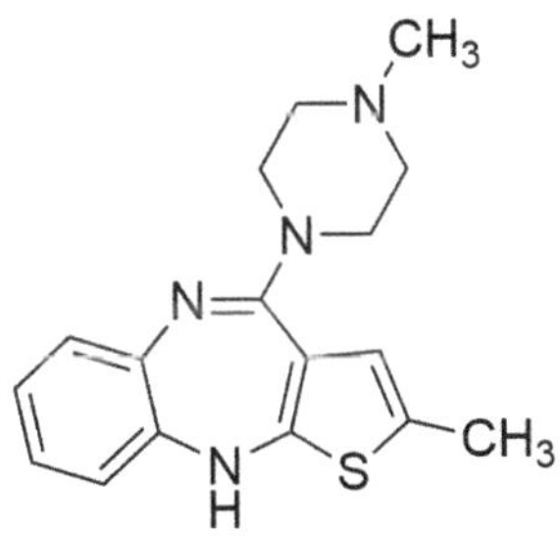

Olanzapine

c) Monoamine Oxidase Inhibitors (MAOIs)

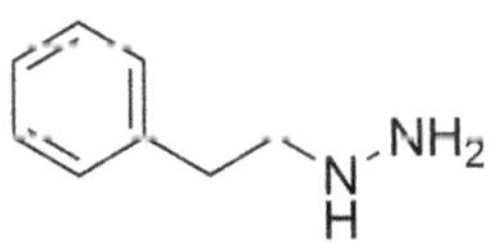

Phenelzine

8.2.6. Monoamine Oxidase Inhibitors (MAOIs)

MAOIs, such as phenelzine, are a less commonly prescribed class of antidepressants (Figure 7). They work by inhibiting the breakdown of neurotransmitters like serotonin, norepinephrine, and dopamine. MAOIs are considered when other treatments have been ineffective, but their use requires careful monitoring due to dietary and medication interactions.

It is important to note that medication management should be individualized, and the decision to prescribe pharmacological interventions for PTSD should involve a thorough assessment by a qualified healthcare provider. The choice of medication depends on the specific symptoms, overall health, and potential interactions with other medications. Additionally, pharmacological interventions are often used in conjunction with psychotherapeutic approaches, such as cognitive-behavioural therapy (CBT), exposure therapy, or eye movement desensitization and reprocessing (EMDR), for a more comprehensive and synergistic treatment plan. Regular monitoring and follow-up with a healthcare provider are essential to assess the effectiveness of the medication and make any necessary adjustments. Table 2 describes the current PTSD guidelines (Ehret, 2019; APA, 2004; APA, 2009; Baldwin et al., 2005; Australian Centre for Posttraumatic Mental Health, 2013; Katzman et al., 2014; Veterans Health Administration, Department of Defense, 2017; National Institute for Health and Care Excellence, 2018; Hoffman et al. 2018; APA, 2019).

Table 2. Current PTSD guidelines

Guideline	Treatment Level			
	Process	First Line	Second Line	Third Line
APA (2004)	Systematic review and clinical consensus	Psy SSRI: Fluoxetine, paroxetine, sertraline SNRI: Venlafaxine Prazosin (combat-related PTSD)	TCA: Amitriptyline, imipramine, desipramine Nefazodone Mirtazapine	SGA: Risperidone, olanzapine
BAP (2014)	Systematic review and expert opinion/ clinical experience	TF: CBT and EMDR SSRI: Paroxetine, sertraline SNRI: Venlafaxine	Augmentation with: olanzapine, risperidone, prazosin	–
ACPMH (2014)	Systematic review	TF: CBT or EMDR SSRI: Clinical choice	Other antidepressants Risperidone Olanzapine Prazosin	–
ADAC (2014)	Systematic review and clinical consensus	CBT SSRI: Fluoxetine, paroxetine, sertraline SNRI: Venlafaxine XR Trauma nightmares and improving sleep quality: Prazosin	Fluvoxamine, mirtazapine, phenelzine Adjunctive SGA: Risperidone, olanzapine Adjunctive: Eszopiclone	Amitriptyline, aripiprazole, bupropion SR, buspirone, carbamazepine, desipramine, duloxetine, escitalopram, imipramine, lamotrigine, memantine, quetiapine, risperidone, topiramate, trazodone Adjunctive: Clonidine, gabapentin, levetiracetam, pregabalin, quetiapine, tiagabine
VA/DoD (2017)	Systematic review and weighted recommendations	TF: Psy or SM	Non-TF Psy SSRI: Paroxetine, sertraline, fluoxetine SNRI: Venlafaxine	Imipramine Nefazodone Phenelzine

continued on following page

Table 2. Continued

Guideline	Treatment Level			
	Process	**First Line**	**Second Line**	**Third Line**
NICE (2018)	Systematic review and expert testimony, including costs	TF: CBT EMDR: Non-combat trauma if a preference for EMDR TF: Computerized CBT: preference versus face-to-face CBT for specific symptoms: sleep disturbance or anger	Medication treatments: Venlafaxine, SSRI, antipsychotics	–
AHRQ (2018)	Systematic review and weighted recommendations with peer review and public commentary	CBT (exposure and mixed therapies) SSRI: Fluoxetine, paroxetine SNRI: Venlafaxine	CPT, CT, EMDR, and NET	BE Psy, imagery rehearsal therapy, trauma affect regulation Prazosin Topiramate Olanzapine Risperidone Sertraline
APA (2017)	Systematic review; compared to previous recommendations	Strongly recommends: TF: Psy interventions: CBT, CPT, CT, PET Suggests or conditionally recommends: BE Psy, EMDR, NET Supports: Fluoxetine, paroxetine, sertraline, venlafaxine	–	–

ACPMH = Australian Centre for Posttraumatic Mental Health; ADAC = Anxiety Disorders Association of Canada; AHRQ = Agency for Healthcare Research and Quality; APA = American Psychiatric Association; BAP = British Association of Psychopharmacology; BE Psy = brief eclectic psychotherapy; CBT = cognitive behavioural therapy; CPT = cognitive processing therapy; CT = cognitive therapy; EMDR = eye movement desensitization and reprocessing; NET = narrative exposure therapy; NICE = National Institute for Clinical Excellence; PET = prolonged exposure therapy; Psy = psychotherapy; PTSD = posttraumatic stress disorder; SGA = second generation antipsychotic; SM = stress management; SSRI = selective serotonin reuptake inhibitors; SNRI = serotonin norepinephrine reuptake inhibitors; TCA = tri-cyclic antidepressant; TF = trauma-focused; VA/DoD = Veterans Association/Department of Defense

8.3. Innovative Approaches

In recent years, the landscape of treating PTSD has expanded beyond traditional therapeutic modalities, giving rise to innovative and multidimensional approaches that aim to address the complex and diverse nature of this condition. These innovative approaches leverage advancements in technology, creative arts, nature-based, and alternative therapies, offering new avenues for healing and resilience (Figure 5). These approaches recognize the diverse needs of individuals and offer alternative pathways to recovery that extend beyond traditional therapeutic methods. Here is a glimpse into some of these cutting-edge interventions (Bourla et al., 2018).

8.3.1. Technology-Assisted Therapies

a) Virtual Reality (VR) Therapy

Virtual Reality (VR) therapy has emerged as a powerful tool for treating PTSD, particularly in the context of exposure therapy. VR therapy provides a simulated environment where individuals can safely confront and process traumatic memories. This immersive experience offers a controlled and customizable setting, allowing therapists to tailor exposure scenarios to individual needs (Kothgassner et al., 2019).

b) Telehealth and Online Platforms

Advances in telehealth and online therapy platforms facilitate access to mental health support, especially for those facing barriers like geographical distance or physical limitations. Telehealth services provide a convenient and flexible way for individuals to engage in therapy, promoting continuity of care (Morland et al., 2017).

8.3.2. Art and Expressive Therapies

Art therapy, music therapy, and other expressive modalities offer alternative channels for individuals to explore and communicate their experiences. Artistic expression can facilitate healing and self-discovery in ways that traditional talk therapies may not fully capture (Green, 2011).

a) Visual Arts

Painting, drawing, and other visual arts offer a creative outlet for individuals to express and process emotions related to trauma. Art therapies provide a non-verbal means of communication, allowing individuals to explore their experiences in a symbolic and metaphorical way.

b) Music Therapy

Music has the power to evoke emotions and memories. Music therapy involves creating, listening to, or discussing music as a therapeutic tool. It can help individuals explore and express complex feelings, reduce anxiety, and enhance emotional regulation.

8.3.3. Nature-Based Therapies

a) Ecotherapy

Also known as nature therapy, ecotherapy involves outdoor activities and interactions with natural environments to promote healing. Spending time in nature has been linked to reduced stress, improved mood, and enhanced overall well-being. Ecotherapy may include activities such as hiking, gardening, or simply spending time in natural settings (Joschko et al., 2023; Chalquist, 2009).

b) Adventure Therapy

Adventure therapy incorporates outdoor and experiential activities, such as wilderness trips, rock climbing, or team-building exercises, into the therapeutic process. These activities encourage individuals to step outside their comfort zones, promoting personal growth, resilience, and a sense of accomplishment. Adventure therapy can be particularly effective for enhancing self-esteem and fostering a connection with nature (Trundle & Hutchinson, 2021; Pringle et al., 2023).

8.3.4. Mindfulness and Meditation

Mindfulness-based interventions, including mindfulness meditation and Mindfulness-Based Stress Reduction (MBSR), have shown promise in reducing PTSD symptoms. These practices emphasize present-moment awareness and non-judgmental acceptance, providing individuals with tools to manage distressing thoughts and emotions. Mindfulness has been integrated into various therapeutic approaches, promoting emotional regulation and resilience. Nowadays, mobile applications focused on mindfulness and meditation provide accessible tools for individuals to manage stress and enhance emotional well-being. These apps often include guided meditation sessions, breathing exercises, and relaxation techniques that can be easily incorporated into daily routines (Boyd et al., 2018; Hofmann & Gomez, 2017).

8.3.5. Biofeedback and Neurofeedback

Biofeedback and neurofeedback utilize real-time monitoring of physiological and neurological responses to help individuals gain control over their bodily functions (Frank et al., 2010; Chiba et al., 2019). These approaches can be employed to address symptoms such as hyperarousal and physiological reactivity. By providing immediate feedback, individuals learn to modulate their physiological responses, promoting a sense of control and relaxation.

a) Biofeedback Apps

Mobile applications and devices that offer biofeedback enable individuals to monitor and gain control over physiological responses such as heart rate, muscle tension, and skin conductance. These tools can be used to enhance self-awareness and develop skills for managing stress and anxiety.

b) Neurofeedback Apps

Some applications use neurofeedback to measure and provide feedback on brainwave activity. While still evolving, these apps aim to help individuals regulate brain function and improve aspects of cognitive and emotional well-being.

8.3.6. Equine-Assisted Therapy

Equine-assisted therapy involves interactions with horses as a therapeutic medium. The unique bond between humans and horses can facilitate emotional regulation, trust-building, and communication skills. Equine-assisted therapy is particularly beneficial for individuals who may find traditional therapy settings challenging or for those seeking a novel and experiential approach to healing (Li & Sanchez-Gracia, 2023; Palomar-Ciria & Bello, 2023).

8.3.7. Cannabis-Assisted Therapy

Research is exploring the potential benefits of cannabinoids, such as cannabidiol (CBD), for managing symptoms of PTSD. While the field is evolving, some studies suggest that cannabinoids may have an impact on anxiety, sleep disturbances, and emotional regulation. However, the use of cannabis for PTSD remains a complex and evolving area, requiring careful consideration of individual factors and legal regulations (Ragnhildstveit et al., 2023).

8.3.8. Biochemical Restoration

Some emerging approaches focus on nutritional and biochemical interventions to support overall mental health. This may include addressing nutritional deficiencies, optimizing gut health, and considering the role of specific supplements. While still evolving, this approach recognizes the interconnectedness of physical and mental well-being (Norwitz & Naidoo, 2021).

These innovative approaches underscore the dynamic nature of PTSD treatment and the importance of tailoring interventions to individual needs. As the field continues to evolve, a holistic and personalized approach that integrates traditional and innovative modalities holds promise for promoting recovery and resilience in individuals affected by PTSD.

8.4. Mind-Body Practices

Mind-body practices including yoga, meditation, and breathwork have emerged as powerful, holistic, and integrative approach in the management and treatment of PTSD (Kim et al., 2013; Laplaud et al., 2023). Incorporating mind-body practices into the treatment of PTSD fosters a comprehensive approach to healing (Figure 5). These practices offer individuals a versatile toolkit to navigate the complex terrain of trauma, helps to recognize the intricate connection between mental and physical well-being, offering individuals coping tools that promote relaxation, self-awareness, and emotional regulation. These mind-body techniques contribute to a more nuanced and personalized approach to supporting individuals on their journey towards recovery from PTSD. Various key mind-body practices have shown promise in supporting individuals with PTSD (Figure 5).

8.4.1. Yoga

Yoga, an ancient practice originating from India, is a mind-body practice that combines physical postures (asanas), breath control (pranayama), and meditation. Its integrative approach can help individuals with PTSD manage symptoms related to both hyperarousal and avoidance. Yoga has been shown to reduce anxiety, improve sleep, and enhance overall mood. For individuals with PTSD, trauma-sensitive yoga approaches prioritize safety and choice, creating an environment where participants can explore movement and breath at their own pace (Kim et al., 2013; Laplaud et al., 2023). The benefits of yoga for PTSD include:

a) Physical Well-Being

Yoga helps improve flexibility, strength, and balance, addressing the somatic manifestations of trauma.

b) Emotional Regulation

Mindful movement in yoga encourages individuals to connect with their bodies, fostering emotional regulation and self-awareness.

c) Grounding and Centering

Yoga emphasizes present-moment awareness, providing a grounding experience for individuals who may feel disconnected or overwhelmed.

8.4.2. Mindfulness Meditation

Mindfulness meditation involves cultivating non-judgmental awareness of the present moment. By focusing on breath, sensations, or thoughts without attachment, individuals develop a heightened sense of presence (Kim et al., 2013). Key benefits of meditation for individuals with PTSD include:

a) Reduced Hyperarousal

Mindfulness meditation helps individuals regulate the autonomic nervous system, reducing symptoms of hyperarousal and anxiety.

b) Intrusive Thoughts Management

By training the mind to focus on the present moment, meditation supports individuals in managing intrusive thoughts and memories associated with trauma.

c) Enhanced Emotional Resilience

Regular meditation practice contributes to emotional resilience, allowing individuals to respond to stressors with greater equanimity.

8.4.3. Breathwork and Deep Relaxation Techniques

Breathwork involves intentional control of the breath to influence physiological and psychological states. Various breathwork techniques, such as diaphragmatic breathing and paced breathing, can help regulate the autonomic nervous system. Deep relaxation practices, including progressive muscle relaxation and guided imagery, promote a sense of calmness and reduce physiological arousal. These techniques are valuable tools for managing anxiety and stress associated with PTSD (Kim et al., 2013). Besides, specific breathwork techniques can be particularly beneficial for individuals with PTSD, addressing symptoms such as hypervigilance and panic attacks. Key aspects of breathwork in PTSD include:

a) Calming the Nervous System

Deep and rhythmic breathing activates the parasympathetic nervous system, promoting relaxation and reducing physiological arousal.

b) Mind-Body Connection

Breathwork enhances awareness of the mind-body connection, helping individuals recognize and regulate physical sensations associated with trauma.

c) Immediate Coping Tool

Breathwork provides individuals with a portable and accessible tool for managing stress and anxiety in real-time.

8.4.4. Tai Chi

Tai Chi is a gentle and slow-moving martial art that incorporates flowing movements and focused breathwork. This mind-body practice has been associated with improvements in mood, sleep, and overall psychological well-being. The deliberate and controlled nature of Tai Chi can provide a grounding and centering experience for individuals with PTSD (Kim et al., 2013).

8.4.5. Acupuncture

Acupuncture, an ancient Chinese medicine practice, involves the insertion of thin needles into specific points on the body. While the mechanisms are not fully understood, acupuncture has shown promise in reducing symptoms of PTSD, potentially by influencing the release of neurotransmitters and modulating the stress response (Tang et al., 2023).

8.4.6. Body-Oriented Therapies

Therapies such as Somatic Experiencing and Sensorimotor Psychotherapy focus on the connection between the mind and body in processing trauma. These approaches incorporate awareness of bodily sensations to facilitate the release of physical tension and support the integration of traumatic memories (Kuhfuß et al., 2021).

8.4.7. Mind-Body Integration Programs

Comprehensive mind-body programs, often offered in integrative healthcare settings, combine various practices such as meditation, yoga, and psychoeducation. These programs emphasize the interconnectedness of mental and physical well-being, providing individuals with a structured and supportive environment for healing (Kim et al., 2013).

Thus, mind-body practices for PTSD are not one-size-fits-all, and individuals may find different modalities more resonant with their preferences and needs. Incorporating these practices into a treatment plan, either as standalone interventions or complementary to traditional therapies, empowers individuals to actively participate in their healing journey. The emphasis on self-care, self-awareness, and holistic well-being contributes to a more resilient and empowered approach to navigating the challenges of PTSD.

9. ROLE OF SOCIAL SUPPORT AND COMMUNITY

The role of social support and community is pivotal in the context of PTSD. It serves not only as a source of emotional and practical assistance but also as a catalyst for healing, resilience, and post-traumatic growth (Gros et al., 2016; Johansen et al., 2022; Sherin & Nemeroff, 2011; Matheson et al., 2020). Recognizing and fostering social connections are integral components of a comprehensive approach to supporting individuals affected by trauma and PTSD.

9.1 Building Resilience

Building resilience is a crucial aspect of navigating the challenges posed by PTSD, and the impact of connection and support in this process cannot be overstated. Resilience refers to the ability to bounce back from adversity, adapt to change, and navigate stressors with a sense of empowerment and efficacy. Social connection and support play instrumental roles in cultivating and sustaining resilience for individuals affected by PTSD. The elements contributing to the building of resilience includes:

9.1.1. Social Support as a Protective Factor

Trauma can often lead to a sense of isolation and alienation. Social support acts as a buffer against the negative impacts of trauma. Having a network of reliable and understanding individuals, be it friends, family, or community members, creates a buffer that can mitigate the severity of PTSD symptoms. Knowing that one is not alone in their struggles fosters a sense of belonging and security.

9.1.2. Emotional Support and Understanding

Emotional support is a cornerstone of resilience. Individuals facing PTSD often grapple with a range of intense emotions. Having supportive relationships provides a safe space for the expression of these emotions without judgment. Feeling understood and validated contributes significantly to emotional well-being and resilience.

9.1.3. Sense of Belonging

Connection with others fosters a sense of belonging, which is fundamental to resilience. Feeling a part of a community or social network provides individuals with a source of identity and purpose. This sense of belonging contributes to a positive self-image and reinforces the notion that one is valued and accepted.

9.1.4. Empathy and Shared Understanding

Empathy is a powerful force in building resilience. When individuals with PTSD experience empathy from others who share a similar understanding of trauma, it creates a bond that transcends words. Shared experiences foster a deeper connection, and the knowledge that others have walked a similar path can be a source of strength and encouragement.

9.1.5. Encouraging Help-Seeking Behaviour

Social support encourages individuals to seek help when needed. Whether it is reaching out to mental health professionals, engaging in therapy, or participating in support groups, the encouragement and endorsement of seeking assistance play a vital role in the resilience-building process.

9.1.6. Strengthening Coping Mechanisms

Connection with supportive individuals can contribute to the development and strengthening of coping mechanisms. Friends and family members can offer help with daily tasks, childcare, or other responsibilities, alleviating stressors that may exacerbate PTSD symptoms. Additionally, learning from others who have faced adversity and successfully coped with trauma provides valuable insights and strategies. Shared coping mechanisms become tools for resilience in the face of ongoing challenges.

9.1.7. Collective Strength of Community

Communities, whether small social circles or larger societal networks, can contribute to the collective strength of individuals affected by PTSD. The shared values, norms, and resources within a community provide a foundation for mutual support and resilience. The community becomes a source of encouragement and empowerment.

9.1.7. Fostering a Positive Environment

Supportive relationships and social connections contribute to the creation of a positive environment and post-traumatic growth. A positive environment is conducive to healing, growth, and the cultivation of a resilient mindset. This environment provides the emotional safety necessary for individuals to embark on their journey towards recovery.

9.1.8. Building a Sense of Safety and Trust

Establishing a sense of safety and trust is fundamental in the recovery process. Social support networks contribute to this by providing a reliable foundation where individuals can express themselves authentically, knowing that they are accepted and supported. This sense of safety is foundational for the gradual healing of trauma-related wounds.

9.1.9. Encouraging Engagement in Meaningful Activities

Involvement in community activities and meaningful pursuits can contribute to a sense of purpose and connectedness. Engaging in activities aligned with personal values and interests helps individuals rebuild a positive and fulfilling life beyond the traumatic experience.

In conclusion, nurturing these connections creates a web of support that empowers individuals to face challenges, embrace growth, and find strength in their journey toward healing. By fostering a sense of belonging and encouraging help-seeking behaviour, social support becomes a cornerstone in the resilient foundation of those navigating the complexities of PTSD.

9.2. Reducing Stigma and Facilitating Treatment

Addressing the stigma associated with PTSD is a critical step in fostering understanding, empathy, and support for individuals affected by this mental health condition. Stigma can perpetuate misconceptions, hinder help-seeking behaviours, and contribute to the isolation of those living with PTSD. Creating a stigma-free environment involves raising awareness, challenging stereotypes, and promoting a culture of compassion (Ahmedani, 2011). The various ways of addressing the stigma of PTSD includes:

9.2.1. Challenging Misconceptions

One of the first steps in addressing PTSD stigma is dispelling misconceptions about the condition. Common myths, such as associating PTSD only with combat veterans or assuming that individuals with PTSD are dangerous, contribute to stigma. Education campaigns, public awareness initiatives, and open discussions can challenge these myths and provide accurate information about the diverse causes and manifestations of PTSD.

9.2.2. Emphasizing the Spectrum of Trauma

PTSD can result from various traumatic experiences, including but not limited to combat, sexual assault, natural disasters, and accidents. Acknowledging the wide spectrum of traumatic events that can lead to PTSD helps combat the stereotype that associates the condition solely with military service. Recognizing the diversity of experiences promotes empathy and reduces judgment.

9.2.3. Humanizing Personal Narratives

Sharing personal stories of individuals living with PTSD humanizes the condition and challenges stereotypes. Real-life narratives highlight the complexity of PTSD, emphasizing that it can affect anyone, regardless of age, gender, or background. By listening to and understanding these stories, society can foster empathy and develop a more nuanced perspective on the challenges faced by individuals with PTSD.

9.2.4. Promoting Help-Seeking Behaviour

Stigma can create barriers to seeking mental health support. Encouraging open conversations about mental health, emphasizing the effectiveness of available treatments, and highlighting stories of recovery can motivate individuals to seek help without fear of judgment. Promoting a culture that values mental health and well-being reduces the stigma surrounding help-seeking behaviour.

9.2.5. Creating Supportive Environments

Establishing supportive environments in workplaces, educational institutions, and communities is crucial for individuals with PTSD. This involves implementing policies that accommodate the unique needs of individuals with PTSD, fostering an inclusive atmosphere, and providing resources for mental health support. Supportive environments reduce the fear of judgment and encourage disclosure.

9.2.6. Educating the Public

Public education campaigns play a vital role in addressing PTSD stigma. These campaigns can raise awareness about the prevalence of PTSD, its impact on individuals and communities, and the importance of empathy and understanding. By fostering a culture of mental health literacy, society can contribute to reducing stigma and promoting a more compassionate perspective.

9.2.7. Combatting Stigmatizing Language

Language matters when discussing mental health. Avoiding stigmatizing language and adopting terminology that is respectful and inclusive helps reshape societal attitudes toward PTSD. Encouraging responsible media reporting and avoiding sensationalized portrayals contribute to a more accurate understanding of PTSD.

9.2.8. Promoting Peer Support

Peer support can be a powerful antidote to stigma. Creating spaces for individuals with lived experiences of PTSD to connect, share, and support one another fosters a sense of community and reduces feelings of isolation. Peer support initiatives help break down stereotypes and demonstrate that individuals with PTSD are not defined by their diagnosis.

Thus, addressing the stigma of PTSD is a collective responsibility that requires a multi-faceted approach. Reducing stigma not only benefits those directly affected by PTSD but also creates a more compassionate and empathetic society for everyone.

10. EMERGING TRENDS AND RESEARCH FRONTIERS

Figure 8. Emerging trends and research frontiers in PTSD treatment

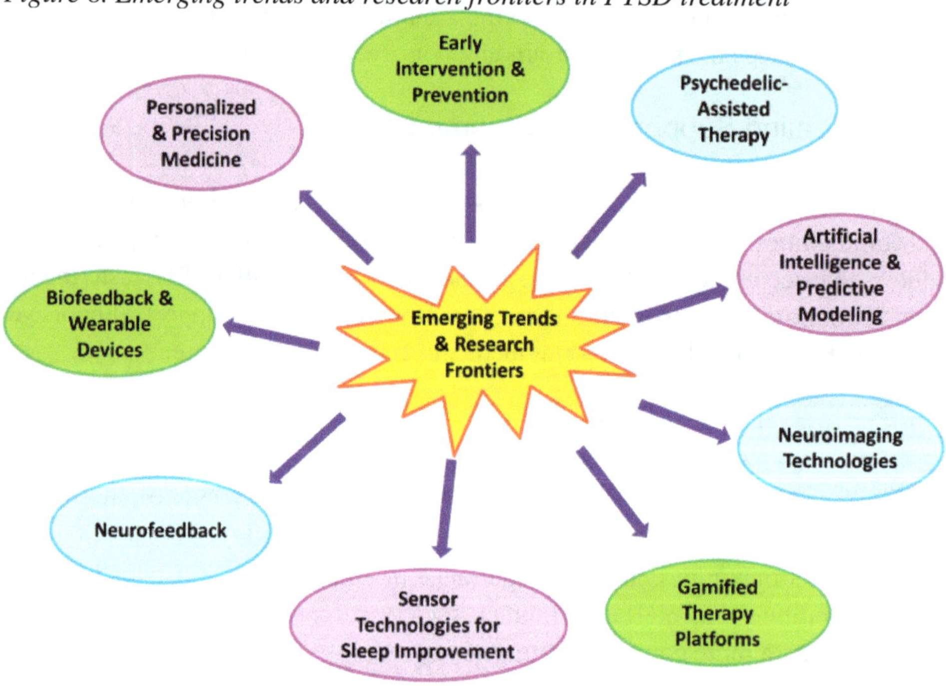

The landscape of PTSD treatment is continually evolving, driven by emerging trends and research frontiers that seek to enhance the effectiveness and accessibility of interventions. The integration of various emerging technologies holds promise for a more nuanced, personalized, and effective approach to addressing the complex and varied challenges associated with trauma (Figure 8). Pioneering studies, including the synergy of traditional and innovative approaches are shaping the comprehensive and holistic paradigm for the treatment of PTSD in the years ahead, offering new perspectives on diagnosis, therapeutic modalities, and preventive strategies.

10.1. Personalized and Precision Medicine

Advancements in genetics, neurobiology, and data analytics are paving the way for personalized and precision medicine approaches in PTSD treatment. Tailoring interventions based on individual differences, including genetic predispositions and neural markers, holds the potential to optimize treatment outcomes. Precision medicine aims to match specific treatments with the unique characteristics of each individual, fostering more targeted and effective interventions (Andreassen et al., 2023).

10.2. Early Intervention and Prevention

Research is increasingly focusing on early intervention strategies and preventive measures to mitigate the long-term impact of trauma. Identifying risk factors, implementing trauma-informed care, and developing resilience-building programs are key components of these efforts (Kearns et al., 2012). Resilience-based prevention and intervention efforts are summarized in Table 3 (Horn & Feder, 2018).

Table 3. Resilience-boosting interventions for children and adults

Intervention type	Program	Population	Intervention summary	Resilience factors targeted
Caregiver- and family-based	Multidimensional Treatment Foster Care for Preschoolers (MTFC-P) Therapist administered	Foster preschool children; foster caregiver(s)	Children's playgroup Facilitate school readiness (supplemented by individual behavioural sessions)	Supportive and consistent parenting Attachment security Parent stress levels
	Attachment and Biobehavioural Catch-Up (ABC) Therapist administered	Foster preschool children; foster caregiver(s) Child protective services involved	10 weekly, in-home sessions	Attachment security Sensitive caregiving Children's regulatory capacity
	Kid's Club and Mom's Empowerment Therapist administered	School-age children and their mothers exposed to intimate partner violence	10-session program over 5 weeks Group format (separate groups for mothers and children)	Social competence Facing fears Social and emotional adjustment for mothers Parenting skills
	FOCUS Therapist administered	Families coping with traumatic exposures and loss; military families; families with chronic illnesses	Narrative sharing process Strengths-based approach	Meaning making Problem solving Social support
School-based	Bounce Back School-based therapist delivered	Multicultural school-age children exposed to traumatic events	10 sessions CBT-based Reduction of PTSD and anxiety symptoms	Cognitive-reappraisal skills
	Mindfulness-based stress reduction Trained instructor delivered	7th and 8th grade males in a low-income urban area	Structured program of mindfulness instruction	Coping skills, emotion awareness

continued on following page

Table 3. Continued

Intervention type	Program	Population	Intervention summary	Resilience factors targeted
Community-based	Positive Youth Development Trained mentors	High-risk and general community youth	Five Cs: competence, confidence, character, connection, caring Engage youth in community (prosocial approach)	Individual strength, positive adult-youth relationships, self-regulation skills
	Communities that care Trained mentors	High-risk and general community youth	Prevalent adolescent behaviour and health problems (e.g. drug abuse prevention)	Family management styles, social support, and academic engagement

10.3. Psychedelic-Assisted Therapy

Research into the therapeutic potential of psychedelics, such as MDMA (3,4-methylenedioxy-methamphetamine) and psilocybin (found in certain mushrooms), is gaining traction. Preliminary studies suggest that these substances, when administered under controlled and supervised conditions, may facilitate breakthroughs in trauma processing and emotional regulation. Psychedelic-assisted therapy is being explored as an adjunct to traditional therapeutic approaches (Mohamed et al., 2022).

10.4. Artificial Intelligence and Predictive Modeling

Artificial Intelligence (AI) and machine learning are being applied to analyze large datasets, including genetic factors, neuroimaging data, and identify patterns, and develop predictive models for PTSD. These tools hold potential for improving diagnostic accuracy, predicting treatment response, and identifying risk factors for the development of PTSD. AI-driven interventions may enhance our understanding of individual variability in PTSD trajectories (Malgaroli & Schultebraucks, 2021; Mentis et al., 2023).

10.5. Neuroimaging Technologies

Technological advancements in neuroimaging, including functional magnetic resonance imaging (fMRI) and positron emission tomography (PET), have allowed researchers to investigate the live brain in unprecedented detail. These imaging techniques provide valuable insights into the neural circuits, connectivity, and activity patterns associated with PTSD, enhancing our understanding of the condition's neurobiological underpinnings. As our neuroscientific understanding of PTSD continues to evolve, these advancements hold promise for the development of targeted interventions, personalized treatments, and novel therapeutic approaches (Prasad et al., 2019).

10.6. Gamified Therapy Platforms

Gamification of therapy involves incorporating game-like elements into therapeutic interventions to enhance engagement and motivation. Gamified therapy platforms for PTSD utilize interactive and immersive experiences to deliver therapeutic content. These platforms can make treatment more engaging, especially for younger individuals, and provide a dynamic and interactive approach to addressing PTSD symptoms (Cheng & Ebrahimi, 2023; Litvin et al., 2020; Drissi et al., 2019).

10.7. Sensor Technologies for Sleep Improvement

Sleep disturbances are common in individuals with PTSD, and emerging sensor technologies are addressing this aspect of treatment. Wearable devices equipped with sensors can monitor sleep patterns, assess sleep quality, and provide insights into sleep-related symptoms. Tailoring interventions based on sleep data contributes to comprehensive PTSD treatment plans (Bourla et al., 2018).

10.8. Neurofeedback

Neurofeedback involves real-time monitoring of brain activity, typically through electroencephalography (EEG), and providing feedback to individuals to help regulate their neural patterns. This technology is being explored as a therapeutic tool for PTSD, aiming to modulate brain activity associated with symptoms such as hyperarousal and intrusive memories. Neurofeedback holds promise for enhancing self-regulation and neural plasticity (Chiba et al., 2019).

10.9. Biofeedback and Wearable Devices

Biofeedback technologies and wearable devices offer real-time monitoring of physiological responses, such as heart rate, skin conductance, and muscle tension. These tools provide individuals with immediate feedback on their stress levels, enabling them to develop self-regulation skills. Wearable devices, such as smartwatches, can also support ongoing monitoring and intervention for PTSD symptoms.

By unravelling the intricacies of the brain's response to trauma, researchers aim to improve diagnostic accuracy, optimize treatment strategies, and ultimately enhance the quality of life for individuals affected by PTSD (Alneyadi et al., 2021).

11. AFTERMATH OF PTSD TREATMENT

Natural disasters like tsunami and man-made disasters like war, killing, terrorist attacks, sexual and physical abuse, robbing, plane crashes, etc. may affect the individual's normal functionalities sometimes leading to PTSD. People require the necessities after surviving such incidents, viz., food, shelter, medical attention, and comfort. For some people these days, psychological treatment has been added to the list of essential demands.

Physicians should be able to determine when and if psychological assistance is required. The National Institute for Clinical Excellence (NICE) has released a new guideline on managing PTSD in primary and secondary care. It contains evidence and recommendations on interventions for adults and children, and it does a great job of summarising the experiences of those who suffer from the condition and those who care for them (NICE, 2005). The guideline emphasizes the wide-ranging effects of trauma in contemporary society and pays particular attention to "disaster planning"; the needs of victims of domestic abuse, refugees, and asylum seekers, as well as the needs of ex-military people and the non-statutory sector.

The guidelines suggest first cautious waiting when symptoms, such as sleep disturbances, emotional instability, difficulties focusing, and flashbacks, are modest and have persisted for fewer than four weeks following traumatic events. The evidence-based conclusion that early psychological assistance, sometimes known as debriefing, has no benefit in preventing PTSD; in fact, despite high satisfaction rates reported, underlies this good counsel. It is obvious that debriefing following tragedies ought to become less common place. However, there is currently no solid data on how a community affected by a tragedy regains control when it comes to handling the turmoil, material losses, grief, and fury, for instance, following a terrorist attack.

The NICE guideline states that when dissociative disorders, depression, suicidality, addiction, medically unexplained physical symptoms, or dissociative disorders develop after trauma, treatment is required. The risk of developing PTSD after trauma is 8-13% for men in contrast to 20-30% in women After experiencing trauma, men are likely to acquire post-traumatic stress disorder (8–13%) than women (20–30%), with a prevalence of 1.3% to 3.9% after 12 months, putting a significant burden on society (Kessler et al., 1995).

A systematic evaluation of the data supporting both pharmaceutical and psychological therapies is included in the NICE guideline. NICE suggests trauma-focused psychological therapy as initial treatment. As a result of the limited effectiveness of both published and unpublished data for a restricted number of pharmacological therapies, NICE advises against the use of pharmaceuticals as first line treatment. Cognitive behavioural therapy is the best method for resetting the fear response (Foa et al., 2000). With gradual exposure to the traumatic experience virtually, the fear response will lessen. Feelings of weakness, guilt, or vulnerability that are generated by the incident are replaced with more grounded thoughts about oneself. The recommendation also endorses, if not as strongly, treatment with eye movement desensitization reprocessing, which reduces the emotional lability associated with the trauma by using bilateral stimulation as a distracting maneuver following exposure.

It is still unclear if the heightened dread associated with PTSD stems from the incident itself or from the repression of incredibly intense feelings of grief and aggression brought on by the traumatic experience (Gersons et al., 2000). Greater focus should be placed on how catastrophic events disrupt the sufferer's perspective on life. Although there is currently little data, the researchers concur with the recommendation to pay attention to the prevalent comorbidities of PTSD, such as anxiety and depression (Summerfield, 2001).

Even with the availability of efficacious psychosocial interventions, one-third of patients do not fully recover (Bradley et al., 2005). Treatment response may be limited because to comorbidity, chronicity, and the build-up of acute and chronic stress. Furthermore, from an evolutionary perspective, it is possible that the ability to recall and learn from danger - what is known as “the gift of nature” - may limit the options available for treating PTSD (Le Doux, 1996). Afterall it is not possible to erase the memories of trauma.

12. RECOVERY PROCESS OF PTSD

It is possible to recover from PTSD. Each person's road to recovery will be unique and dependent on a number of variables, such as the degree of the trauma, the person's level of personal resilience, the calibre of their support networks, and the therapies they have received. Weekly therapy sessions may be the form of treatment for some, while more intense care such as inpatient treatment at a residential facility, medication, or more sophisticated psychotherapy techniques may be necessary for others.

12.1. Stages of PTSD Recovery

Stage 1: The Emergency Stage

This is the stage that immediately follows the trauma and is also occasionally referred to as the impact stage. It is common to have a wide range of strong, perplexing emotions throughout this period. You could struggle to absorb what happened in the moment and feel as though you are in shock or numb. Symptoms can differ based on the trauma's complexity, severity, and effect on you. For instance, compared to someone who watched a vehicle accident but was unharmed, someone who was the victim of a robbery at gunpoint might have more severe, long-lasting anxiety.

In this phase, it is critical to get expert assistance as soon as feasible. Early intervention can help you begin your recovery process sooner by slowing the worsening of your PTSD symptoms.

Stage 2: The Rescue Stage

The "Rescue Stage," which is the second phase of PTSD treatment, is when you start talking about the specifics of the traumatic event that led to your trauma. You might still experience symptoms like hopelessness, rage, or anxiety throughout this period, but as you move forward, you will be able to deal with the trauma's underlying cause more easily.

Stage 3: The Intermediate Recovery Stage

At this stage, your symptoms and general ability to operate in daily activities start to improve more noticeably. You might discover that you can continue some of your regular activities and go back to work or school with less anxiety. Along with starting to build new interactions with people, you might also start to adopt constructive coping strategies. Although it usually takes longer, it is feasible to build a network of people who are sympathetic to your situation with enough time and effort. As you continue to adjust, it will also entail discussing and coming up with coping mechanisms for new difficulties that crop up.

Stage 4: The Reconstruction Stage

When you have advanced significantly in your treatment and start to think about issues related to your future, you are in the final stage of recovery from PTSD. Trauma-related symptoms could still be present, but they are treated in consultation with a therapist in addition to creating new objectives.

13. CONCLUSIONS

In the intricate exploration of PTSD development and the myriad threads that weave through the tapestry of trauma, the conclusion brings us to a profound acknowledgment of the complexities involved in navigating this challenging terrain. The chapter describes journey of PTSD from the inception of trauma to the paths of recovery that requires a comprehensive understanding of the multifaceted factors, *viz.* biological, psychological, and environmental, at play and a personalized approach to treatment. The varied treatment approaches offer a diverse array of interventions, from traditional therapies to innovative technological solutions and holistic practices. These approaches stand as bridges that connect individuals to healing, emphasizing that the path to recovery is as unique as the individuals who traverse it. Thus, the journey from trauma to recovery is not a linear path but a dynamic and evolving process. The insights gained guide us in fostering environments where healing can flourish, and individuals can reclaim their lives with resilience, strength, and the assurance that they are not alone in their journey toward recovery.

REFERENCES

Acheson, D. T., Gresack, J. E., & Risbrough, V. B. (2012). Hippocampal dysfunction effects on context memory: Possible etiology for post-traumatic stress disorder. *Neuropharmacology*, 62(2), 674–685. DOI: 10.1016/j.neuropharm.2011.04.029 PMID: 21596050

Adamowska, S., Adamowski, T., Frydecka, D., & Kiejna, A. (2014). Diagnostic validity polish language version of the questionnaire MINI-KID (Mini international neuropsychiatry interview for children and adolescent). *Comprehensive Psychiatry*, 55(7), 1744–1750. DOI: 10.1016/j.comppsych.2014.05.019 PMID: 25023384

Agustini, E. N., & Matsuo, H. (2012). Children and Adolescents-Survivors of the 2004 Indian Ocean Tsunami: Prevalence of Long-Term PTSD and Coping Strategies. In Lopez, G. I. (Ed.), *Tsunami-Analysis of a Hazard-From Physical Interpretation to Human Impact*. IntechOpen Limited.

Ahmedani, B. K. (2011). Mental health stigma: society, individuals, and the profession. J Soc Work Values Ethics, 8(2), 4-1–4-16.

Alneyadi, M., Drissi, N., Almeqbaali, M., & Ouhbi, S. (2021). Biofeedback-based connected mental health interventions for anxiety: Systematic literature review. *JMIR mHealth and uHealth*, 9(4), e26038. DOI: 10.2196/26038 PMID: 33792548

Ambrosini, P. J. (2000). Historical development and present status of the schedule for affective disorders and schizophrenia for school-age children (K-SADS). *Journal of the American Academy of Child and Adolescent Psychiatry*, 39(1), 49–58. DOI: 10.1097/00004583-200001000-00016 PMID: 10638067

American Psychiatric Association. (1980). *Diagnostic and statistical manual of mental disorders* (3rd ed.). American Psychiatric Association.

American Psychiatric Association. (1994). *Diagnostic and Statistical Manual of Mental Disorders* (4th ed.).

American Psychiatric Association. (2004). *Practice guideline for the treatment of patient with acute stress disorder and posttraumatic stress disorder*. American Psychiatric Association.

American Psychiatric Association. (2009). *Practice guideline for the treatment of patients with acute stress disorder and posttraumatic stress disorder: guideline watch*. American Psychiatric Association.

American Psychiatric Association. (2013). *Diagnostic and statistical manual of mental disorders* (5th ed.). American Psychiatric Association.

American Psychological Association. (2017). Guideline Development Panel for the Treatment of PTSD in Adults. Clinical practice guideline for the treatment of Posttraumatic Stress Disorder (PTSD) in adults [Internet]. Available from: https://www.apa.org/ptsdguidelines/

Andreassen, O. A., Hindley, G. F. L., Frei, O., & Smeland, O. B. (2023). New insights from the last decade of research in psychiatric genetics: Discoveries, challenges and clinical implications. *World Psychiatry; Official Journal of the World Psychiatric Association (WPA)*, 22(1), 4–24. DOI: 10.1002/wps.21034 PMID: 36640404

Asmundson, G. J., & Taylor, S. (2009). PTSD diagnostic criteria: Understanding etiology and treatment. *The American Journal of Psychiatry*, 166(Suppl. 6), 726. DOI: 10.1176/appi.ajp.2009.08121799 PMID: 19487404

Australian Centre for Posttraumatic Mental Health. (2013). *Australian guidelines for the treatment of acute stress disorder and posttraumatic stress disorder*. Australian Centre for Posttraumatic Mental Health.

Averill, L. A., Purohit, P., Averill, C. L., Boesl, M. A., Krystal, J. H., & Abdallah, C. G. (2017). Glutamate dysregulation and glutamatergic therapeutics for PTSD: Evidence from human studies. *Neuroscience Letters*, 649, 147–155. DOI: 10.1016/j.neulet.2016.11.064 PMID: 27916636

Baldwin, D. S., Anderson, I. M., Nutt, D. J., Allgulander, C., Bandelow, B., den Boer, J. A., Christmas, D. M., Davies, S., Fineberg, N., Lidbetter, N., Malizia, A., McCrone, P., Nabarro, D., O'Neill, C., Scott, J., van der Wee, N., & Wittchen, H. U. (2014). Evidence-based pharmacological treatment of anxiety disorders, post-traumatic stress disorder and obsessive-compulsive disorder. A revision of the 2005 guidelines from the British Association for Psychopharmacology. *Journal of Psychopharmacology (Oxford, England)*, 28(5), 403–439. DOI: 10.1177/0269881114525674 PMID: 24713617

Barbui, C., Purgato, M., Abdulmalik, J., Acarturk, C., Eaton, J., Gastaldon, C., Gureje, O., Hanlon, C., Jordans, M., Lund, C., Nose, M., Ostuzzi, G., Papola, D., Tedeschi, F., Tol, W., Turrini, G., Patel, V., & Thornicroft, G. (2020). Efficacy of psychosocial interventions for mental health outcomes in low-income and middle-income countries: An umbrella review. *The Lancet. Psychiatry*, 7(2), 162–172. DOI: 10.1016/S2215-0366(19)30511-5 PMID: 31948935

Blank, A. A. (1985). The unconscious flashback to the war in Vietnam veterans: clinical mystery, legal defense, and community problem. In Sonnenberg, S. M., & Talbot, J. A. (Eds.), *The Trauma of War: Stress and Recovery in Vietnam Veterans* (pp. 293–308). American Psychiatric Association.

Bomyea, J., Risbrough, V., & Lang, A. J. (2012). A consideration of select pre-trauma factors as key vulnerabilities in PTSD. *Clinical Psychology Review*, 32(7), 630–641. DOI: 10.1016/j.cpr.2012.06.008 PMID: 22917742

Bourla, A., Mouchabac, S., Hage, W. E., & Ferreri, F. (2018). e-PTSD: an overview on how new technologies can improve prediction and assessment of posttraumatic stress disorder (PTSD). Eur J Psychotraumatol, 9(sup1), 1424448.

Boyd, J. E., Lanius, R. A., & McKinnon, M. C. (2018). Mindfulness-based treatments for posttraumatic stress disorder: A review of the treatment literature and neurobiological evidence. *Journal of Psychiatry & Neuroscience*, 43(1), 7–25. DOI: 10.1503/jpn.170021 PMID: 29252162

Bradley, R., Greene, J., Russ, E., Dutra, L., & Westen, D. (2005). A multidimensional meta-analysis of psychotherapy for PTSD. *The American Journal of Psychiatry*, 162(2), 214–227. DOI: 10.1176/appi.ajp.162.2.214 PMID: 15677582

Bradley, R., Greene, J., Russ, E., Dutra, L., & Westen, D. (2005). A multidimensional meta-analysis of psychotherapy for post traumatic stress disorder. *The American Journal of Psychiatry*, 162, 214–227. DOI: 10.1176/appi.ajp.162.2.214 PMID: 15677582

Bremner, J. D. (2006). Traumatic stress: Effects on the brain. *Dialogues in Clinical Neuroscience*, 8(4), 445–461. DOI: 10.31887/DCNS.2006.8.4/jbremner PMID: 17290802

Chalquist, C. (2009). A look at the ecotherapy research evidence. *Ecopsychology*, 1(2), 64–74. DOI: 10.1089/eco.2009.0003

Cheng, C., & Ebrahimi, O. V. (2023). Gamification: A Novel Approach to Mental Health Promotion. *Current Psychiatry Reports*, 25(11), 577–586. DOI: 10.1007/s11920-023-01453-5 PMID: 37801212

Chiba, T., Kanazawa, T., Koizumi, A., Ide, K., Taschereau-Dumouchel, V., Boku, S., Hishimoto, A., Shirakawa, M., Sora, I., Yoneda, H., & Kawato, M. (2019). Current status of neurofeedback for post-traumatic stress disorder: A systematic review and the possibility of decoded neurofeedback. *Frontiers in Human Neuroscience*, 13, 233. DOI: 10.3389/fnhum.2019.00233 PMID: 31379538

Christiansen, D. M., & Hansen, M. (2015). Accounting for sex differences in PTSD: A multi-variable mediation model. *European Journal of Psychotraumatology*, 6(1), 26068. DOI: 10.3402/ejpt.v6.26068 PMID: 25604705

Creamer, M., Bell, R., & Failla, S. (2003). Psychometric properties of the impact of event scale - Revised. *Behaviour Research and Therapy*, 41(12), 1489–1496. DOI: 10.1016/j.brat.2003.07.010 PMID: 14705607

Cruz, D., Lichten, M., Berg, K., & George, P. (2022). Developmental trauma: Conceptual framework, associated risks and comorbidities, and evaluation and treatment. *Frontiers in Psychiatry*, 13, 800687. DOI: 10.3389/fpsyt.2022.800687 PMID: 35935425

D'Souza, D. (1995). Post-traumatic stress disorder – A scar for life. *The British Journal of Clinical Practice*, 49(Suppl 6), 309–313. DOI: 10.1111/j.1742-1241.1995.tb09994.x PMID: 8554955

Davidson, J. R., Hughes, D., Blazer, D. G., & George, L. K. (1991). Post-traumatic stress disorder in the community: An epidemiological study. *Psychological Medicine*, 21(Suppl 3), 713–721. DOI: 10.1017/S0033291700022352 PMID: 1946860

Davidson, P., & Parker, K. (2001). Eye movement desensitization and reprocessing (EMDR): A meta-analysis. *Journal of Consulting and Clinical Psychology*, 69(2), 305–316. DOI: 10.1037/0022-006X.69.2.305 PMID: 11393607

Drissi, N., Ouhbi, S., Idtissi, M. A. J., & Ghogho, M. (2019). Gamification-based apps for PTSD: An analysis of functionality and characteristics. 2019 IEEE/ACS 16th International Conference on Computer Systems and Applications (AICCSA), Abu Dhabi, United Arab Emirates, pp. 1-6.

Ehret, M. (2019). Treatment of posttraumatic stress disorder: Focus on pharmacotherapy. *The Mental Health Clinician*, 9(6), 373–382. DOI: 10.9740/mhc.2019.11.373 PMID: 31857933

Foa, E., Rothbaum, B., & Furr, J. (2003). Augmenting exposure therapy with other CBT procedures. *Psychiatric Annals*, 33(1), 47–53. DOI: 10.3928/0048-5713-20030101-08

Foa, E. B., Keane, T., & Friedman, M. (2000). *Effective treatments for post traumatic stress disorder: practice guidelines from the International Society for Traumatic Stress Studies*. Guilford Press.

Ford, J. D., Grasso, D. J., Elhai, J. D., & Courtois, C. A. (2015). Social, cultural, and other diversity issues in the traumatic stress field. Posttraumatic Stress Disorder, 503-546.

Forman-Hoffman, V., Middleton, J. C., Feltner, C., Gaynes, B. N., Weber, R. P., Bann, C., Viswanathan, M., Lohr, K. N., Baker, C., & Green, J. (2018). Psychological and pharmacological treatments for adults with posttraumatic stress disorder: a systematic review update. AHRQ Comparative Effectiveness Reviews, Rockville (MD): Agency for Healthcare Research and Quality (US), Report No.: 18-EHC011-EFReport No.: 2018-SR-01. DOI: 10.23970/AHRQEPCCER207

Francati, V., Vermetten, E., & Bremner, J. D. (2007). Functional neuroimaging studies in posttraumatic stress disorder: Review of current methods and findings. *Depression and Anxiety*, 24(3), 202–218. DOI: 10.1002/da.20208 PMID: 16960853

Frank, D. L., Khorshid, L., Kiffer, J. F., Moravec, C. S., & McKee, M. G. (2010). Biofeedback in medicine: Who, when, why and how? *Mental Health in Family Medicine*, 7(2), 85–91. PMID: 22477926

Frijling, J. L. (2017). Preventing PTSD with oxytocin: Effects of oxytocin administration on fear neurocircuitry and PTSD symptom development in recently trauma-exposed individuals. *European Journal of Psychotraumatology*, 8(1), 1302652. DOI: 10.1080/20008198.2017.1302652 PMID: 28451068

Gersons, B. P. R., Carlier, I. V. E., Lamberts, R. D., & van der Kolk, B. (2000). A randomized clinical trial of brief eclectic psychotherapy in police officers with posttraumatic stress disorder. *Journal of Traumatic Stress*, 13(2), 333–437. DOI: 10.1023/A:1007793803627 PMID: 10838679

Green, A. (2011). Art and music therapy for trauma survivors. *Canadian Art Therapy Association Journal*, 24(2), 14–19. DOI: 10.1080/08322473.2011.11415547

Green, B. L. (1982). Assessing levels of psychological impairment following disaster: Consideration of actual and methodological dimensions. *The Journal of Nervous and Mental Disease*, 170(9), 544–552. DOI: 10.1097/00005053-198209000-00005 PMID: 7108503

Gros, D. F., Flanagan, J. C., Korte, K. J., Mills, A. C., Brady, K. T., & Back, S. E. (2016). Relations between social support, PTSD symptoms, and substance use in veterans. *Psychology of Addictive Behaviors*, 30(7), 764–770. DOI: 10.1037/adb0000205 PMID: 27786511

Hansford, M., & Jobson, L. (2021). Social support and self-construal as moderators of lifetime trauma exposure on posttraumatic stress disorder symptoms. *Traumatology*, 27(2), 205–214. DOI: 10.1037/trm0000281

Hembree, E. A., & Foa, E. B. (2000). Posttraumatic stress disorder: Psychological factors and psychosocial interventions. *The Journal of Clinical Psychiatry*, 61S, 33–39. PMID: 10795607

Herman, J. L. (1992). *Trauma and Recovery*. Basic Books.

Herman, J. P., McKlveen, J. M., Ghosal, S., Kopp, B., Wulsin, A., Makinson, R., Scheimann, J., & Myers, B. (2016). Regulation of the hypothalamic-pituitary-adrenocortical stress response. *Comprehensive Physiology*, 6(2), 603–621. DOI: 10.1002/cphy.c150015 PMID: 27065163

Hofmann, S. G., & Gomez, A. F. (2017). Mindfulness-based interventions for anxiety and depression. *The Psychiatric Clinics of North America*, 40(4), 739–749. DOI: 10.1016/j.psc.2017.08.008 PMID: 29080597

Horn, S. R., & Feder, A. (2018). Understanding resilience and preventing and treating PTSD. *Harvard Review of Psychiatry*, 26(3), 158–174. DOI: 10.1097/HRP.0000000000000194 PMID: 29734229

Hu, J., Feng, B., Zhu, Y., Wang, W., Xie, J., & Zheng, X. (2017). Gender Differences in PTSD: Susceptibility and Resilience. In Alvinus, A. (Ed.), *Gender Differences in Different Contexts*. IntechOpen Limited. DOI: 10.5772/65287

Jiang, S., Postovit, L., Cattaneo, A., Binder, E. B., & Aitchison, K. J. (2019). Epigenetic modifications in stress response genes associated with childhood trauma. *Frontiers in Psychiatry*, 10, 808. DOI: 10.3389/fpsyt.2019.00808 PMID: 31780969

Johansen, V. A., Milde, A. M., Nilsen, R. M., Breivik, K., Nordanger, D. Ø., Stormark, K. M., & Weisæth, L. (2022). The relationship between perceived social support and PTSD symptoms after exposure to physical assault: An 8 years longitudinal study. *Journal of Interpersonal Violence*, 37(9-10), NP7679–NP7706. DOI: 10.1177/0886260520970314 PMID: 33140665

Joschko, L., Palsdottir, A. M., Grahn, P., & Hinse, M. (2023). Nature-based therapy in individuals with mental health disorders, with a focus on mental well-being and connectedness to nature-a pilot study. *International Journal of Environmental Research and Public Health*, 20(3), 2167. DOI: 10.3390/ijerph20032167 PMID: 36767534

Karatzias, T., Murphy, P., Cloitre, M., Bisson, J., Roberts, N., Shevlin, M., Hyland, P., Maercker, A., Ben-Ezra, M., Coventry, P., Mason-Roberts, S., Bradley, A., & Hutton, P. (2019). Psychological interventions for ICD-11 complex PTSD symptoms: Systematic review and meta-analysis. *Psychological Medicine*, 49(11), 1761–1775. DOI: 10.1017/S0033291719000436 PMID: 30857567

Katzman, M. A., Bleau, P., Blier, P., Chokka, P., Kjernisted, K., & van Ameringen, M. (2014). Canadian clinical practice guidelines for the management of anxiety, posttraumatic stress and obsessive compulsive disorders. *BMC Psychiatry*, 14(Suppl 1), S1. DOI: 10.1186/1471-244X-14-S1-S1 PMID: 25081580

Kearns, M. C., Ressler, K. J., Zatzick, D., & Rothbaum, B. O. R. (2012). Early interventions for PTSD: A review. *Depression and Anxiety*, 29(10), 833–842. DOI: 10.1002/da.21997 PMID: 22941845

Kessler, R. C., Sonnega, A., Bromet, E., Hughes, M., & Nelson, C. B. (1995). Posttraumatic stress disorder in the national comorbidity survey. *Archives of General Psychiatry*, 52(12), 1048–1060. DOI: 10.1001/archpsyc.1995.03950240066012 PMID: 7492257

Kim, S. H., Schneider, S. M., Kravitz, L., Mermier, C., & Burge, M. R. (2013). Mind-body practices for posttraumatic stress disorder. *Journal of Investigative Medicine*, 61(5), 827–834. DOI: 10.2310/JIM.0b013e3182906862 PMID: 23609463

Kothgassner, O. D., Goreis, A., Kafka, J. X., Eickels, R. L. V., Plener, P. L., & Felnhofer, A. (2019). Virtual reality exposure therapy for posttraumatic stress disorder (PTSD): A meta-analysis. *European Journal of Psychotraumatology*, 10(1), 1654782. DOI: 10.1080/20008198.2019.1654782 PMID: 31489138

Kuhfuß, M., Maldei, T., Hetmanek, A., & Baumann, N. (2021). Somatic experiencing-effectiveness and key factors of a body-oriented trauma therapy: A scoping literature review. *European Journal of Psychotraumatology*, 12(1), 1929023. DOI: 10.1080/20008198.2021.1929023 PMID: 34290845

Kulka, R. A., Schlenger, W. E., Fairbank, J. A., Hough, R. L., Jordan, B. K., Marmar, C. R., & Weiss, D. S. (1990). *Trauma and the Vietnam War Generation: Report of findings from the National Vietnam Veterans Readjustment Study*. Brunner/Mazel.

La Greca, A. M., Taylor, C. J., & Herge, W. M. (2012). Traumatic stress disorders in children and adolescents. In Beck, J. G., & Sloan, D. M. (Eds.), *The Oxford Handbook of Traumatic Stress Disorders*. Oxford University Press. DOI: 10.1093/oxfordhb/9780195399066.013.0008

Laplaud, N., Perrochon, A., Gallou-Guyot, M., Moens, M., Goudman, L., David, R., Rigoard, P., & Billot, M. (2023). Management of post-traumatic stress disorder symptoms by yoga: An overview. *BMC Complementary Medicine and Therapies*, 23(1), 258. DOI: 10.1186/s12906-023-04074-w PMID: 37480017

Le Doux, J. E. (1996). *The emotional brain*. Simon and Schuster.

Lely, J. C. G., Smid, G. E., Jongedijk, R. A., Knipscheer, J. W., & Kleber, R. J. (2019). The effectiveness of narrative exposure therapy: A review, meta-analysis and meta-regression analysis. *European Journal of Psychotraumatology*, 10(1), 1550344. DOI: 10.1080/20008198.2018.1550344 PMID: 31007868

Li, J., & Sanchez-Garcia, R. (2023). Equine-assisted interventions for veterans with posttraumatic stress disorder: A systematic review. *Frontiers in Psychiatry*, 14, 1277338. DOI: 10.3389/fpsyt.2023.1277338 PMID: 38025432

Li, Y., Zhou, Y., Chen, X., Fan, F., Musa, G., & Hoven, C. (2020). Post-Traumatic Stress Disorder in Children and Adolescents: Some Recent Research Findings. In Lobera, I. J. (Ed.), *Pyschosomatic Medicine*. IntechOpen Limited. DOI: 10.5772/intechopen.92284

Litvin, S., Saunders, R., Maier, M. A., & Luttke, S. (2020). Gamification as an approach to improve resilience and reduce attrition in mobile mental health interventions: A randomized controlled trial. *PLoS One*, 15(9), e0237220. DOI: 10.1371/journal.pone.0237220 PMID: 32877425

Maercker, A., & Horn, A. B. (2013). A socio-interpersonal perspective on PTSD: The case for environments and interpersonal processes. *Clinical Psychology & Psychotherapy*, 20(6), 465–481. DOI: 10.1002/cpp.1805 PMID: 22730216

Malgaroli, M., & Schultebraucks, K. (2021). Artificial intelligence and posttraumatic stress disorder. *European Psychologist*, 25(4), 272–282. DOI: 10.1027/1016-9040/a000423

Mann, S. K., & Marwaha, R. (2023). Posttraumatic Stress Disorder. [Updated 2023 Jan 30] In *StatPearls* [Internet]. StatPearls Publishing., Available from https://www.ncbi.nlm.nih.gov/books/NBK559129/

Matheson, K., Asokumar, A., & Anisman, H. (2020). Resilience: Safety in the aftermath of traumatic stressor experiences. *Frontiers in Behavioral Neuroscience*, 14, 596919. DOI: 10.3389/fnbeh.2020.596919 PMID: 33408619

Mattson, E., James, L., & Engdahl, B. (2018). Personality factors and their impact on PTSD and post-traumatic growth is mediated by coping style among OIF/OEF veterans. *Military Medicine*, 183(9-10), e475–e480. DOI: 10.1093/milmed/usx201 PMID: 29590428

Mentis, A. F. A., Lee, D., & Roussos, P. (2023). Applications of artificial intelligence-machine learning for detection of stress: A critical overview. *Molecular Psychiatry*. Advance online publication. DOI: 10.1038/s41380-023-02047-6 PMID: 37020048

Mohamed, A., Touheed, S., Ahmed, M., Hor, M., & Fatima, S. (2022). The efficacy of psychedelic-assisted therapy in managing post-traumatic stress disorder (PTSD): A new frontier? *Cureus*, 14(10), e30919. DOI: 10.7759/cureus.30919 PMID: 36465766

Monson, C. M., Schnurr, P. P., Resick, P. A., Friedman, M. J., Young-Xu, Y., & Stevens, S. P. (2006). Cognitive processing therapy for veterans with military-related posttraumatic stress disorder. *Journal of Consulting and Clinical Psychology*, 74(5), 898–907. DOI: 10.1037/0022-006X.74.5.898 PMID: 17032094

Morland, L. A., Greene, C. J., Rosen, C. S., Kuhn, E., Hoffman, J., & Sloan, D. M. (2017). Telehealth and eHealth interventions for posttraumatic stress disorder. *Current Opinion in Psychology*, 14, 102–108. DOI: 10.1016/j.copsyc.2016.12.003 PMID: 28813306

Motlagh, H. (2010). Impact of event scale revised. *Journal of Physiotherapy*, 56(3), 203. DOI: 10.1016/S1836-9553(10)70029-1 PMID: 20795930

Mueller, J., Orth, U., Wang, J., & Maercker, A. (2009). Disclosure attitudes and social acknowledgement as predictors of posttraumatic stress disorder symptom severity in Chinese and German crime victims. *Canadian Journal of Psychiatry*, 54(8), 547–556. DOI: 10.1177/070674370905400807 PMID: 19726007

National Institute for Clinical Excellence. (2005). *The management of post-traumatic stress disorder in primary and secondary care*. NICE.

National Institute for Health and Care Excellence. (2018). Post-traumatic stress disorder (NICE Quality Standard NG116) [Internet]. Available from: https://www.nice.org.uk.guidance/ng116/evidenc.

Nickerson, A., Cloitre, M., Bryant, R. A., Schnyder, U., Morina, N., & Schick, M. (2016). The factor structure of complex posttraumatic stress disorder in traumatized refugees. *European Journal of Psychotraumatology*, 7(1), 33253. DOI: 10.3402/ejpt.v7.33253 PMID: 27989268

Nie, Y., Wen, L., Song, J., Wang, N., Huang, L., Gao, L., & Qu, M. (2022). Emerging trends in epigenetic and childhood trauma: Bibliometrics and visual analysis. *Frontiers in Psychiatry*, 13, 925273. DOI: 10.3389/fpsyt.2022.925273 PMID: 36458128

Nixon, R. D., Meiser-Stedman, R., Dalgleish, T., Yule, W., Clark, D. M., Perrin, S., & Smith, P. (2013). The Child PTSD Symptom Scale: An update and replication of its psychometric properties. *Psychological Assessment*, 25(3), 1025–1031. DOI: 10.1037/a0033324 PMID: 23815109

Norwitz, N. G., & Naidoo, U. (2021). Nutrition as metabolic treatment of anxiety. *Frontiers in Psychiatry*, 12, 598119. DOI: 10.3389/fpsyt.2021.598119 PMID: 33643090

Olff, M. (2017). Sex and gender differences in post-traumatic stress disorder: an update. Eur J Psychotraumatol, 8(sup4), 1351204.

Palomar-Ciria, N., & Bello, H. J. (2023). Equine-assisted therapy in post-traumatic stress disorder: A systematic review and meta-analysis. *Journal of Equine Veterinary Science*, 128, 104871. DOI: 10.1016/j.jevs.2023.104871 PMID: 37355148

Perrin, S., Meiser-Stedman, R., & Smith, P. (2005). The Children's Revised Impact of Event Scale (CRIES): Validity as a screening instrument for PTSD. *Behavioural and Cognitive Psychotherapy*, 33(4), 487–498. DOI: 10.1017/S1352465805002419

Prasad, A., Chaichi, A., Kelley, D. P., Francis, J., & Gartia, M. R. (2019). Current and future functional imaging techniques for post-traumatic stress disorder. *RSC Advances*, 9(42), 24568–24594. DOI: 10.1039/C9RA03562A PMID: 35527877

Pringle, G., Boddy, J., Slattery, M., & Harris, P. (2023). Adventure therapy for adolescents with complex trauma: A scoping review and analysis. *Journal of Experimental Education*, 46(4), 433–454.

Ragnhildstveit, A., Kaiyo, M., Snyder, M. B., Jackson, L. K., Lopez, A., Mayo, C., Miranda, A. C., August, R. J., Seli, P., Robison, R., & Averill, L. A. (2023). Cannabis-assisted psychotherapy for complex dissociative posttraumatic stress disorder: A case report. *Frontiers in Psychiatry*, 14, 1051542. DOI: 10.3389/fpsyt.2023.1051542 PMID: 36846226

Regier, D. A., Kuhl, E. A., & Kupfer, D. J. (2013). The DSM-5: Classification and criteria changes. *World Psychiatry; Official Journal of the World Psychiatric Association (WPA)*, 12(2), 92–98. DOI: 10.1002/wps.20050 PMID: 23737408

Ressler, K. J. (2010). Amygdala activity, fear, and anxiety: Modulation by stress. *Biological Psychiatry*, 67(12), 1117–1119. DOI: 10.1016/j.biopsych.2010.04.027 PMID: 20525501

Rivers, W. H. R. (1918). The repression of war experience. *Lancet*, 1, 73–177. PMID: 19980290

Sareen, J. (2014). Posttraumatic stress disorder in adults: Impact, comorbidity, risk factors, and treatment. *Canadian Journal of Psychiatry*, 59(9), 460–467. DOI: 10.1177/070674371405900902 PMID: 25565692

Sherin, J. E., & Nemeroff, C. B. (2011). Post-traumatic stress disorder: The neurobiological impact of psychological trauma. *Dialogues in Clinical Neuroscience*, 13(3), 263–278. DOI: 10.31887/DCNS.2011.13.2/jsherin PMID: 22034143

Skolariki, K., Vrahatis, A. G., Krokidis, M. G., Exarchos, T. P., & Vlamos, P. (2023). Assessing and modelling of post-traumatic stress disorder using molecular and functional biomarkers. *Biology (Basel)*, 12(8), 1050. DOI: 10.3390/biology12081050 PMID: 37626936

Smith, P., Perrin, S., Yule, W., & Rabe-Hesketh, S. (2001). War exposure and maternal reactions in the psychological adjustment of children from Bosnia-Hercegovina. *Journal of Child Psychology and Psychiatry, and Allied Disciplines*, 42(3), 395–404. DOI: 10.1111/1469-7610.00732 PMID: 11321208

Steinberg, A. M., Brymer, M. J., Decker, K. B., & Pynoos, R. S. (2004). The University of California at Los Angeles posttraumatic stress disorder reaction index. *Current Psychiatry Reports*, 6(2), 96–100. DOI: 10.1007/s11920-004-0048-2 PMID: 15038911

Summerfield, D. (2001). The invention of post-traumatic stress disorder and the social usefulness of a psychiatric category. *BMJ (Clinical Research Ed.)*, 322(7278), 95–98. DOI: 10.1136/bmj.322.7278.95 PMID: 11154627

Tang, X., Lin, S., Fang, D., Lin, B., Yao, L., Wang, L., Xu, Q., Lu, L., & Xu, N. (2023). Efficacy and underlying mechanisms of acupuncture therapy for PTSD: Evidence from animal and clinical studies. *Frontiers in Behavioral Neuroscience*, 17, 1163718. DOI: 10.3389/fnbeh.2023.1163718 PMID: 37200784

Tripathi, K. D. (2013). Essentials of Medical Pharmacology. Jaypee Brothers Medical Publishers (P) Ltd. Seventh edition.

Trundle, G., & Hutchinson, R. (2021). The phased model of adventure therapy: Trauma-focussed, low arousal, & positive behavioural support. *Journal of Adventure Education and Outdoor Learning*, 21(1), 82–92. DOI: 10.1080/14729679.2020.1736109

Turner, S., Beidel, D., & Frueh, B. (2005). Multicomponent behavioral treatment for chronic combat-related posttraumatic stress disorder: Trauma management therapy. *Behavior Modification*, 29(1), 39–69. DOI: 10.1177/0145445504270872 PMID: 15557478

van der Kolk, B. (2000a). Posttraumatic stress disorder and the nature of trauma. *Dialogues in Clinical Neuroscience*, 2(1), 7–22. DOI: 10.31887/DCNS.2000.2.1/bvdkolk PMID: 22034447 van der Kolk, B. (2000b). The diagnosis and treatment of Complex PTSD. In Yehuda, R. (Ed.), *Current Treatment of PTSD*. American Psychiatric Press.

van der Kolk, B. A., van der Hart, O., & Marmar, C. R. (1996). Dissociation and information processing in posttraumatic stress disorder. In van der Kolk, B. A., McFarlane, A. C., & Weisaeth, L. (Eds.), *Traumatic Stress: The Effects of Overwhelming Experience on Mind, Body and Society* (pp. 303–327). Guilford Press.

Veith, I. (1965). Hysteria. The history of a disease. Chicago University: Press of Chicago, pp. 1-301.

Veterans Health Administration, Department of Defense. (2017). *VA/DoD clinical practice guideline for the management of posttraumatic stress*. Veterans Health Administration, Department of Defense.

Chapter 5

Unveiling the Path to Healing: A Comprehensive Examination of Current PTSD Treatment Strategies

Ranjit Barua
https://orcid.org/0000-0003-2236-3876
OmDayal Group of Institutions, India

Sumit Bhowmik
OmDayal Group of Institutions, India

Sudipto Datta
https://orcid.org/0000-0003-2161-6878
Indian Institute of Science, Bangalore, India

ABSTRACT

Post-Traumatic Stress Disorder (PTSD) is a mental health condition that can develop after exposure to a traumatic event, such as combat, sexual assault, natural disasters, or serious accidents. Individuals with PTSD often experience intrusive memories, nightmares, hyperarousal, and avoidance of stimuli associated with the trauma, leading to significant distress and impairment in daily life. Treatment plans are tailored to individual needs, often combining various strategies for optimal effectiveness. Regular assessment and collaboration between mental health professionals and individuals with PTSD are essential to monitor progress and refine treatment approaches. As ongoing research continues to explore new avenues, the landscape of PTSD treatment evolves, offering hope for improved outcomes and enhanced quality of life for those affected by this challenging condition.

DOI: 10.4018/979-8-3693-2089-1.ch005

INTRODUCTION

Post-Traumatic Stress Disorder (PTSD) is a mental health condition that can develop after exposure to a traumatic event (Schrader et al., 2021). Various treatment strategies aim to alleviate symptoms and improve the overall well-being of individuals with PTSD (Kip et al., 2018). Current PTSD treatment strategies encompass a range of therapeutic approaches (Kaczkurkin et al., 2015). Psychotherapy, particularly Cognitive-Behavioral Therapy (CBT), is a cornerstone of treatment. CBT helps individuals identify and modify negative thought patterns and behaviors related to the trauma (Solan et al., 2019). Prolonged Exposure (PE) and Eye Movement Desensitization and Reprocessing (EMDR) are specialized forms of therapy that focus on gradually processing traumatic memories to reduce their emotional impact (Van Minnen et al., 2020). Medications, such as selective serotonin reuptake inhibitors (SSRIs) and serotonin-norepinephrine reuptake inhibitors (SNRIs), are commonly prescribed to alleviate symptoms like anxiety and depression associated with PTSD (Banzi et al., 2015). Mindfulness techniques, relaxation exercises, and complementary therapies, including yoga and acupuncture, are also employed to address physiological and psychological aspects of PTSD (Barua., 2024). Figure 1 shows the mechanisms of PTSD-related elevated inflammation. Advancements in technology have introduced innovative treatments like Virtual Reality (VR) therapy, which exposes individuals to controlled, immersive environments related to their trauma (Barua et al., 2022). Mobile apps and online programs offer accessible resources for self-help, guided meditation, and stress management. Group therapy and peer support play crucial roles, providing individuals with a sense of understanding and community (Schraderet al., 2021) (Barua et al., 2023). Additionally, service and support animals, such as therapy dogs, contribute to emotional well-being.

Figure 1. Mechanisms that contribute to PTSD's elevated inflammatory response. The pituitary, adrenal, and hypothalamic axis are all impacted by the immune system. The dotted line indicates inhibition based on the process, the red arrow shows the ultimate outcome of neuroinflammation, and the black arrow shows a sequence of sequential processes. NF-κB, nuclear factor-κB; adrenocorticotropin; AVP, arginine vasopressin; CRH, corticotropin-releasing hormone; GR, glucocorticoid receptor; IL, interleukin; TNF-α, tumor necrosis factor α; ACTH, NE, norepinephrine (Lee et al., 2022)

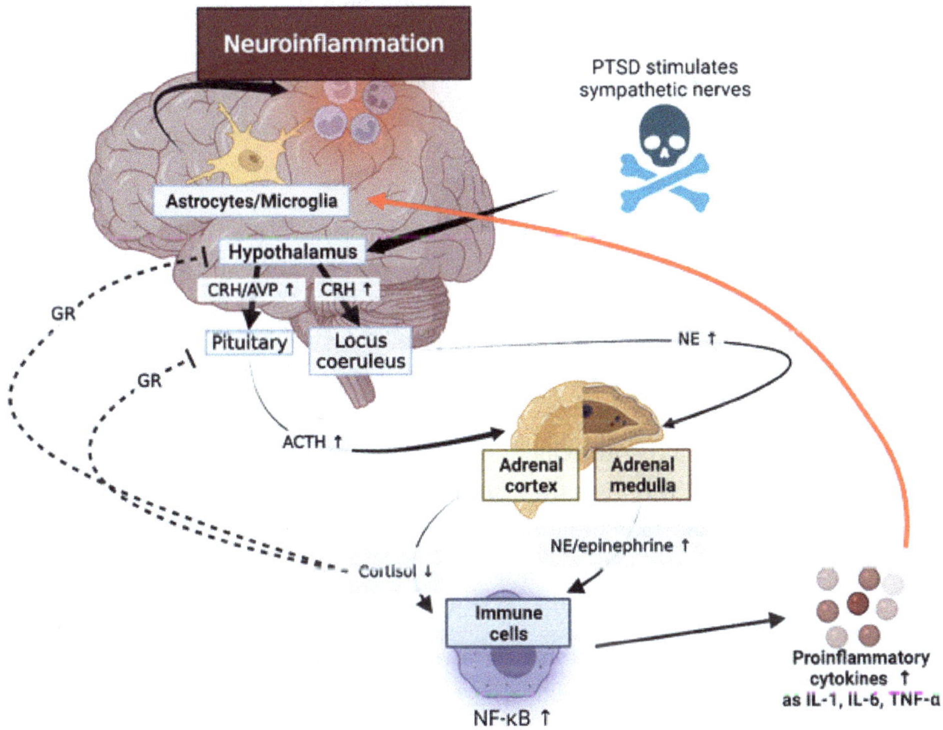

1. THE POST-TRAUMATIC STRESS DISORDER (PTSD) CONCEPTION IN CONTEMPORARY PERSPECTIVE

Post-Traumatic Stress Disorder (PTSD) is a complex and debilitating mental health condition that arises in response to exposure to traumatic events (Solan et al., 2019). Historically, the understanding of trauma-related conditions has evolved, leading to the conceptualization and recognition of PTSD as a distinct diagnosis (Kip et al., 2018). Figure 2 shows the influence of early emotional abuse, neglect, or care on the ability of the mind to cope with traumatic stress in later life, and Figure 3 shows the In a CT scan, the cortisol levels in the brains of healthy individuals and those suffering from PTSD are contrasted. This scan gauges the brain's inflammatory response to cortisol, a stress hormone that triggers the "fight or flight" response. Therefore observe, individuals with PTSD have elevated cortisol inflammation, which may have negative effects on brain function, reduced pain sensitivity, and emotional regulation. A person with post-traumatic stress disorder (PTSD) has cortisol strewn all over their brain. Because it is readily misled into an alerted state, this leads to the "fight or flight" panic reflex more frequently than a healthy brain. This essay explores the modern concept of PTSD, tracing its historical roots, diagnostic criteria, prevalence, etiology, and contemporary approaches to treatment.

2.1. Historical Context

Before the formal recognition of PTSD, historical accounts describe various manifestations of psychological distress in response to traumatic events. During World War I, the term "shell shock" was used to characterize symptoms experienced by soldiers exposed to the trauma of warfare. However, these early conceptualizations lacked the specificity and diagnostic criteria that define PTSD in the contemporary context (Zhou et al., 2021).The term "Post-Traumatic Stress Disorder" itself gained prominence with the introduction of the Diagnostic and Statistical Manual of Mental Disorders (DSM) in its third edition (DSM-III) in 1980. The inclusion of PTSD marked a pivotal moment in the recognition of trauma-related mental health conditions as distinct entities deserving specialized attention and treatment.

Figure 2. The effect of early emotional care, emotional abuse, or neglect on the way the mind reacts to catastrophic stress in later life (Jowf et al., 2022)

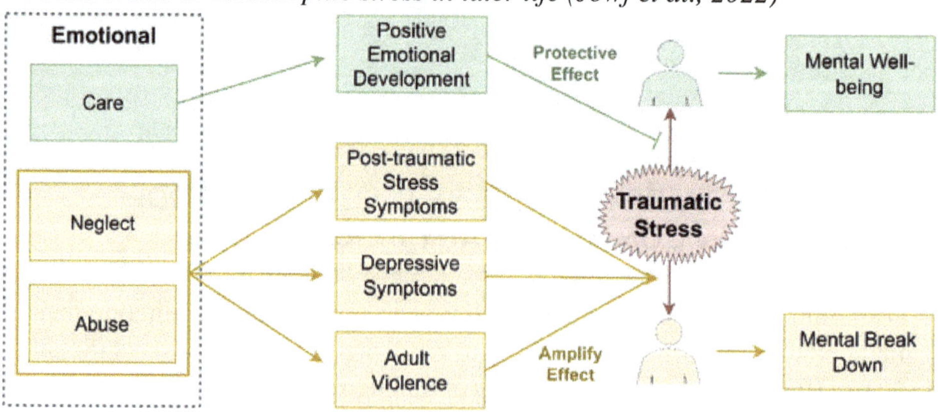

2.2. Diagnostic Criteria

The DSM-5, the latest edition of the diagnostic manual, outlines specific criteria for diagnosing PTSD (First et al., 2021). To meet the criteria, an individual must have been exposed to a traumatic event involving actual or threatened death, serious injury, or sexual violence (Du et al., 2022). The diagnostic criteria include the presence of intrusive symptoms (e.g., flashbacks, nightmares), avoidance of trauma-related stimuli, negative alterations in cognition and mood, and alterations in arousal and reactivity (van Ginneken et al., 2021) (Barua et al., 2024).

The diagnostic criteria acknowledge that the impact of trauma extends beyond the immediate aftermath, recognizing that symptoms may not manifest until months or even years after the traumatic event. Additionally, the DSM-5 introduced a significant shift by recognizing that trauma exposure can occur through indirect means, such as repeated exposure to distressing details of traumatic events (e.g., first responders, healthcare professionals) (First et al., 2021).

2.3. Prevalence

PTSD can affect individuals of all ages, ethnicities, and backgrounds, with a lifetime prevalence estimated to be around 6.8% in the general population according to the National Institute of Mental Health (NIMH) (Stein et al, 2020). Certain populations, such as military veterans, survivors of sexual assault, and individuals in high-risk professions, may be more vulnerable to developing PTSD (Purgato et al., 2023).

The prevalence of PTSD varies globally, influenced by factors such as sociocultural context, access to mental health care, and the nature of trauma exposure (Maihofer et al., 2022). Armed conflicts, natural disasters, and community violence are among the environmental stressors that can contribute to higher rates of PTSD in certain regions (First et al., 2021).

Figure 3. A comparison of the cortisol levels in a healthy brain and a PTSD sufferer's brain using a CT scan (PTSD & the Brain, n.d.)

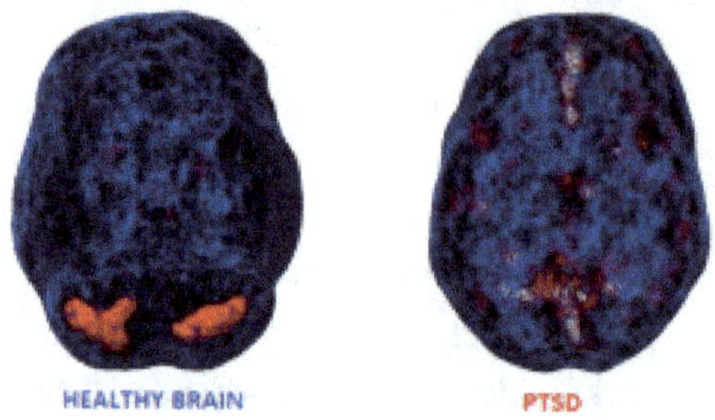

2.4. Etiology

The development of PTSD is multifaceted, involving a complex interplay of biological, psychological, and environmental factors (Wilson et al., 2019). Neurobiological research has identified alterations in brain regions involved in fear processing and emotion regulation among individuals with PTSD. Genetic factors may also contribute to susceptibility, influencing an individual's response to trauma (Solan et al., 2019). Psychological factors, such as prior trauma history, pre-existing mental health conditions, and coping mechanisms, play a role in the onset and maintenance of PTSD (Maihofer et al., 2022). The severity and nature of the traumatic event, as well as the level of perceived threat, contribute to the likelihood of developing PTSD (Figure 4). Trauma elements linked to PTSD (post-traumatic stress disorder). Gender, intelligence, genetic background, and a variety of neurological characteristics are pre-trauma parameters; the kind and length of trauma exposure are peri-trauma factors. Furthermore, social support networks, coping mechanisms, and cognitive flexibility are examples of post-trauma aspects.

Environmental factors, including social support and the availability of mental health resources, influence the trajectory of PTSD (Wilson et al., 2019). A lack of support or exposure to ongoing stressors can exacerbate symptoms, while a strong support network and access to effective interventions can contribute to resilience and recovery (Stein et al, 2020).

2.5. Contemporary Approaches to Treatment

The contemporary treatment landscape for PTSD is diverse, reflecting an understanding of the condition as complex and multifaceted. (Ben-Zion et al., 2020) Modern drug and clinical therapies for Post-Traumatic Stress Disorder (PTSD) encompass a variety of approaches aimed at alleviating symptoms and improving overall well-being (Barua et al., 2022). Both pharmacologic and psychotherapeutic interventions are commonly employed in the contemporary treatment of PTSD.

Figure 4. Post-traumatic stress disorder (PTSD) is linked to trauma factors (Nisar et al., 2020)

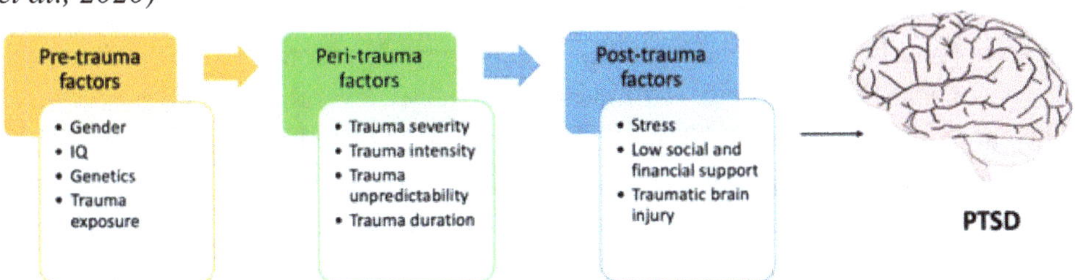

2.6. Pharmacologic Therapies:

a. **Selective Serotonin Reuptake Inhibitors (SSRIs):**
    - *Sertraline (Zoloft), Paroxetine (Paxil):* These SSRIs are FDA-approved for the treatment of PTSD. They help regulate serotonin levels, addressing symptoms such as anxiety, depression, and intrusive thoughts (Eissazade et al., 2023).

b. **Serotonin-Norepinephrine Reuptake Inhibitors (SNRIs):**
    - *Venlafaxine (Effexor XR):* SNRIs like venlafaxine may be prescribed to alleviate symptoms of PTSD by affecting both serotonin and norepinephrine levels (Song et al., 2020) (Arakawa et al., 2019).

c. **Prazosin:**
    - *Prazosin is an alpha-1 adrenergic receptor antagonist:* It is sometimes used off-label to address nightmares and sleep disturbances associated with PTSD by blocking the effects of norepinephrine (Mansbart et al., 2022).

d. **Atypical Antipsychotics:**
    - *Risperidone, Quetiapine:* In some cases, atypical antipsychotics may be prescribed to manage symptoms such as hyperarousal and irritability (Gómez Revuelta et al., 2020).

e. **Benzodiazepines:**
    - *Not typically recommended:* While benzodiazepines may provide short-term relief for anxiety symptoms, they are generally avoided in PTSD

treatment due to the risk of dependence and potential for worsening PTSD symptoms (Muzaale et al., 2020).

2.7. Non-pharmacologic Therapies:

Non-pharmacologic treatments for Post-Traumatic Stress Disorder (PTSD) focus on therapeutic interventions and techniques that do not involve medication. These approaches aim to address the psychological, emotional, and behavioral aspects of PTSD, promoting healing and recovery. Several evidence-based non-pharmacologic treatments have shown efficacy in helping individuals manage PTSD symptoms.Treatment approaches often involve a combination of psychotherapy, pharmacotherapy, and complementary interventions. Here are key components of contemporary PTSD treatment:

a. **Psychotherapy:**
    - *Cognitive-Behavioral Therapy (CBT):* CBT, particularly Prolonged Exposure (PE) and Cognitive Processing Therapy (CPT), is considered a first-line treatment for PTSD. PE involves gradual exposure to trauma-related memories and situations, while CPT focuses on identifying and challenging maladaptive thoughts (Taguchi et al., 2021).
    - *Prolonged Exposure (PE):* PE involves gradually confronting and processing traumatic memories and reminders to reduce anxiety and avoidance behaviors (Harned et al., 2021).
    - *Eye Movement Desensitization and Reprocessing (EMDR):* EMDR integrates bilateral stimulation with exposure to trauma-related memories, facilitating the processing and integration of distressing experiences (Winkler et al., 2021).

b. **Pharmacotherapy:**
    - *Antidepressants:* Selective serotonin reuptake inhibitors (SSRIs) (Eissazade et al., 2023), and serotonin-norepinephrine reuptake inhibitors (SNRIs) are commonly prescribed to alleviate symptoms of depression and anxiety associated with PTSD (Arakawa et al., 2019).

c. **Neurostimulation Therapies:**
    - *Transcranial Magnetic Stimulation (TMS):* TMS involves the application of magnetic fields to stimulate brain regions associated with PTSD symptoms. This emerging treatment shows promise in modulating neural activity (Siebner et al., 2022).

d. **Mindfulness and Yoga:**
    - *Mindfulness-Based Interventions:* Mindfulness practices, such as Mindfulness-Based Stress Reduction (MBSR), aim to enhance aware-

ness of the present moment, reducing symptoms of hyperarousal and improving overall well-being (Tian et al., 2022).

- *Yoga and Tai Chi:* Integrating physical activity with mindfulness, these practices promote relaxation and can be effective in reducing symptoms (Deuel et al., 2020).

e. **Virtual Reality (VR) Therapy:**
   - VR therapy allows individuals to confront and process traumatic memories in a controlled, virtual environment. This immersive approach has shown promise in the treatment of PTSD, particularly in addressing avoidance behaviors (Liu et al., 2022).

f. **Group Therapy and Peer Support:**
   - *Group Therapy:* Group sessions provide a supportive environment for individuals to share their experiences, reduce isolation, and learn coping strategies (Pries et al., 2022).
   - *Peer Support Programs:* Connecting with others who have experienced similar traumas fosters a sense of community and understanding.

g. **Complementary Therapies:**
   - *Art and Music Therapy:* These creative therapies provide alternative avenues for expression and can be beneficial in addressing emotional trauma (van Bruggen-Rufi et al., 2023).
   - *Equine-Assisted Therapy:* Interactions with horses in a therapeutic setting can help individuals build trust, improve emotional regulation, and enhance self-esteem (Arnon et al., 2022).

h. **Service and Support Animals:**
   - *Animal-Assisted Therapy:* The use of trained service animals or therapy animals, such as dogs, can provide emotional support and companionship, reducing symptoms of anxiety and depression (Chen et al., 2022).

2.7. Integrated Approaches:

Modern approaches often involve an integrated and personalized combination of pharmacologic and clinical therapies. The choice of treatment depends on individual preferences, the severity of symptoms, and the presence of co-occurring conditions (Nievergelt et al., 2019). Ongoing research continues to explore new therapeutic modalities and refine existing interventions to enhance the effectiveness of PTSD treatment in the modern clinical landscape. It is essential that treatment regimens are frequently customized, and a mix of these approaches may be employed according to the unique requirements and inclinations of any individual (Barua., 2024) (Jones et al., 2022) To find the most efficient and individualized treatment plan, mental health experts and people with PTSD must regularly assess each other. Strategies for treating PTSD are also evolving as a result of continued study and developments in the area.

2. IMPACT OF COVID 19 ON PTSD

The COVID-19 pandemic has left an indelible mark on global health and society (Barua et al., 2021), influencing various aspects of daily life(Taguchi et al., 2021) (Barua et al., 2024). Beyond its immediate impact on physical health, the pandemic has taken a toll on mental health, contributing to the development and exacerbation of mental health conditions, including Post-Traumatic Stress Disorder (PTSD) (Schrader et al., 2021). Understanding the complex interplay between COVID-19 and PTSD is crucial for addressing the mental health challenges arising from this unprecedented global crisis (Delanerolle et al., 2022).One significant factor contributing to the potential rise in PTSD cases is the direct exposure to trauma associated with COVID-19 (Barua et al., 2022). Individuals who have contracted the virus, experienced severe illness, or lost loved ones may be at an increased risk of developing PTSD. The sudden and overwhelming nature of the pandemic, coupled with the fear of severe health consequences, can lead to persistent distressing memories, nightmares, and hyperarousal symptoms characteristic of PTSD (Solan et al., 2019).

Healthcare workers and first responders, on the front lines of the pandemic, have faced unique challenges that elevate their risk of PTSD. The chronic stress, exhaustion, and exposure to traumatic events in healthcare settings can contribute to the development or exacerbation of PTSD symptoms. These essential workers often grapple with the emotional toll of witnessing significant suffering and loss, coupled with the constant fear of infection.The widespread fear of infection has been a pervasive element of the pandemic, impacting individuals across the globe. The uncertainty surrounding the virus, coupled with the potential severity of illness, has led to heightened anxiety and stress (First et al., 2021). The constant worry about personal health and the health of loved ones can contribute to PTSD symptoms, particularly in individuals with pre-existing mental health conditions or a history of trauma.Social isolation and disruptions to daily life have been key features of the pandemic, contributing to mental health challenges. Lockdowns, social distancing measures, and restrictions on social gatherings have led to increased loneliness and reduced opportunities for social support. The disruption of routines and the loss of familiar coping mechanisms can exacerbate feelings of anxiety and depression, potentially contributing to the development of PTSD (Solan et al., 2019).

Economic instability and uncertainty have added another layer of stress during the pandemic. Job losses, financial hardships, and economic downturns have created significant challenges for many individuals and families. The economic impact of the pandemic can contribute to the development of PTSD symptoms, especially for those facing housing insecurity, unemployment, and financial strain.The disruption of mental health services during the pandemic has been a significant concern (Solan et al., 2019).The strain on healthcare systems and shifting priorities have led to delays or limitations in accessing mental health care. This disruption may hinder individuals seeking help for PTSD symptoms, creating additional barriers to adequate support (Barua et al., 2021).Media exposure and information overload have played a role in shaping public perceptions and responses to the pandemic. Constant exposure to distressing news, images, and statistics can contribute to heightened anxiety and stress. For individuals with a history of trauma, media exposure may act as a trigger, potentially exacerbating PTSD symptoms.Efforts to address the mental health impact of COVID-19 include increased awareness, accessibility of mental health services, and support for individuals and communities facing heightened stressors. Long-term research is ongoing to understand the lasting effects of the pandemic on mental health and to develop effective interventions for those experiencing PTSD symptoms. The recognition of the intricate relationship between COVID-19 and PTSD is fundamental to implementing comprehensive strategies that address both the immediate and long-term mental health consequences of the pandemic.The COVID-19 pandemic has had significant and widespread effects on mental health, including an impact on the prevalence and exacerbation of Post-Traumatic Stress Disorder (PTSD) (Chauhan et al., 2021). Several factors associated with the pandemic contribute to the potential for increased PTSD symptoms among individuals. Here are some ways in which COVID-19 has impacted PTSD:

a. **Direct Exposure to Trauma:**
    - Individuals directly affected by COVID-19, such as those who contracted the virus, experienced severe illness, or lost loved ones, may be at risk of developing PTSD. The trauma associated with the virus's direct impact can lead to persistent distressing memories, nightmares, and hyperarousal symptoms.

b. **Healthcare Workers and First Responders:**
    - Healthcare workers and first responders have faced unprecedented challenges during the pandemic, including high patient volumes, limited resources, and the constant risk of exposure to the virus. This chronic stress and exposure to traumatic events can contribute to the development or exacerbation of PTSD symptoms among these essential workers.

c. **Fear of Infection:**
    - The pervasive fear of contracting the virus, especially during the early stages of the pandemic, has led to heightened anxiety and stress for

many individuals. Constant worry about personal health and the health of loved ones can contribute to PTSD symptoms, particularly in those with pre-existing mental health conditions (Banzi et al., 2015).

d. **Social Isolation and Disruption:**
   - Lockdowns, social distancing measures, and restrictions on social gatherings have led to increased social isolation and disruption of daily routines. These changes can contribute to feelings of loneliness, depression, and anxiety, which may further impact mental health and increase the risk of PTSD symptoms (Solan et al., 2019).

e. **Economic Uncertainty:**
   - Job losses, financial instability, and economic uncertainty have been widespread during the pandemic. Economic stressors can contribute to the development of PTSD symptoms, as individuals may face challenges related to housing, food insecurity, and overall financial well-being.

f. **Loss of Support Systems:**
   - Restrictions on travel and social interactions have limited access to traditional support systems. The loss of in-person social connections and reduced access to mental health resources may contribute to the exacerbation of PTSD symptoms, particularly for those who rely on social support.

g. **Disruption of Mental Health Services:**
   - The strain on healthcare systems and the shift in priorities during the pandemic have led to disruptions in mental health services. Delayed or limited access to therapy and psychiatric care may hinder individuals seeking help for PTSD symptoms.

h. **Media Exposure and Information Overload:**
   - Constant exposure to news and information about the pandemic, often depicting distressing scenes and statistics, can contribute to heightened anxiety and stress. Media exposure may act as a trigger for individuals with a history of trauma, potentially exacerbating PTSD symptoms.

It's crucial to remember that not everyone who experiences heightened stress and anxiety during a pandemic will go on to acquire post-traumatic stress disorder (PTSD). On the other hand, those who already have mental health issues, have experienced trauma in the past, or have other risk factors may be more susceptible to the psychological effects of COVID-19. The pandemic's effects on mental health are being addressed via raising awareness, making mental health services more accessible, and providing support to communities and people dealing with pressures. Long-term studies are being conducted to comprehend the pandemic's long-term consequences on mental health and to provide efficient therapies for people who are suffering from PTSD symptoms.

3. ARTIFICIAL INTELLIGENCE (AI) AND PTSD

Artificial Intelligence (AI) has the potential to offer valuable support in the diagnosis, treatment, and management of Post-Traumatic Stress Disorder (PTSD). While AI cannot replace human interaction and expertise, it can complement existing approaches by providing innovative solutions and improving accessibility to mental health care (Huckins et al., 2020). Here are several ways in which AI can contribute to helping individuals with PTSD:

a. **Early Detection and Screening:**
    - AI algorithms can analyze large datasets, including electronic health records and self-reported symptoms, to identify potential indicators of PTSD. Early detection allows for timely intervention and support, preventing the escalation of symptoms (Lee et al., 2021).

b. **Personalized Treatment Plans:**
    - AI can analyze diverse data sources, including genetic information, brain imaging, and behavioral patterns, to tailor treatment plans to individual needs. This personalized approach enhances the effectiveness of interventions by considering the unique characteristics and responses of each person (Masoumian Hosseini et al., 2023).

c. **Virtual Therapeutic Interventions:**
    - Virtual reality (VR) therapy, powered by AI, can create immersive environments to expose individuals to controlled and therapeutic scenarios related to their trauma. This allows for gradual desensitization and processing of traumatic memories in a safe and controlled setting.

d. **Chatbots for Support:**
    - AI-driven chatbots can provide immediate and accessible support for individuals with PTSD. These virtual assistants use natural language processing to engage in conversations, offer coping strategies, and provide information about mental health resources. Chatbots can be available 24/7, offering continuous support (Abd-Alrazaq et al., 2021).

c. **Predictive Analytics:**
    - AI algorithms can analyze patterns in patient data to predict potential triggers or times of increased vulnerability for individuals with PTSD. This information can be used to implement proactive interventions or preventive strategies.

f. **Monitoring Symptoms and Progress:**
    - Wearable devices and sensors equipped with AI capabilities can monitor physiological and behavioral markers associated with PTSD. This continuous monitoring provides real-time data, allowing healthcare providers to assess symptom severity and track progress over time.

g. **Natural Language Processing in Therapy Sessions:**
    - AI-driven natural language processing tools can assist therapists during sessions by analyzing verbal and written communication. This technology can help identify underlying patterns, emotions, and cognitive distortions, aiding therapists in tailoring their approach to individual patient needs.

h. **Data-Driven Research and Insights:**
    - AI facilitates the analysis of vast datasets to uncover patterns, correlations, and insights related to PTSD. This data-driven research can enhance our understanding of the disorder, inform the development of new interventions, and contribute to evidence-based practices.

i. **Mobile Apps for Self-Help:**
    - AI-powered mobile applications can provide self-help tools for individuals with PTSD. These apps may include features such as mood tracking, guided meditation, and stress management exercises, offering users practical ways to manage symptoms on their own.

j. **Enhanced Accessibility to Mental Health Resources:**
    - AI-powered platforms can improve accessibility to mental health resources by providing information, virtual support, and self-help tools. This is particularly beneficial for individuals who may face barriers to traditional mental health care, such as geographical constraints or stigma.

While AI holds promise in supporting individuals with PTSD, it is essential to approach its integration with caution, ensuring ethical considerations, data privacy, and the need for a human touch in mental health care are prioritized. Collaborative efforts between mental health professionals, researchers, and technologists are crucial to harness the full potential of AI in the service of improving outcomes for individuals affected by PTSD.

4. CONCLUSIONS

The modern concept of PTSD reflects a nuanced understanding of the impact of trauma on mental health. From its historical roots as "shell shock" to its formal recognition in the DSM-5, PTSD has evolved as a distinct diagnosis with specific diagnostic criteria. The prevalence of PTSD underscores the widespread impact of trauma, affecting diverse populations globally.

Etiological factors encompass a complex interplay of genetics, neurobiology, psychology, and environment. Treatment approaches have evolved to address the multifaceted nature of PTSD, emphasizing a combination of psychotherapeutic, pharmacological, and complementary interventions. Emerging technologies, such as virtual reality therapy, contribute to innovative treatment options.

While progress has been made in the understanding and treatment of PTSD, ongoing research and advocacy are essential to further refine diagnostic criteria, enhance treatment efficacy, and reduce barriers to accessing mental health care. The modern conceptualization of PTSD acknowledges the resilience of individuals in the face of trauma while recognizing the importance of comprehensive and individualized approaches to promote healing and recovery.

ACKNOWLEDGMENT

The authors would like to thank Mrs. NibeditaBardhan for language proof reading.

REFERENCES

Abd-Alrazaq, A. A., Alajlani, M., Ali, N., Denecke, K., Bewick, B. M., & Househ, M. (2021). Perceptions and Opinions of Patients About Mental Health Chatbots: Scoping Review. *Journal of Medical Internet Research*, 23(1), e17828. DOI: 10.2196/17828 PMID: 33439133

Arakawa, R., Stenkrona, P., Takano, A., Svensson, J., Andersson, M., Nag, S., Asami, Y., Hirano, Y., Halldin, C., & Lundberg, J. (2019). Venlafaxine ER Blocks the Norepinephrine Transporter in the Brain of Patients with Major Depressive Disorder: A PET Study Using [18F]FMeNER-D2. *The International Journal of Neuropsychopharmacology*, 22(4), 278–285. DOI: 10.1093/ijnp/pyz003 PMID: 30649319

Arnon, S., Fisher, P. W., Pickover, A., Lowell, A., Turner, J. B., Hilburn, A., Jacob-McVey, J., Malajian, B. E., Farber, D. G., Hamilton, J. F., Hamilton, A., Markowitz, J. C., & Neria, Y. (2020). Equine-Assisted Therapy for Veterans with PTSD: Manual Development and Preliminary Findings. *Military Medicine*, 185(5-6), e557–e564. DOI: 10.1093/milmed/usz444 PMID: 32034416

Banzi, R., Cusi, C., Randazzo, C., Sterzi, R., Tedesco, D., & Moja, L. (2015). Selective serotonin reuptake inhibitors (SSRIs) and serotonin-norepinephrine reuptake inhibitors (SNRIs) for the prevention of migraine in adults. *Cochrane Database of Systematic Reviews*, 4(4), CD002919. Advance online publication. DOI: 10.1002/14651858.CD002919.pub3 PMID: 25829028

Barua, R. (2024). An Investigation of AI Techniques for Detecting Kidney Stones in CT Scan Images Through Advanced Image Processing. In Sharma, A., Chanderwal, N., Tyagi, S., Upadhyay, P., & Tyagi, A. (Eds.), *Enhancing Medical Imaging with Emerging Technologies* (pp. 133–150). IGI Global., DOI: 10.4018/979-8-3693-5261-8.ch008

Barua, R. (2024). An In-Depth Exploration of AI and Humanoid Robotics' Role in Contemporary Healthcare. In V. Grover, B. Balusamy, N. M.K., V. Anand, & M. Milanova (Eds.), *Approaches to Human-Centered AI in Healthcare* (pp. 42-61). IGI Global. https://doi.org/DOI: 10.4018/979-8-3693-2238-3.ch003

Barua, R., & Bardhan, N. (2021). Downfall of the Sports Industry Due to the Pandemic of COVID-19. In Faganel, A., Rižnar, I., & Baruca, A. (Eds.), *Impacts and Implications for the Sports Industry in the Post-COVID-19 Era* (pp. 60–72). IGI Global., DOI: 10.4018/978-1-7998-6780-7.ch004

Barua, R., Das, D., & Biswas, N. (2024). Revolutionizing Drug Discovery With Artificial Intelligence: Enhancing Efficiency, Addressing Ethical Concerns, and Overcoming Limitations. In V. Grover, B. Balusamy, N. M.K., V. Anand, & M. Milanova (Eds.), *Approaches to Human-Centered AI in Healthcare* (pp. 62-85). IGI Global. https://doi.org/DOI: 10.4018/979-8-3693-2238-3.ch004

Barua, R., & Das, S. (2022). Improvements of Virtual and Augmented Reality for Advanced Treatments in Urology. In Coelho, L., Queirós, R., & Reis, S. (Eds.), *Emerging Advancements for Virtual and Augmented Reality in Healthcare* (pp. 117–131). IGI Global., DOI: 10.4018/978-1-7998-8371-5.ch008

Barua, R., Datta, P., & Chowdhury, A. R. (2022). The Impact of 3D Printing Technology on the COVID-19 Pandemic. In Moumtzoglou, A. (Ed.), *Quality of Healthcare in the Aftermath of the COVID-19 Pandemic* (pp. 135–154). IGI Global., DOI: 10.4018/978-1-7998-9198-7.ch008

Barua, R., & Datta, S. (2023). Artificial Intelligence in Modern Medical Science: A Promising Practice. In Rajest, S., Singh, B., Obaid, A. J., Regin, R., & Chinnusamy, K. (Eds.), *Recent Developments in Machine and Human Intelligence* (pp. 1–12). IGI Global., DOI: 10.4018/978-1-6684-9189-8.ch001

Barua, R., & Datta, S. (2024). An Extensive Evaluation of New Federated Learning Approaches for COVID-19 Identification. In Hassan, A., Prasad, V., Bhattacharya, P., Dutta, P., & Damaševičius, R. (Eds.), *Pioneering Smart Healthcare 5.0 with IoT, Federated Learning, and Cloud Security* (pp. 246–257). IGI Global., DOI: 10.4018/979-8-3693-2639-8.ch014

Barua, R., Datta, S., & Bardhan, N. (2021). Impact of Social Media on Pandemic COVID-19 Outbreak. In G. Sarı (Ed.), *Handbook of Research on Representing Health and Medicine in Modern Media* (pp. 422-435). IGI Global. https://doi.org/DOI: 10.4018/978-1-7998-6825-5.ch025

Barua, R., Datta, S., Datta, P., & Chowdhury, A. R. (2022). The Study of Traditional Medicine for the Treatment of COVID-19. In El Hiba, O., Radhakrishnan, J., Balzano, T., & Isbaine, F. (Eds.), *Handbook of Research on Pathophysiology and Strategies for the Management of COVID-19* (pp. 221–241). IGI Global., DOI: 10.4018/978-1-7998-8225-1.ch014

Barua, R., Datta, S., & Sarkar, A. (2023). Artificial Intelligence and Robotics-Based Minimally Invasive Surgery: Innovations and Future Perceptions. In Karthick, G., & Karupusamy, S. (Eds.), *Contemporary Applications of Data Fusion for Advanced Healthcare Informatics* (pp. 350–368). IGI Global., DOI: 10.4018/978-1-6684-8913-0.ch015

Ben-Zion, Z., Zeevi, Y., Keynan, N. J., Admon, R., Kozlovski, T., Sharon, H., Halpern, P., Liberzon, I., Shalev, A. Y., Benjamini, Y., & Hendler, T. (2020). Multi-domain potential biomarkers for post-traumatic stress disorder (PTSD) severity in recent trauma survivors. *Translational Psychiatry*, 10(1), 208. DOI: 10.1038/s41398-020-00898-z PMID: 32594097

Chauhan, N., Soni, S., & Jain, U. (2021). Optimizing testing regimes for the detection of COVID-19 in children and older adults. *Expert Review of Molecular Diagnostics*, 21(10), 999–1016. DOI: 10.1080/14737159.2021.1962708 PMID: 34324823

Chen, C. R., Hung, C. F., Lee, Y. W., Tseng, W. T., Chen, M. L., & Chen, T. T. (2022). Functional Outcomes in a Randomized Controlled Trial of Animal-Assisted Therapy on Middle-Aged and Older Adults with Schizophrenia. *International Journal of Environmental Research and Public Health*, 19(10), 6270. DOI: 10.3390/ijerph19106270 PMID: 35627807

Delanerolle, G., Zeng, Y., Shi, J. Q., Yeng, X., Goodison, W., Shetty, A., Shetty, S., Haque, N., Elliot, K., Ranaweera, S., Ramakrishnan, R., Raymont, V., Rathod, S., & Phiri, P. (2022). Mental health impact of the Middle East respiratory syndrome, SARS, and COVID-19: A comparative systematic review and meta-analysis. *World Journal of Psychiatry*, 12(5), 739–765. DOI: 10.5498/wjp.v12.i5.739 PMID: 35663292

Deuel, L. M., & Seeberger, L. C. (2020). Complementary Therapies in Parkinson Disease: A Review of Acupuncture, Tai Chi, Qi Gong, Yoga, and Cannabis. *Neurotherapeutics; the Journal of the American Society for Experimental NeuroTherapeutics*, 17(4), 1434–1455. DOI: 10.1007/s13311-020-00900-y PMID: 32785848

. Du, J., Diao, H., Zhou, X., Zhang, C., Chen, Y., Gao, Y., & Wang, Y. (2022). Post-traumatic stress disorder: a psychiatric disorder requiring urgent attention. *Medical review (2021), 2*(3), 219–243. https://doi.org/DOI: 10.1515/mr-2022-0012

Eissazade, N., Mosavari, H., Eghdami, S., Boroon, M., Ashrafi, F., & Shalbafan, M. (2023). Efficacy and safety of 5-hydroxytryptamine-3 (5-HT3) receptor antagonists in augmentation with selective serotonin reuptake inhibitors (SSRIs) in the treatment of moderate to severe obsessive-compulsive disorder: A systematic review and meta-analysis of randomized clinical trials. *Scientific Reports*, 13(1), 20837. DOI: 10.1038/s41598-023-47931-x PMID: 38012263

First, M. B., Gaebel, W., Maj, M., Stein, D. J., Kogan, C. S., Saunders, J. B., Poznyak, V. B., Gureje, O., Lewis-Fernández, R., Maercker, A., Brewin, C. R., Cloitre, M., Claudino, A., Pike, K. M., Baird, G., Skuse, D., Krueger, R. B., Briken, P., Burke, J. D., & Reed, G. M. (2021). An organization- and category-level comparison of diagnostic requirements for mental disorders in ICD-11 and DSM-5. *World Psychiatry; Official Journal of the World Psychiatric Association (WPA)*, 20(1), 34–51. DOI: 10.1002/wps.20825 PMID: 33432742

Gómez-Revuelta, M., Pelayo-Terán, J. M., Juncal-Ruiz, M., Vázquez-Bourgon, J., Suárez-Pinilla, P., Romero-Jiménez, R., Setién Suero, E., Ayesa-Arriola, R., & Crespo-Facorro, B. (2020). Antipsychotic Treatment Effectiveness in First Episode of Psychosis: PAFIP 3-Year Follow-Up Randomized Clinical Trials Comparing Haloperidol, Olanzapine, Risperidone, Aripiprazole, Quetiapine, and Ziprasidone. *The International Journal of Neuropsychopharmacology*, 23(4), 217–229. DOI: 10.1093/ijnp/pyaa004 PMID: 31974576

Harned, M. S., Schmidt, S. C., Korslund, K. E., & Gallop, R. J. (2021). Does Adding the Dialectical Behavior Therapy Prolonged Exposure (DBT PE) Protocol for PTSD to DBT Improve Outcomes in Public Mental Health Settings? A Pilot Nonrandomized Effectiveness Trial With Benchmarking. *Behavior Therapy*, 52(3), 639–655. DOI: 10.1016/j.beth.2020.08.003 PMID: 33990239

Huckins, L. M., Chatzinakos, C., Breen, M. S., Hartmann, J., Klengel, T., da Silva Almeida, A. C., Dobbyn, A., Girdhar, K., Hoffman, G. E., Klengel, C., Logue, M. W., Lori, A., Maihofer, A. X., Morrison, F. G., Nguyen, H. T., Park, Y., Ruderfer, D., Sloofman, L. G., van Rooij, S. J. H., & Daskalakis, N. P.PTSD Working Group of Psychiatric Genomics Consortium. (2020). Analysis of Genetically Regulated Gene Expression Identifies a Prefrontal PTSD Gene, SNRNP35, Specific to Military Cohorts. *Cell Reports*, 31(9), 107716. DOI: 10.1016/j.celrep.2020.107716 PMID: 32492425

Jones, K. A., Freijah, I., Carey, L., Carleton, R. N., Devenish-Meares, P., Dell, L., Rodrigues, S., Madden, K., Johnson, L., Hosseiny, F., & Phelps, A. J. (2022). Moral Injury, Chaplaincy and Mental Health Provider Approaches to Treatment: A Scoping Review. *Journal of Religion and Health*, 61(2), 1051–1094. DOI: 10.1007/s10943-022-01534-4 PMID: 35290554

Jowf, G. I. A., Ahmed, Z. T., An, N., Reijnders, R. A., Ambrosino, E., Rutten, B. P. F., De Nijs, L., & Eijssen, L. (2022, May 26). *A Public Health Perspective of Post-Traumatic Stress Disorder*. International Journal of Environmental Research and Public Health. *International Journal of Environmental Research and Public Health*, 19(11), 6474. Advance online publication. DOI: 10.3390/ijerph19116474 PMID: 35682057

Kaczkurkin, A. N., & Foa, E. B. (2015). Cognitive-behavioral therapy for anxiety disorders: An update on the empirical evidence. *Dialogues in Clinical Neuroscience*, 17(3), 337–346. DOI: 10.31887/DCNS.2015.17.3/akaczkurkin PMID: 26487814

Kip, K. E., & Diamond, D. M. (2018). Clinical, Empirical, and Theoretical Rationale for Selection of Accelerated Resolution Therapy for Treatment of Post-traumatic Stress Disorder in VA and DoD Facilities. *Military Medicine*, 183(9-10), e314–e321. DOI: 10.1093/milmed/usy027 PMID: 29635395

Lee, D. H., Lee, J., Hong, D. Y., Lee, E. C., Park, S. W., Lee, M. R., & Oh, J. S. (2022, April 20). Neuroinflammation in Post-Traumatic Stress Disorder. *Biomedicines*. Advance online publication. DOI: 10.3390/biomedicines10102518 PMID: 35625690

Lee, E. E., Torous, J., De Choudhury, M., Depp, C. A., Graham, S. A., Kim, H. C., Paulus, M. P., Krystal, J. H., & Jeste, D. V. (2021). Artificial Intelligence for Mental Health Care: Clinical Applications, Barriers, Facilitators, and Artificial Wisdom. *Biological Psychiatry: Cognitive Neuroscience and Neuroimaging*, 6(9), 856–864. DOI: 10.1016/j.bpsc.2021.02.001 PMID: 33571718

Liu, Z., Ren, L., Xiao, C., Zhang, K., & Demian, P. (2022). Virtual Reality Aided Therapy towards Health 4.0: A Two-Decade Bibliometric Analysis. *International Journal of Environmental Research and Public Health*, 19(3), 1525. DOI: 10.3390/ijerph19031525 PMID: 35162546

Maihofer, A. X., Choi, K. W., Coleman, J. R. I., Daskalakis, N. P., Denckla, C. A., Ketema, E., Morey, R. A., Polimanti, R., Ratanatharathorn, A., Torres, K., Wingo, A. P., Zai, C. C., Aiello, A. E., Almli, L. M., Amstadter, A. B., Andersen, S. B., Andreassen, O. A., Arbisi, P. A., Ashley-Koch, A. E., & Nievergelt, C. M. (2022). Enhancing Discovery of Genetic Variants for Posttraumatic Stress Disorder Through Integration of Quantitative Phenotypes and Trauma Exposure Information. *Biological Psychiatry*, 91(7), 626–636. DOI: 10.1016/j.biopsych.2021.09.020 PMID: 34865855

Mansbart, F., Kienberger, G., Sönnichsen, A., & Mann, E. (2022). Efficacy and safety of adrenergic alpha-1 receptor antagonists in older adults: A systematic review and meta-analysis supporting the development of recommendations to reduce potentially inappropriate prescribing. *BMC Geriatrics*, 22(1), 771. DOI: 10.1186/s12877-022-03415-7 PMID: 36171560

Masoumian Hosseini, M., Masoumian Hosseini, S. T., Qayumi, K., Ahmady, S., & Koohestani, H. R. (2023). The Aspects of Running Artificial Intelligence in Emergency Care; a Scoping Review. *Archives of Academic Emergency Medicine*, 11(1), e38. DOI: 10.22037/aaem.v11i1.1974 PMID: 37215232

Muzaale, A. D., Daubresse, M., Bae, S., Chu, N. M., Lentine, K. L., Segev, D. L., & McAdams-DeMarco, M. (2020). Benzodiazepines, Codispensed Opioids, and Mortality among Patients Initiating Long-Term In-Center Hemodialysis. *Clinical Journal of the American Society of Nephrology; CJASN*, 15(6), 794–804. DOI: 10.2215/CJN.13341019 PMID: 32457228

Nievergelt, C. M., Maihofer, A. X., Klengel, T., Atkinson, E. G., Chen, C. Y., Choi, K. W., Coleman, J. R. I., Dalvie, S., Duncan, L. E., Gelernter, J., Levey, D. F., Logue, M. W., Polimanti, R., Provost, A. C., Ratanatharathorn, A., Stein, M. B., Torres, K., Aiello, A. E., Almli, L. M., & Koenen, K. C. (2019). International meta-analysis of PTSD genome-wide association studies identifies sex- and ancestry-specific genetic risk loci. *Nature Communications*, 10(1), 4558. DOI: 10.1038/s41467-019-12576-w PMID: 31594949

Nisar, S., Bhat, A. A., Hashem, S., Syed, N., Yadav, S. K., Uddin, S., Fakhro, K., Bagga, P., Thompson, P. M., Reddy, R., Frenneaux, M., & Haris, M. (2020, June 24). Genetic and Neuroimaging Approaches to Understanding Post-Traumatic Stress Disorder. *International Journal of Molecular Sciences*, 21(12), 4503. Advance online publication. DOI: 10.3390/ijms21124503 PMID: 32599917

Pries, J., Niecke, A., Vetter, A., & Schultz-Venrath, U. (2022). More than one way home - Student raters' impressions of interventions and group processes in mentalisation based group psychotherapy and group analytic psychotherapy. *Research in Psychotherapy*, 25(3), 642. DOI: 10.4081/ripppo.2022.642 PMID: 36629759

PTSD & the Brain. (n.d.). PTSD. https://ptsdvietnam1.weebly.com/ptsd--the-brain.html

Purgato, M., Prina, E., Ceccarelli, C., Cadorin, C., Abdulmalik, J. O., Amaddeo, F., Arcari, L., Churchill, R., Jordans, M. J., Lund, C., Papola, D., Uphoff, E., van Ginneken, N., Tol, W. A., & Barbui, C. (2023). Primary-level and community worker interventions for the prevention of mental disorders and the promotion of well-being in low- and middle-income countries. *Cochrane Database of Systematic Reviews*, 10(10), CD014722. Advance online publication. DOI: 10.1002/14651858.CD014722.pub2 PMID: 37873968

Schrader, C., & Ross, A. (2021). A Review of PTSD and Current Treatment Strategies. *Missouri Medicine*, 118(6), 546–551. PMID: 34924624

Siebner, H. R., Funke, K., Aberra, A. S., Antal, A., Bestmann, S., Chen, R., Classen, J., Davare, M., Di Lazzaro, V., Fox, P. T., Hallett, M., Karabanov, A. N., Kesselheim, J., Beck, M. M., Koch, G., Liebetanz, D., Meunier, S., Miniussi, C., Paulus, W., & Ugawa, Y. (2022). Transcranial magnetic stimulation of the brain: What is stimulated? - A consensus and critical position paper. *Clinical Neurophysiology*, 140, 59–97. DOI: 10.1016/j.clinph.2022.04.022 PMID: 35738037

Sloan, D. M., Marx, B. P., Resick, P. A., Young-McCaughan, S., Dondanville, K. A., Mintz, J., Litz, B. T., & Peterson, A. L.STRONG STAR Consortium. (2019). Study design comparing written exposure therapy to cognitive processing therapy for PTSD among military service members: A noninferiority trial. *Contemporary Clinical Trials Communications*, 17, 100507. DOI: 10.1016/j.conctc.2019.100507 PMID: 31890987

Song, S. Y., Ko, Y. B., Kim, H., Lee, G. W., Yang, J. B., Chang, H. K., Kwak, S. M., Jung, J., Lee, S., Lee, S. Y., & Yoo, H. J. (2020). Effect of serotonin-norepinephrine reuptake inhibitors for patients with chemotherapy-induced painful peripheral neuropathy: A meta-analysis. *Medicine*, 99(1), e18653. DOI: 10.1097/MD.0000000000018653 PMID: 31895829

Stein, D. J., Harris, M. G., Vigo, D. V., Tat Chiu, W., Sampson, N., Alonso, J., Altwaijri, Y., Bunting, B., Caldas-de-Almeida, J. M., Cía, A., Ciutan, M., Degenhardt, L., Gureje, O., Karam, A., Karam, E. G., Lee, S., Medina-Mora, M. E., Mneimneh, Z., Navarro-Mateu, F., & Kessler, R. C.WHO World Mental Health Survey Collaborators. (2020). Perceived helpfulness of treatment for posttraumatic stress disorder: Findings from the World Mental Health Surveys. *Depression and Anxiety*, 37(10), 972–994. DOI: 10.1002/da.23076 PMID: 32667096

Taguchi, K., Numata, N., Takanashi, R., Takemura, R., Yoshida, T., Kutsuzawa, K., Yoshimura, K., & Shimizu, E. (2021). Integrated cognitive behavioral therapy for chronic pain: An open-labeled prospective single-arm trial. *Medicine*, 100(6), e23859. DOI: 10.1097/MD.0000000000023859 PMID: 33578513

Tian, X., Yi, L. J., Liang, C. S., Gu, L., Peng, C., Chen, G. H., & Jiménez-Herrera, M. F. (2022). The Impact of Mindfulness-Based Stress Reduction (MBSR) on Psychological Outcomes and Quality of Life in Patients With Lung Cancer: A Meta-Analysis. *Frontiers in Psychology*, 13, 901247. DOI: 10.3389/fpsyg.2022.901247 PMID: 35837627

van Ginneken, N., Chin, W. Y., Lim, Y. C., Ussif, A., Singh, R., Shahmalak, U., Purgato, M., Rojas-García, A., Uphoff, E., McMullen, S., Foss, H. S., Thapa Pachya, A., Rashidian, L., Borghesani, A., Henschke, N., Chong, L.-Y., & Lewin, S. (2021). Primary-level worker interventions for the care of people living with mental disorders and distress in low- and middle-income countries. *Cochrane Database of Systematic Reviews*, 8(8), CD009149. Advance online publication. DOI: 10.1002/14651858.CD009149.pub3 PMID: 34352116

Van Minnen, A., Voorendonk, E. M., Rozendaal, L., & de Jongh, A. (2020). Sequence matters: Combining Prolonged Exposure and EMDR therapy for PTSD. *Psychiatry Research*, 290, 113032. DOI: 10.1016/j.psychres.2020.113032 PMID: 32454314

vanBruggen-Rufi, M., & van der Stouw, G. (2023). Music Therapy and Korsakoff'sSyndrome: The State of the Art. *Journal of Clinical Medicine*, 12(14), 4609. DOI: 10.3390/jcm12144609 PMID: 37510723

Wilson, M. A., Liberzon, I., Lindsey, M. L., Lokshina, Y., Risbrough, V. B., Sah, R., Wood, S. K., Williamson, J. B., & Spinale, F. G. (2019). Common pathways and communication between the brain and heart: Connecting post-traumatic stress disorder and heart failure. *Stress (Amsterdam, Netherlands)*, 22(5), 530–547. DOI: 10.1080/10253890.2019.1621283 PMID: 31161843

Winkler, O., Dhaliwal, R., Greenshaw, A., O'Shea, K., Abba-Aji, A., Chima, C., Purdon, S. E., & Burback, L. (2021). Web Based Eye Movement Desensitization and Reprocessing for Adults With Suicidal Ideation: Protocol for a Randomized Controlled Trial. *JMIR Research Protocols*, 10(11), e30711. DOI: 10.2196/30711 PMID: 34734835

. Zhou, Y. G., Shang, Z. L., Zhang, F., Wu, L. L., Sun, L. N., Jia, Y. P., Yu, H. B., & Liu, W. Z. (2021). PTSD: Past, present and future implications for China. *Chinese journal of traumatology = Zhonghuachuangshangzazhi, 24*(4), 187–208. DOI: 10.1016/j.cjtee.2021.04.011

KEY TERMS AND DEFINITIONS

AI: Artificial Intelligence or AI refers to the simulation of human intelligence in machines programmed to think and act like humans. It encompasses a broad range of technologies, including machine learning, neural networks, and natural language processing. AI systems are designed to perform tasks that typically require human intelligence, such as problem-solving, learning, planning, and decision-making. These systems can analyze large amounts of data, recognize patterns, and make predictions or recommendations. AI is used in various industries and applications, from healthcare and finance to transportation and entertainment, aiming to enhance efficiency, accuracy, and automation.

Aging: Basically a natural and inevitable process of physical, psychological, and social changes over time. It involves a gradual decline in bodily functions, such as muscle strength, vision, and cognitive abilities. While aging is a universal experience, the rate and impact can vary widely among individuals due to genetics, lifestyle, and environmental factors. As people age, they may face challenges like chronic diseases, reduced mobility, and social isolation, but also opportunities for wisdom, experience, and personal growth. Proper healthcare, a balanced diet, regular exercise, and social engagement can help individuals age gracefully and maintain a good quality of life.

PTSD: Post-Traumatic Stress Disorder (PTSD) is a mental health condition that can develop after experiencing or witnessing a traumatic event. Symptoms often include flashbacks, nightmares, severe anxiety, and uncontrollable thoughts about the event. People with PTSD may also experience emotional numbness, detachment from others, and heightened reactions to triggers that remind them of the trauma. It can significantly impact daily life, relationships, and overall well-being. Treatment typically involves psychotherapy, medication, or a combination of both to help manage symptoms and improve quality of life.

Stress: Stress is the body's natural response to challenges or demands, often referred to as a "fight or flight" reaction. It's a physiological and psychological reaction to perceived threats or pressure. While short-term stress can be beneficial, motivating us to act or perform, prolonged or chronic stress can have negative effects on both mental and physical health. Common symptoms of stress include irritability, fatigue, difficulty concentrating, and changes in sleep or appetite. Managing stress is important for overall well-being and can be achieved through various techniques such as relaxation exercises, time management, and seeking social support.

Trauma: Trauma refers to a deeply distressing or disturbing experience that overwhelms an individual's ability to cope. It can result from a single event or a series of events that pose a threat to one's physical or emotional well-being. Traumatic experiences often lead to intense feelings of fear, helplessness, or horror. The impact of trauma can be long-lasting and may manifest in various ways, including flashbacks, nightmares, anxiety, and emotional numbness. Individuals may also develop post-traumatic stress disorder (PTSD) or other mental health conditions as a result. Treatment often involves therapy and support to help process the trauma and rebuild resilience.

Chapter 6
Exploring Diverse Interventions in Treating PTSD

Sameer Saharan
https://orcid.org/0000-0002-7487-6297
Mody University of Science and Technology, India

Sanchi Vardawat
Mody University of Science and Technology, India

Jitendra Binwal
Mody University of Science and Technology, India

Tilak Ram Chandrakar
Mody University of Science and Technology, India

Mridu Sharma
Mody University of Science and Technology, India

ABSTRACT

Post-Traumatic Stress Disorder (PTSD) poses significant challenges, demanding a multifaceted approach to treatment. This chapter aims to explore non-traditional interventions, psychoactive substances, and medical procedures in managing PTSD. From yoga, meditation, and exercise to the role of outdoor environments, psychoactive substances, and innovative medical procedures like stellate ganglion blocking and trans-cranial stimulation. This chapter delves into the efficacy, mechanisms, and potential integration of these interventions in PTSD treatment.

DOI: 10.4018/979-8-3693-2089-1.ch006

INTRODUCTION

Post-Traumatic Stress Disorder (PTSD) is a complex mental health condition triggered by experiencing or witnessing a traumatic event. It manifests in various ways and poses significant challenges in treatment due to its multifaceted nature. PTSD is characterized by a range of symptoms, including intrusive memories, flashbacks, nightmares, hypervigilance, avoidance of trauma-related stimuli, negative mood alterations, and alterations in arousal and reactivity (Cameron & Gusman, 2003). These symptoms often persist long after the traumatic event, affecting a person's daily life, relationships, and overall well-being. The treatment landscape for PTSD is diverse, acknowledging the intricate nature of the disorder. Evidence-based therapies like Cognitive Behavioral Therapy (CBT), particularly Prolonged Exposure (PE) and Cognitive Processing Therapy (CPT), have shown efficacy in addressing PTSD symptoms by helping individuals process traumatic memories and modify maladaptive beliefs (Datta et al., 2023; Kaidesoja et al., 2023). Eye Movement Desensitization and Reprocessing (EMDR) is another therapy involving guided eye movements that have demonstrated effectiveness in reducing PTSD symptoms (Carlini et al., 2023).

However, the complexity of PTSD lies in its variability among individuals and the co-occurrence of other mental health conditions such as depression, anxiety, substance abuse, and physical health issues (Khwaja et al., 2023). Comorbidities often complicate treatment strategies, requiring a comprehensive approach that considers both PTSD symptoms and associated conditions. Pharmacotherapy, involving antidepressants and other medications, is sometimes used to manage specific symptoms like depression or sleep disturbances (Carlini et al., 2023). However, medications might not target the core symptoms of PTSD directly and can have varying effects among individuals. Furthermore, cultural factors, socio-economic status, and access to care significantly influence the treatment journey for those with PTSD. Stigma, lack of awareness, and barriers to mental health services often hinder individuals from seeking or receiving adequate treatment.

In recent years, emerging approaches such as mindfulness-based therapies, yoga, animal-assisted therapies, and innovative technologies like virtual reality exposure therapy have shown promise in complementing traditional treatments (Morina et al., 2023). These approaches aim to address specific symptoms or provide alternative means of processing trauma. The complexities in treating PTSD emphasize the importance of personalized, holistic care. Integrative treatment models that combine various therapeutic modalities, peer support, family involvement, and community resources offer a comprehensive approach tailored to individual needs. Early intervention, education about coping strategies, and resilience-building programs can also play a crucial role in preventing the chronicity of PTSD (Niles et al., 2023).

Research into the neurobiology of trauma and the individualized responses to treatment continues to advance our understanding of PTSD. Identifying biomarkers, genetic predispositions, and neural pathways associated with PTSD may lead to more targeted and effective interventions in the future.

Challenges in traditional therapeutic approaches

Traditional therapeutic approaches, while foundational in mental health care, encounter several challenges that impact their effectiveness and relevance in contemporary practice (Sciarrino & Myers, 2023). These challenges span various dimensions, from limitations in treatment accessibility to evolving patient needs and therapeutic methodologies. One significant challenge is the issue of accessibility. Traditional therapies often require skilled professionals, which can lead to limited availability, especially in remote or underserved areas. This lack of access exacerbates disparities in mental health care, preventing many individuals from receiving timely and adequate treatment (Salome et al., 2023).

Additionally, the cost associated with traditional therapy sessions and the duration of treatment pose financial challenges for many individuals. Long-term therapy can be expensive, making it inaccessible for those with limited financial resources or inadequate insurance coverage (Metcalf et al., 2023). Another critical challenge lies in the evolving landscape of mental health needs. Traditional therapeutic models may not always align with the diverse needs of contemporary society (Salome et al., 2023). The rise of digital technology, changing social dynamics, and the increasing prevalence of certain mental health conditions demand more versatile and adaptable approaches. Moreover, traditional therapeutic methodologies might face limitations in addressing complex or multifaceted mental health issues. Conditions like personality disorders, complex trauma, or severe mood disorders often require more specialized and nuanced interventions that may not fit within the framework of traditional approaches (Metcalf et al., 2023; Salome et al., 2023).

Cultural competency and inclusivity are also challenges in traditional therapy. Therapists may not always have the cultural understanding or sensitivity needed to effectively connect with and address the needs of diverse populations. This can lead to a lack of trust or misunderstanding between the therapist and the client, hindering the therapeutic process. The one-size-fits-all approach in traditional therapies might not fully cater to individual differences and preferences. Some individuals may seek alternative or complementary therapies that align better with their beliefs, values, or cultural practices, which may not always be integrated into traditional therapeutic models (Ehrenstein & Shipa, 2023; Magill et al., 2023; Midyett, 2023).

Furthermore, the stigma associated with mental health care remains a significant barrier. Many individuals feel hesitant or ashamed to seek traditional therapy due to societal perceptions or fear of being labeled, impacting their willingness to engage in treatment. The ongoing advancements in neuroscience and the understanding of brain-behavior relationships have led to a deeper comprehension of mental health conditions (Merkley et al., 2023). However, traditional therapeutic approaches might not always incorporate the latest scientific findings or evidence-based practices, potentially limiting their effectiveness in addressing certain mental health concerns.

Addressing these challenges requires a multi-faceted approach. Integrating technology into therapy, such as telehealth and digital interventions, can enhance accessibility and reach for individuals in remote areas or those with mobility issues. Implementing sliding-scale fees or insurance coverage reforms can improve affordability and inclusivity. Culturally competent training for therapists, along with diversification and adaptation of therapeutic approaches, is crucial to cater to the diverse needs of clients. Collaboration between traditional therapeutic models and complementary approaches, such as mindfulness-based therapies, art therapy, or peer support networks, can broaden the spectrum of care and offer more tailored options.

The need for exploring alternative interventions and innovative treatments

Exploring alternative interventions and innovative treatments for PTSD is pivotal due to the limitations inherent in conventional approaches. PTSD, a complex mental health condition, manifests with a diverse array of symptoms and responses, making a one-size-fits-all approach ineffective. Conventional treatments, including psychotherapy and medications, although beneficial for many, might not adequately address the multifaceted nature of PTSD for all individuals. Thus, diversifying treatment options becomes imperative to offer a more comprehensive and personalized approach to care (Burback et al., 2023; Fu, 2023; Nie et al., 2023).

The complexity of PTSD symptoms often leads to treatment-resistant cases. Some individuals do not respond optimally to existing treatments or experience persistent symptoms despite therapeutic interventions. This phenomenon highlights the necessity for innovative and alternative approaches that can potentially address these gaps in care. By exploring novel methods, such as non-traditional therapies, emerging technologies, and innovative pharmacotherapies, there's an opportunity to create more effective interventions and improve therapeutic outcomes for those with PTSD (Fu, 2023; McGorrill, 2023).

Furthermore, emerging technologies present a new frontier in PTSD treatment. Innovations like virtual reality (VR) therapy, biofeedback systems, and neurofeedback techniques are gaining attention for their potential in desensitizing individuals to traumatic memories or environments and retraining neural responses. VR therapy, for instance, recreates trauma-related scenarios in a controlled environment, providing a safe space for individuals to process and confront their traumatic experiences under therapeutic guidance (Calcerano & Ciurlia, 2023; Choi et al., 2023; Kerr et al., 2023).

This exploration into alternative interventions and innovative treatments seeks to individualize care for those grappling with PTSD. Tailoring treatments to suit individual needs and symptom presentations is crucial, considering the diverse responses seen in individuals experiencing traumatic stress. By providing a spectrum of treatment options, healthcare providers can offer more personalized care, thereby improving therapeutic outcomes and quality of life for individuals navigating the challenges of PTSD. Moreover, bridging the gaps in existing treatments is a paramount goal of this exploration. While traditional approaches have shown efficacy, there's recognition of the need for more comprehensive treatments that address the multifaceted nature of PTSD (Moser et al., 2023). Innovative interventions aim to complement existing therapies, providing additional tools and strategies to manage symptoms that might not respond optimally to conventional treatments alone.

The research and development of alternative interventions and innovative treatments represent a commitment to advancing mental health care. It's a testament to the evolving understanding of PTSD and the determination to alleviate the burden of this condition on individuals and society. By continuously exploring and integrating new approaches, the field of PTSD treatment strives to evolve, offering hope and improved outcomes for those affected by this debilitating condition.

Non-Traditional Interventions:

Non-traditional interventions for PTSD encompass diverse approaches like mindfulness therapies, yoga, art therapy, and acupuncture. These holistic methods go beyond conventional talk therapy, focusing on mind-body connections to empower individuals and offer coping strategies. Their emphasis on holistic well-being aims to complement traditional treatments, providing diverse avenues for individuals grappling with PTSD to address their symptoms and enhance their overall quality of life (Wagner & Cáceres-Melillo, 2023).

Yoga and Meditation:

Mind-body practices, notably yoga and meditation, have emerged as promising adjunctive therapies in managing PTSD symptoms, offering a holistic approach to healing. These practices delve into the interconnectedness of mental and physical well-being, providing individuals coping with PTSD a path toward stress reduction, emotional regulation, and overall improved quality of life. The evidence supporting their efficacy lies in their ability to address various symptoms associated with PTSD, promoting resilience and fostering a sense of well-being (Laplaud et al., 2023).

Yoga, a centuries-old practice originating in ancient India, combines physical postures (asanas), breathing techniques (pranayama), and meditation (dhyana). The holistic nature of yoga aligns with the core aspects of PTSD recovery, emphasizing the mind-body connection and promoting self-awareness (Davis et al., 2023). Several studies highlight the benefits of yoga in managing PTSD symptoms. Research indicates that yoga interventions significantly reduce stress, anxiety, and depression, common comorbidities in PTSD. The practice of asanas and controlled breathing in yoga induces relaxation responses, alleviating physiological arousal associated with PTSD and promoting emotional regulation. Moreover, yoga fosters mindfulness, the state of being present and aware of one's thoughts and sensations without judgment. This aspect is particularly valuable in PTSD management, as individuals often experience intrusive thoughts and heightened reactivity. Through mindfulness techniques incorporated in yoga, individuals learn to cultivate a non-judgmental awareness of their experiences, enhancing their capacity to manage distressing symptoms (Davis et al., 2023; Haller et al., 2023; Laplaud et al., 2023).

Meditation, a central component of many mind-body practices, encompasses various techniques such as mindfulness meditation, loving-kindness meditation, and transcendental meditation. These techniques center on cultivating a focused and calm state of mind, fostering relaxation and mental clarity. Studies exploring meditation's impact on PTSD report promising results. Meditation practices have been associated with reduced symptoms of hyperarousal, intrusive thoughts, and avoidance behaviors characteristic of PTSD. Additionally, meditation's neurobiological effects on the brain, particularly in areas associated with stress response and emotional regulation, contribute to its therapeutic benefits for individuals with PTSD (Jamil et al., 2023).

The evidence supporting the benefits of yoga and meditation in PTSD management underscores their role in enhancing overall well-being. Beyond symptom reduction, these practices offer individuals a sense of empowerment, self-regulation, and improved coping mechanisms. The holistic approach of mind-body practices aligns with the complex nature of PTSD, addressing not only the symptoms but also fostering resilience and promoting a sense of control over one's experiences. Furthermore, the accessibility and adaptability of yoga and meditation make them suitable for various populations affected by PTSD. These practices can be tailored to accommodate individuals' physical abilities, making them inclusive and adaptable in diverse therapeutic settings (Burback et al., 2023; Freese, 2023; Jamil et al., 2023; Wahid et al., 2023).

The exploration of mind-body practices like yoga and meditation unveils their profound potential in managing PTSD symptoms. The evidence supporting their efficacy in stress reduction, emotional regulation, and overall well-being highlights their role as valuable adjunctive therapies in the comprehensive treatment of PTSD. Integrating these practices into therapeutic interventions offers a holistic approach to healing, empowering individuals to navigate the challenges of PTSD and fostering a path toward recovery and improved quality of life.

Exercise and Physical Activity:

Physical activity and exercise have emerged as influential components in managing PTSD symptoms, offering a multifaceted approach to alleviating the challenges individuals face post-trauma. The impact of physical activity extends beyond mere fitness, playing a significant role in reducing anxiety, enhancing mood, improving sleep quality, and contributing to overall well-being. Understanding the profound effects of exercise on PTSD symptoms sheds light on its therapeutic potential and underscores its importance as a complementary intervention in the holistic management of this condition. Numerous studies have explored the benefits of physical activity in mitigating PTSD symptoms. Engaging in regular exercise has been linked to reductions in anxiety and stress levels, both of which are prevalent in individuals with PTSD. The release of endorphins during physical exertion contributes to an improved mood and a sense of well-being, counteracting the negative emotional impact of trauma (Bryant et al., 2023; Crombie et al., 2023; Ha et al., 2023; Shafia et al., 2023; Vancampfort et al., 2023).

Moreover, the relationship between physical activity and sleep quality is noteworthy in the context of PTSD management. Sleep disturbances are common among those with PTSD and can exacerbate other symptoms. Regular exercise has been associated with better sleep patterns, including increased sleep duration and improved sleep quality. The regulation of circadian rhythms and the reduction of stress hormones through exercise play a pivotal role in fostering restorative sleep. The neurobiological effects of exercise further elucidate its impact on PTSD symptoms. Physical activity stimulates the production of neurotransmitters like serotonin and dopamine, which are integral in regulating mood and emotions (Vancampfort et al., 2023). Additionally, exercise has been found to positively affect brain-derived neurotrophic factor (BDNF), promoting neuroplasticity and potentially mitigating some of the neurological changes associated with PTSD (Zhang et al., 2023).

The type and intensity of exercise also play a role in its therapeutic impact on PTSD. While any form of physical activity can be beneficial, aerobic exercises like running, swimming, or cycling have shown pronounced effects on mental health. These exercises elevate heart rate and oxygen consumption, facilitating the release of endorphins and promoting relaxation responses in the body. Furthermore, the social aspect of certain physical activities contributes to their therapeutic value. Group exercises or team sports foster social support networks, reducing feelings of isolation and enhancing social connections, which are essential in mitigating PTSD symptoms (Vancampfort et al., 2023).

The role of physical activity in PTSD management extends beyond symptom reduction. Its integration into daily routines promotes a sense of structure, routine, and discipline, empowering individuals and offering a sense of control over their lives. Engaging in regular exercise serves as a coping mechanism, providing a healthy outlet for managing stress and anxiety associated with PTSD (Neuner, 2023; Vancampfort et al., 2023).

Importantly, the accessibility and adaptability of exercise make it a versatile intervention for individuals with varying levels of physical fitness or mobility limitations. Tailoring exercise programs to individuals' abilities ensures inclusivity and encourages sustained engagement in physical activity as part of a holistic approach to PTSD recovery.

Outdoor Environments and Nature Therapy:

The therapeutic benefits of nature exposure in PTSD treatment offer a profound avenue for healing, encompassing ecotherapy, wilderness therapy, and the rejuvenating effects of natural environments on mental health. The healing potential of nature on individuals coping with PTSD lies in its ability to provide solace, restoration, and a sense of connection, offering a complementary approach to traditional treatments.

Ecotherapy, also known as nature therapy or green therapy, utilizes the healing properties of nature to improve mental well-being. It involves structured activities or interventions in natural settings, aiming to promote relaxation, reduce stress, and foster emotional healing. Nature's inherent ability to induce calmness and reduce physiological arousal becomes instrumental in managing PTSD symptoms. Research has demonstrated the therapeutic benefits of ecotherapy in mitigating PTSD symptoms. Immersion in natural environments has been linked to reductions in anxiety, depression, and rumination—common features of PTSD. The tranquility and sensory stimulation offered by natural surroundings contribute to a sense of emotional balance and well-being (Putri et al., 2023).

Wilderness therapy, a form of adventure-based therapy, employs outdoor activities in natural settings to facilitate personal growth and emotional healing. This immersive approach involves engaging in activities like hiking, camping, or outdoor challenges, promoting self-reflection, resilience, and coping skills development among individuals with PTSD.The healing effects of natural environments on mental health are attributed to various factors. Biophilia, the innate human connection to nature, underscores the comfort and solace individuals find in natural settings. Exposure to green spaces, forests, or open landscapes triggers positive emotional responses and encourages a sense of connectedness to the natural world, fostering emotional restoration and reducing symptoms of stress and anxiety (Pringle et al., 2023; Vella et al., 2023).

Moreover, the sensory experiences offered by nature, such as the sight of greenery, the sound of flowing water, or the touch of natural elements, stimulate relaxation responses in the body. This sensory engagement promotes mindfulness and a sense of grounding, diverting attention away from intrusive thoughts or hyperarousal associated with PTSD.The concept of attention restoration theory further supports the therapeutic benefits of nature exposure. Natural environments, characterized by soft fascination and effortless attention, provide a respite from cognitive overload and promote mental restoration (Bell et al., 2023; Fisher, 2023). This restoration of cognitive resources contributes to stress reduction and emotional well-being, offering individuals with PTSD a reprieve from the overwhelming effects of trauma

Additionally, the role of nature in promoting physical activity cannot be overlooked. Engaging in outdoor activities amidst natural settings encourages exercise, which has been shown to have positive effects on mental health, including symptom reduction in PTSD. The combination of physical activity and nature exposure creates a synergistic effect, enhancing the therapeutic outcomes for individuals with PTSD (Putri et al., 2023).

The accessibility and inclusivity of nature-based therapies make them valuable in PTSD treatment. These interventions can be tailored to accommodate individuals with diverse abilities, providing opportunities for everyone to benefit from the healing aspects of nature. The therapeutic benefits of nature exposure in PTSD treatment offer a complementary and holistic approach to conventional therapies. Ecotherapy, wilderness therapy, and the healing effects of natural environments on mental health present opportunities for emotional healing, stress reduction, and promoting overall well-being. Embracing nature as a therapeutic tool empowers individuals coping with PTSD, offering them solace, restoration, and a pathway toward recovery and improved quality of life.

Psychoactive Substances

Cannabinoids and PTSD:

Post-Traumatic Stress Disorder (PTSD) is a complex mental health condition that can develop after experiencing or witnessing a traumatic event. Traditional treatments, including psychotherapy and medications, may not always provide adequate relief for all individuals with PTSD. As a result, alternative approaches, including cannabinoids, have been increasingly studied for their potential therapeutic benefits (Wolfgang & Hoge, 2023).

Cannabinoids are chemical compounds found in the cannabis plant. CBD and THC are the two primary cannabinoids that have garnered significant attention for their potential effects on mental health (Nacasch et al., 2023).

1. Cannabidiol (CBD): CBD is a non-psychoactive compound, meaning it does not produce the "high" associated with cannabis. It has gained attention for its purported anxiolytic (anxiety-reducing) and neuroprotective properties (Martínez et al., 2020).
2. Tetrahydrocannabinol (THC): THC is the psychoactive compound in cannabis responsible for the euphoric sensation. It's known for its potential impact on modulating fear responses and emotional memory (Martínez et al., 2020).

Potential Benefits of Cannabinoids in PTSD Management

1. CBD in PTSD Treatment: Research suggests that CBD may offer several potential benefits for individuals with PTSD:
   a. Anxiety Reduction: CBD, a non-psychoactive component of Cannabis, has garnered attention for its anxiolytic properties. Research indicates that CBD interacts with the endocannabinoid system, influencing serotonin receptors and other neurotransmitter systems involved in stress response. Preclinical and clinical studies suggest that CBD may modulate fear-related memories and reduce anxiety levels in individuals with PTSD. By regulating emotional responses and blunting hyperarousal, CBD showcases potential in mitigating core symptoms of PTSD without inducing the psychoactive effects associated with THC (Martínez et al., 2020; Nacasch et al., 2023).
   b. Sleep Improvement: Sleep disturbances, including insomnia and nightmares, are prevalent among individuals with PTSD. CBD has shown promise in addressing these sleep-related issues. Studies suggest that CBD may influence sleep architecture by prolonging the time spent in deep sleep and reducing REM sleep, thereby potentially alleviating nightmares. Its anxiolytic and calming effects might contribute to improved sleep quality, offering individuals with PTSD better restorative sleep (Martínez et al., 2020; Nacasch et al., 2023).
   c. Fear Extinction: One hallmark of PTSD is the persistence of distressing memories related to the traumatic event. CBD's impact on fear extinction processes is of particular interest. Preclinical studies propose that CBD may facilitate fear extinction and disrupt the reconsolidation of traumatic memories. By modulating the retrieval and consolidation of aversive memories,

CBD could aid in the modification of traumatic experiences, potentially reducing the emotional intensity and intrusiveness of these memories.

d. Mood Regulation and Antidepressant Effects: The co-occurrence of depression with PTSD presents a significant challenge in treatment. CBD's interaction with serotonin receptors and its influence on neural circuits associated with mood regulation suggest potential antidepressant effects. By enhancing serotonin signaling and regulating emotional responses, CBD might alleviate depressive symptoms commonly observed in individuals with PTSD, contributing to improved overall emotional well-being.
e. Neuroprotective and Anti-Inflammatory Properties: Chronic stress and trauma exposure in PTSD can lead to neurobiological alterations and inflammatory responses in the brain. CBD's anti-inflammatory and antioxidant properties have garnered interest for their potential neuroprotective effects. By reducing neuroinflammation and oxidative stress, CBD might mitigate neurobiological changes associated with PTSD. This could potentially protect against neuronal damage and promote neural repair mechanisms, offering prospects for addressing the neurobiological consequences of trauma (Martínez et al., 2020).

2. THC and Trauma Processing: Tetrahydrocannabinol (THC), the psychoactive component of Cannabis, interacts with the endocannabinoid system, influencing various neural pathways involved in emotion, memory, and stress response. Research suggests that THC might modulate fear responses and emotional memory, potentially affecting trauma processing in individuals with PTSD (Martínez et al., 2020; Zabik et al., 2022).
   a. Impact on Fear Responses: THC's influence on fear responses is a subject of interest in PTSD research. Preclinical studies propose that THC, acting on cannabinoid receptors in the brain, might affect fear extinction processes. By altering the retrieval and consolidation of fear-related memories, THC could potentially influence the emotional intensity and persistence of traumatic memories. This modulation of fear responses might contribute to attenuating the emotional impact of traumatic experiences, aiding in trauma processing.
   b. Emotional Memory Modulation: Emotional memory consolidation and retrieval are intricate processes affected by THC. Studies indicate that THC's interaction with the endocannabinoid system may impact the encoding and retrieval of emotional memories. In the context of PTSD, where intrusive and distressing memories are a hallmark, THC's effects on memory modulation raise intriguing possibilities. It might alter the salience and emotional valence of traumatic memories, potentially diminishing their emotional grip and intrusive nature.

c. Potential Assisting Role in Trauma Processing: The potential role of THC in trauma processing revolves around its impact on fear responses and emotional memory. By modifying the emotional charge and retrieval of traumatic memories, THC could theoretically facilitate exposure-based therapies, aiding individuals in confronting and processing traumatic experiences. This assistance in trauma processing might offer relief from intrusive thoughts and emotional distress associated with PTSD.
d. Concerns Surrounding THC Use in Vulnerable Populations: Despite its potential benefits, several concerns arise regarding THC's use, particularly in vulnerable populations:
   i. Psychoactive Effects: THC's psychoactive properties can induce alterations in perception, cognition, and mood. These effects might exacerbate anxiety or induce paranoia, potentially intensifying distress in individuals already grappling with PTSD symptoms.
   ii. Dependency Risks: Chronic THC use raises concerns about dependency and addiction. Vulnerable populations, including those with PTSD, may be at heightened risk of developing substance use disorders, warranting caution in THC administration.
   iii. Psychiatric Vulnerability: Individuals with a predisposition to psychotic disorders or other psychiatric vulnerabilities might be susceptible to exacerbation of symptoms due to THC's psychoactive effects. The potential for adverse psychological reactions necessitates careful consideration in vulnerable populations.
   iv. Regulatory Constraints: The legal status and regulatory restrictions on THC pose challenges in its clinical application. Differing legal frameworks and accessibility issues further complicate its use in therapeutic contexts.

Challenges and Limitations

1. Regulatory Restrictions: Legal and regulatory constraints limit comprehensive research on cannabinoids, resulting in fragmented studies and varied access to cannabis-related products.
2. Variations in CBD/THC Ratios: The optimal ratio of CBD to THC for PTSD treatment remains unclear. Different ratios may yield varying effects, making standardized treatment challenging.
3. Dosing and Long-Term Effects: Determining optimal doses and understanding the long-term effects of cannabinoids on individuals with PTSD require further exploration. Variability in individual responses adds complexity to establishing standardized treatment protocols.

4. Efficacy Variability: Individual responses to cannabinoids can vary significantly. Factors such as genetics, metabolism, and the severity of PTSD symptoms contribute to diverse responses among patients. This variability makes it challenging to predict the efficacy of cannabinoids and necessitates personalized treatment approaches.
5. Psychiatric Comorbidities: PTSD commonly coexists with other psychiatric conditions such as depression, anxiety disorders, or substance use disorders. Understanding how cannabinoids interact with these comorbidities and their potential impact on symptom exacerbation or remission is complex and requires comprehensive evaluation.
6. Potential Adverse Effects: While CBD is generally considered well-tolerated, it can cause side effects such as fatigue, diarrhea, or changes in appetite in some individuals. THC, with its psychoactive properties, presents additional concerns, including cognitive impairment, increased heart rate, and potential exacerbation of psychiatric symptoms.
7. Dependency Risks: Chronic use of THC raises concerns about dependency and addiction. Individuals with PTSD, already susceptible to maladaptive coping mechanisms, may face an increased risk of developing dependency on cannabinoids for symptom management.
8. Interactions with Medications: Cannabinoids, particularly CBD, can interact with other medications, impacting their metabolism and efficacy. Understanding potential drug interactions and their implications for individuals with PTSD who might be on multiple medications is crucial for safe and effective treatment.
9. Lack of Longitudinal Studies: Long-term studies examining the sustained effects, safety profiles, and tolerability of cannabinoids in individuals with PTSD are scarce. Longitudinal research is essential to assess the persistence of therapeutic effects and monitor potential adverse effects over time.
10. Stigma and Perception: Societal perceptions and stigma surrounding cannabis use, especially in medical contexts, can influence patient acceptance and healthcare provider willingness to prescribe cannabinoids as part of PTSD treatment. Addressing misconceptions and educating stakeholders is vital to fostering acceptance and understanding of cannabinoid therapies.
11. Standardization and Quality Control: Ensuring the consistency and quality of cannabinoid-based products remains a challenge. Standardization of formulations, quality control measures, and establishing reliable sources of cannabinoids are crucial for reliable and reproducible treatment outcomes.

Navigating these challenges and limitations requires a multidisciplinary approach, involving rigorous research, regulatory adaptations, healthcare provider education, and ethical considerations. Addressing these complexities is pivotal in advancing the understanding and application of cannabinoids within comprehensive PTSD treatment frameworks (Perez Alday et al., 2023; Punski-Hoogervorst et al., 2023; Zaccari et al., 2022).

Considerations for Cannabinoid Use in PTSD Treatment

1. Individual Responses: Responses to cannabinoids can vary significantly among individuals. Factors like genetic predispositions, dosage, and method of consumption influence their efficacy and tolerability.
2. Ethical and Legal Concerns: Ethical considerations, especially regarding vulnerable populations such as veterans or individuals with comorbid conditions, necessitate cautious and regulated use of cannabinoids in PTSD treatment.
3. Evidence-Based Practice: The integration of cannabinoids into PTSD treatment should be grounded in evidence-based practice. Robust clinical trials and empirical data supporting their efficacy, safety, and optimal dosing are essential before widespread adoption in clinical settings.
4. Patient Education and Informed Consent: Comprehensive education of patients regarding the potential benefits, risks, and uncertainties surrounding cannabinoid therapies is crucial. Ensuring informed consent involves transparent discussions about psychoactive effects, possible side effects, and long-term implications.
5. Healthcare Provider Training: Healthcare providers require adequate training and education to understand the complexities of cannabinoid therapies. Knowledge about cannabinoid pharmacology, interactions, and their role in PTSD management is crucial for safe and effective use.
6. Monitoring and Surveillance: Regular monitoring and surveillance are necessary when incorporating cannabinoids into PTSD treatment. Assessing treatment responses, tracking potential side effects, and adjusting dosages based on individual tolerability are integral to ensuring patient safety and treatment optimization.
7. Comprehensive Care Approach: Cannabinoids should be considered as part of a comprehensive care approach rather than standalone treatment. Integrating them into multidisciplinary treatment plans, including psychotherapy, behavioral interventions, and social support, enhances their potential efficacy and addresses the multifaceted nature of PTSD.
8. Regulatory Compliance and Quality Control: Adherence to regulatory standards and quality control measures is paramount. Ensuring that cannabinoid-based products comply with established regulations and undergo rigorous quality testing is crucial for their safe and reliable use in clinical settings.
9. Continual Research and Adaptation: Given the evolving nature of cannabinoid research, continual evaluation and adaptation of treatment protocols based on emerging evidence are essential. Keeping abreast of new findings and refining

treatment strategies based on scientific advancements is critical for optimizing patient outcomes.

10. Potential for Drug Interactions: Considering the potential for interactions between cannabinoids and other medications used in PTSD treatment is crucial. Healthcare providers must carefully assess and manage potential drug interactions to prevent adverse effects or reduced efficacy of concomitant medications.
11. Patient Population and Vulnerability: Tailoring cannabinoid treatments while considering the diverse needs and vulnerabilities of specific patient populations is essential. For instance, elderly patients or those with compromised health may have different tolerances or susceptibilities that require individualized approaches.
12. Long-term Safety and Efficacy: Long-term studies evaluating the safety and efficacy of cannabinoids in individuals with PTSD are essential. Assessing the sustained benefits and potential risks over extended periods is critical for establishing their role in long-term PTSD management.

Integrating these considerations into clinical practice facilitates a cautious, evidence-based, and patient-centered approach to the use of cannabinoids in PTSD treatment, ensuring maximal benefit while minimizing potential risks and uncertainties (Martínez et al., 2020; Nacasch et al., 2023; Pacitto et al., 2022; Wolfgang & Hoge, 2023).

Research Gaps and Future Directions

1. Need for Rigorous Studies: While promising, existing research on cannabinoids and PTSD is limited and fragmented. Rigorous randomized controlled trials (RCTs) are imperative to comprehensively understand their efficacy, safety, and long-term impacts on PTSD symptomatology.
2. Informed and Regulated Use: Comprehensive research outcomes will inform regulations and treatment guidelines, facilitating safe and informed use of cannabinoids as adjunctive therapies within comprehensive PTSD treatment frameworks.
3. Subtypes of PTSD: Research should investigate whether specific subtypes of PTSD (e.g., dissociative subtype, complex PTSD) exhibit differential responses to cannabinoids. Understanding how cannabinoids impact distinct symptom clusters or presentations of PTSD could guide personalized treatment approaches.
4. Optimal Formulations and Delivery Methods: Further exploration is needed to determine the most effective formulations (e.g., oils, capsules, tinctures) and delivery methods (oral, sublingual, inhalation) for delivering cannabinoids in

PTSD treatment. Evaluating bioavailability, absorption rates, and sustained effects is crucial for optimizing therapeutic outcomes.

5. Long-term Follow-up Studies: Longitudinal studies tracking individuals over extended periods are essential to assess the sustained effects, tolerability, and potential risks associated with prolonged cannabinoid use in PTSD management. Understanding any delayed or cumulative effects is critical for long-term treatment planning.
6. Biomarkers and Predictors of Treatment Response: Identifying biomarkers or genetic predictors that indicate responsiveness to cannabinoid therapy in PTSD could revolutionize treatment personalization. Research focusing on identifying potential markers for treatment response or adverse reactions is imperative.
7. Mechanistic Studies: Deeper exploration into the underlying mechanisms of action of cannabinoids in PTSD is necessary. Investigating their effects on neurobiological pathways, such as the endocannabinoid system, stress response systems, and neural circuitry implicated in PTSD, can offer insights into their therapeutic potential.
8. Comparative Effectiveness Studies: Comparative studies comparing cannabinoids with existing pharmacotherapies or psychotherapies for PTSD are essential. Comparative effectiveness research would elucidate the relative efficacy, safety profiles, and cost-effectiveness of cannabinoids in relation to standard treatments.
9. Special Populations and Vulnerabilities: Research focusing on specific populations, such as pediatric or geriatric patients, individuals with treatment-resistant PTSD, or those with significant comorbidities, is vital. Tailoring cannabinoid interventions to address unique vulnerabilities and needs within these populations requires dedicated investigation.
10. Economic and Health Outcomes Research: Evaluating the economic impact and cost-effectiveness of integrating cannabinoids into PTSD treatment is crucial. Studying health outcomes, including quality of life measures, functional improvements, and reduction in healthcare utilization, provides a comprehensive understanding of their overall benefits.
11. Psycho-Social Implications: Exploring the psycho-social implications of using cannabinoids in PTSD treatment is essential. Understanding patient perspectives, stigma reduction, and the impact on social and occupational functioning is crucial for holistic treatment planning.
12. Safety and Tolerance in Vulnerable Groups: Comprehensive studies examining the safety and tolerability of cannabinoids in vulnerable groups, such as pregnant individuals, individuals with substance use history, or those with medical comorbidities, are necessary to ensure safe and responsible use.

Addressing these research gaps will contribute to a more nuanced understanding of cannabinoids' role in PTSD treatment, providing evidence-based guidelines and optimizing their integration within comprehensive therapeutic approaches.

Psychedelics and Emerging Research

Psychedelics have re-emerged as a focal point in psychiatric research, especially concerning mental health conditions like depression, anxiety, and PTSD. This resurgence in interest stems from a growing body of research exploring the therapeutic potential of substances like psilocybin (found in "magic mushrooms"), LSD, MDMA (commonly known as ecstasy), and ayahuasca (Lowe et al., 2022). The exploration of psychedelics, including substances like LSD, psilocybin, MDMA, and ayahuasca, gained traction in the mid-20th century for their potential in psychiatric treatment. However, due to cultural shifts and regulatory crackdowns in the late 1960s, these substances were classified as illegal drugs, stalling research for decades. Recently, a paradigm shift in societal attitudes and regulatory frameworks has sparked a renaissance in psychedelic research, opening doors for studying their potential therapeutic benefits.

Therapeutic Applications of Psychedelics

1. Psilocybin and Depression: Psilocybin, found in certain mushrooms, has shown promise in treating depression. Clinical trials exploring psilocybin-assisted therapy have reported significant reductions in depressive symptoms, potentially due to the substance's ability to induce transformative experiences and alter negative thought patterns (N.-X. Li et al., 2022).
2. LSD and Anxiety Disorders: Early investigations into LSD-assisted therapy suggest its potential in alleviating anxiety in specific individuals. The substance's profound effects on consciousness may facilitate emotional processing and enable individuals to confront deeply rooted anxieties (Lowe et al., 2022).
3. MDMA and PTSD: MDMA, commonly known as ecstasy, has garnered attention for its potential in treating PTSD. Clinical trials using MDMA-assisted therapy have demonstrated promising results in reducing PTSD symptoms, fostering trust, and facilitating emotional processing of traumatic memories (Lowe et al., 2022).
4. Ayahuasca and Healing: Ayahuasca, a traditional Amazonian brew, is being explored for its potential therapeutic effects. Research suggests that the substance might aid in addiction treatment, alleviate depression, and promote spiritual healing experiences (Lowe et al., 2022).

Mechanisms and Challenges in Research

1. Neurobiological Effects: Psychedelics interact with serotonin receptors in the brain, leading to altered states of consciousness and increased neural plasticity. These substances might induce changes in brain connectivity that underlie their therapeutic effects.
2. Regulatory Constraints: Despite promising findings, regulatory hurdles pose significant challenges. The classification of psychedelics as Schedule I substances restricts research opportunities, funding, and access to these substances for clinical studies.
3. Safety and Ethical Considerations: Ensuring the safety of participants in psychedelic studies is paramount. Managing potential adverse effects and ethical considerations, especially in vulnerable populations, requires stringent protocols and comprehensive monitoring.
4. Psychological Effects and Therapeutic Mechanisms: Understanding the psychological effects of psychedelics, such as ego dissolution, altered perception of time, and mystical experiences, is crucial. Investigating how these experiences correlate with therapeutic outcomes and their impact on psychological well-being and introspection is an important research avenue.
5. Dosage and Treatment Protocols: Determining optimal dosages and treatment protocols for different psychedelic substances in therapeutic settings is a critical research focus. Studying the effects of various dosing regimens, frequency of administration, and their impact on sustained therapeutic benefits is necessary for treatment standardization.
6. Psychedelic-Assisted Psychotherapy Models: Research should focus on developing and refining models of psychedelic-assisted psychotherapy. Investigating the integration of psychedelics with psychotherapeutic approaches, setting, preparation, and integration sessions is essential for maximizing therapeutic outcomes.
7. Neuroimaging and Biomarkers: Utilizing neuroimaging techniques and identifying potential biomarkers to elucidate the neurobiological underpinnings of psychedelic effects is imperative. Studying changes in brain activity, functional connectivity, and identifying potential biomarkers associated with therapeutic responses could enhance understanding and treatment optimization.
8. Risk of Misuse and Abuse Potential: Investigating the potential for misuse or abuse of psychedelics in therapeutic settings is crucial. Understanding the risk factors for misuse, addiction potential, and strategies for preventing misuse while ensuring access for therapeutic purposes is a significant research challenge.

9. Cross-Cultural Considerations: Recognizing and addressing cultural, social, and contextual factors that influence the reception and efficacy of psychedelic treatments is important. Researching how different cultural contexts impact therapeutic outcomes and tailoring interventions accordingly is essential for global implementation.
10. Long-Term Effects and Safety Profile: Conducting longitudinal studies to assess the long-term effects, safety, and tolerability of psychedelic treatments is vital. Examining potential adverse effects, including persistent perceptual changes or psychological distress, over extended periods is critical for ensuring patient safety.
11. Placebo and Blinding Challenges: Developing robust placebo-controlled designs that account for the unique and identifiable subjective effects of psychedelics presents challenges. Addressing blinding issues while ensuring scientific rigor in clinical trials is essential for reliable outcome measurements.
12. Health Economics and Accessibility: Evaluating the economic implications of psychedelic therapies and their accessibility within healthcare systems is important. Studying cost-effectiveness, insurance coverage, and strategies to ensure equitable access to these treatments is crucial for their integration into mainstream healthcare.
13. Addressing these mechanisms and challenges will contribute to a more comprehensive understanding of psychedelics' therapeutic potential and facilitate their responsible and effective utilization in clinical settings (Eder-Moreau et al., 2022; Levesque et al., 2023).

Future Outlook and Controversies

1. Clinical Integration and Education: Advocates suggest that psychedelics could become part of psychiatric care. However, concerns regarding potential misuse, long-term effects, and societal attitudes necessitate a balanced approach with extensive education and public discourse.
2. Potential for Stigma Reduction: Educating the public about the potential benefits of psychedelics in therapeutic settings is essential. Clear communication about the risks, benefits, and ongoing research can help reduce stigma and misconceptions surrounding these substances.
3. Policy Reforms and Regulatory Shifts: Anticipated shifts in regulatory frameworks could impact the future of psychedelic research and clinical integration. Advocates emphasize the need for policy reforms to facilitate research, expand access, and enable responsible use while mitigating potential risks.

4. Diverse Therapeutic Applications: Beyond PTSD and mental health, exploring the potential of psychedelics in treating other psychiatric disorders (e.g., depression, addiction, OCD) and conditions like cluster headaches or chronic pain presents a promising avenue. Research diversification broadens their potential therapeutic landscape.
5. Public Health and Harm Reduction Strategies: Developing harm reduction strategies and public health initiatives is crucial to mitigate potential risks associated with recreational use or unguided self-administration of psychedelics. Educating individuals about safe use, dosage, and risks is imperative.
6. Ethical Considerations in Research and Practice: Ethical dilemmas regarding consent, vulnerability, and the use of psychedelics in vulnerable populations necessitate ongoing ethical discussions and guidelines. Ethical frameworks need to evolve alongside scientific advancements to ensure responsible research and clinical practice.
7. Economic and Societal Impact: Assessing the broader societal and economic implications of integrating psychedelics into mental healthcare systems is necessary. Evaluating healthcare costs, societal attitudes, workforce training, and economic feasibility contributes to informed decision-making.
8. Cultural and Indigenous Knowledge: Acknowledging the cultural significance and traditional use of psychedelics in various indigenous cultures is essential. Respectful engagement with indigenous knowledge holders and integrating cultural perspectives in research and practice ensures cultural sensitivity and ethical practice.
9. Commercialization and Industry Influence: Balancing commercial interests with ethical considerations and patient welfare is a concern. Regulating industry involvement, avoiding profit-driven agendas, and safeguarding patient interests amid commercialization are critical.
10. Global Harmonization and Research Collaboration: Establishing international collaboration and harmonizing guidelines for psychedelic research ensures standardized protocols, data sharing, and collective advancements. Global cooperation facilitates broader insights and reduces research redundancies.
11. Public Perception and Media Influence: Addressing sensationalism and misrepresentation of psychedelic research in media is crucial. Providing accurate information, dispelling myths, and promoting balanced discussions within the media sphere helps shape informed public perceptions.
12. Integration into Traditional Medicine: Exploring the integration of psychedelic therapies into holistic and traditional healing practices presents both opportunities and challenges. Understanding compatibility, synergy, and cultural contexts enhances therapeutic approaches.

Navigating these future outlooks and controversies demands a multidisciplinary approach, including scientific rigor, ethical considerations, policy reforms, community engagement, and ongoing education. Addressing these complex aspects is pivotal in realizing the potential benefits of psychedelics while safeguarding patient safety and societal well-being (Fantasia et al., 2023; Makhdoomi et al., 2022).

Innovative Medical Procedures:

Innovative medical procedures for PTSD explore novel approaches beyond traditional therapies. Emerging techniques like psychedelic-assisted therapy, virtual reality exposure therapy, and transcranial magnetic stimulation are being investigated. These methods aim to address symptoms by altering neural pathways, fostering emotional processing, or inducing therapeutic experiences. These innovative procedures signify a frontier in mental health treatment, offering potential alternatives for individuals with treatment-resistant PTSD, aiming to alleviate symptoms and improve overall well-being.

Stellate Ganglion Blockade

Stellate Ganglion Blockade (SGB) stands as an interventional procedure that involves the targeted injection of a local anesthetic near the stellate ganglion, a cluster of nerves situated in the neck. This region plays a pivotal role within the sympathetic nervous system, which governs various bodily functions, notably the body's response to stress and trauma. SGB aims to modulate this system, addressing the heightened arousal and hyperactivity often observed in individuals grappling with PTSD.One of the proposed mechanisms behind SGB revolves around its ability to influence the sympathetic nervous system. By administering an anesthetic in proximity to the stellate ganglion, the procedure intends to modulate the signaling of this system, thereby potentially alleviating symptoms associated with PTSD. The disruption of these signaling pathways could lead to a dampening of the physiological stress response, potentially reducing hyperarousal, anxiety, and intrusive thoughts often experienced by individuals with PTSD.

Clinical studies and preliminary research have shown promising outcomes regarding SGB's impact on PTSD symptoms. Reports suggest a reduction in hyperarousal, decreased anxiety levels, and a mitigation of intrusive thoughts following this intervention. These positive outcomes signify a potential avenue for alleviating distressing manifestations linked to trauma. Moreover, its minimally invasive nature and outpatient procedure design contribute to its appeal as an alternative to traditional therapeutic approaches for certain individuals.

However, while initial findings are promising, further research is imperative to understand the broader efficacy and long-term sustainability of SGB in PTSD treatment. Substantial variation in individual responses necessitates a deeper understanding of factors influencing diverse reactions to the procedure. Ongoing studies aim to clarify optimal protocols, potential side effects, and the integration of SGB into comprehensive PTSD treatment frameworks.

Ethical and safety considerations remain critical in the administration of SGB. Despite being minimally invasive, ensuring patient safety, addressing potential side effects, and determining appropriate patient selection are paramount. The variability in responses and the need for cautious ethical considerations underscore the importance of further research to delineate SGB's applicability and limitations within the spectrum of PTSD treatment options.

Stellate Ganglion Blockade presents a promising avenue in exploring alternative treatments for PTSD, particularly in addressing symptoms like hyperarousal and anxiety. Its potential to alleviate specific manifestations of trauma highlights a need for comprehensive research, including larger clinical trials and long-term assessments, to substantiate its efficacy, safety profile, and broader utility in PTSD treatment paradigms (T.-T. Li et al., 2022).

Trans-cranial Stimulation

Transcranial stimulation techniques, encompassing methods like Transcranial Magnetic Stimulation (TMS) and Transcranial Direct Current Stimulation (tDCS), offer non-invasive approaches to modulate brain activity. These interventions target specific brain regions implicated in mood regulation, memory processing, and emotional responses, showing promise as potential alternatives or adjuncts to traditional PTSD treatments.TMS, involving the application of magnetic pulses to specific brain areas, is theorized to alter neural pathways associated with PTSD symptoms. By targeting regions like the prefrontal cortex or limbic system, TMS may regulate emotional responses and memory processing linked to trauma. Conversely, tDCS delivers low-intensity electrical currents to the scalp, potentially modulating cortical excitability and neural plasticity. By enhancing or inhibiting neuronal activity in particular brain regions, tDCS might regulate mood and emotional reactivity in individuals with PTSD.Preliminary studies suggest encouraging outcomes regarding transcranial stimulation techniques and their impact on PTSD symptoms. Reports indicate potential reductions in anxiety, depressive symptoms, and intrusive thoughts, demonstrating their potential in addressing emotional dysregulation linked to trauma. These interventions are proposed as complementary therapies, potentially augmenting the effects of established treatments like psychotherapy or medications for individuals facing treatment-resistant symptoms.

However, challenges persist in utilizing transcranial stimulation for PTSD. Individual responses vary, impacting treatment efficacy and necessitating the determination of optimal stimulation parameters. Ensuring safety, monitoring for potential adverse effects, and addressing ethical considerations concerning vulnerable populations are paramount in the application of these techniques. Looking ahead, personalized treatment approaches based on neuroimaging and biomarker identification hold promise for tailoring stimulation protocols to individual brain circuitry and symptomatology. Additionally, longitudinal studies assessing treatment durability and exploring maintenance protocols are crucial for understanding the sustained benefits of transcranial stimulation in PTSD.

Transcranial stimulation techniques represent an emerging paradigm in PTSD treatment. While early findings suggest their potential in mitigating certain symptoms, extensive research, including large-scale clinical trials and long-term evaluations, is necessary. Understanding individual responses, optimizing protocols, ensuring safety, and addressing ethical considerations will be pivotal in fully leveraging the therapeutic potential of transcranial stimulation for individuals navigating the complexities of PTSD (Tedla et al., 2023).

CONCLUSION

Post-Traumatic Stress Disorder (PTSD) presents complex challenges that often resist conventional treatments. This comprehensive exploration delves into a spectrum of interventions, encompassing psychotherapies, pharmacotherapies, emerging therapies, and alternative approaches, aiming to unveil their efficacy, mechanisms, limitations, and future potentials in addressing PTSD.

Psychotherapies, notably Cognitive-Behavioral Therapy (CBT), such as Prolonged Exposure (PE) and Cognitive Processing Therapy (CPT), stand as established treatments for PTSD. They confront traumatic memories, modify maladaptive beliefs, and reduce avoidance behaviors, showcasing considerable effectiveness in symptom alleviation. Eye Movement Desensitization and Reprocessing (EMDR), incorporating targeted eye movements during memory recall, also exhibit efficacy, albeit its underlying mechanisms remain debated.

In the pharmacotherapy domain, Selective Serotonin Reuptake Inhibitors (SSRIs) like sertraline and paroxetine are commonly prescribed for PTSD. While offering symptom relief, not all individuals respond favorably to these medications, emphasizing the necessity for alternative pharmacological approaches. Emerging medications such as MDMA-assisted therapy and ketamine show promise in clinical trials, potentially managing treatment-resistant symptoms and facilitating emotional processing in PTSD.

Innovative therapies like Transcranial Magnetic Stimulation (TMS) and Transcranial Direct Current Stimulation (tDCS) represent non-invasive brain stimulation techniques that modulate neural circuits associated with PTSD symptoms. Preliminary findings suggest their potential, although extensive research is ongoing. Stellate Ganglion Blockade (SGB), an anesthetic injection near the stellate ganglion, displays promise in reducing hyperarousal and anxiety linked to PTSD, providing a minimally invasive alternative.

Beyond conventional treatments, alternative interventions like yoga, mindfulness, and nature exposure therapies present novel avenues in managing PTSD. Mind-body practices contribute to stress reduction and emotional regulation, potentially benefiting individuals with PTSD. Exposure to natural environments, encompassing ecotherapy and wilderness therapy, shows potential therapeutic benefits for improving mental health and alleviating PTSD symptoms.

In conclusion, diverse interventions offer promising avenues in managing the intricate symptoms of PTSD. While established psychotherapies and pharmacotherapies remain integral, emerging and alternative interventions present exciting prospects. Brain stimulation techniques and novel medications offer hope for individuals with treatment-resistant symptoms, while alternative approaches underscore holistic care. Comprehensive integration of these interventions into tailored treatment frameworks, backed by rigorous research, holds the potential to enhance treatment outcomes and improve the lives of those affected by PTSD. Further exploration through controlled trials and mechanistic investigations is crucial to validate and optimize the efficacy, safety, and long-term benefits of these diverse interventions within comprehensive PTSD care paradigms.

REFERENCES

Bell, S. L., Hickman, C., & Houghton, F. (2023). From therapeutic landscape to therapeutic 'sensescape'experiences with nature? A scoping review. *Wellbeing, Space and Society*, 4, 100126. DOI: 10.1016/j.wss.2022.100126

Bryant, R. A., Dawson, K. S., Azevedo, S., Yadav, S., Cahill, C., Kenny, L., Maccallum, F., Tran, J., Rawson, N., Tockar, J., Garber, B., & Keyan, D. (2023). Augmenting trauma-focused psychotherapy for post-traumatic stress disorder with brief aerobic exercise in Australia: A randomised clinical trial. *The Lancet. Psychiatry*, 10(1), 21–29. DOI: 10.1016/S2215-0366(22)00368-6 PMID: 36436532

Burback, L., Brémault-Phillips, S., Nijdam, M. J., McFarlane, A., & Vermetten, E. (2023). Treatment of Posttraumatic Stress Disorder: A State-of-the-art Review. *Current Neuropharmacology*. PMID: 37132142

Calcerano, D., & Ciurlia, G. (2023). *Neurofeedback in Virtual Reality Naturalistic Scenarios for Enhancing Relaxation: Visual and Auditory Stimulation to Promote Brain Entrainment*. Politecnico di Torino.

Cameron, R. P., & Gusman, D. (2003). The primary care PTSD screen (PC-PTSD): Development and operating characteristics. *Primary Care Psychiatry*, 9(1), 9–14.

Carlini, S. V., Osborne, L. M., & Deligiannidis, K. M. (2023). Current pharmacotherapy approaches and novel GABAergic antidepressant development in postpartum depression. *Dialogues in Clinical Neuroscience*, 25(1), 92–100. DOI: 10.1080/19585969.2023.2262464 PMID: 37796239

Choi, Y.-J., Choi, E.-J., & Ko, E. (2023). Neurofeedback Effect on Symptoms of Posttraumatic Stress Disorder: A Systematic Review and Meta-Analysis. *Applied Psychophysiology and Biofeedback*, 48(3), 1–16. DOI: 10.1007/s10484-023-09593-3 PMID: 37314616

Crombie, K. M., Adams, T. G., Dunsmoor, J. E., Greenwood, B. N., Smits, J. A., Nemeroff, C. B., & Cisler, J. M. (2023). Aerobic exercise in the treatment of PTSD: An examination of preclinical and clinical laboratory findings, potential mechanisms, clinical implications, and future directions. *Journal of Anxiety Disorders*, 94, 102680. DOI: 10.1016/j.janxdis.2023.102680 PMID: 36773486

Datta, N., Matheson, B. E., Citron, K., Van Wye, E. M., & Lock, J. D. (2023). Evidence based update on psychosocial treatments for eating disorders in children and adolescents. *Journal of Clinical Child and Adolescent Psychology*, 52(2), 159–170. DOI: 10.1080/15374416.2022.2109650 PMID: 35950931

Davis, L. W., Schmid, A. A., Daggy, J. K., & Yang, Z. (2023). Mediators of improved PTSD symptoms in veterans and civilians following a yoga program. *Acta Neuropsychiatrica*, 35(4), 1–9. DOI: 10.1017/neu.2023.5 PMID: 36710002

Eder-Moreau, E., Zhu, X., Fisch, C. T., Bergman, M., Neria, Y., & Helpman, L. (2022). Neurobiological alterations in females with PTSD: A systematic review. *Frontiers in Psychiatry*, 13, 862476. DOI: 10.3389/fpsyt.2022.862476 PMID: 35770056

Ehrenstein, M. R., & Shipa, M. (2023). SLE is not a one-size-fits-all disease. *The Journal of Experimental Medicine*, 220(6), e20230559. DOI: 10.1084/jem.20230559 PMID: 37097613

Fantasia, A. T., Prybutok, G., & Prybutok, V. (2023). The Impact of Post-Traumatic Stress Disorder on Addiction to Information over Searching and Information Avoidance.

Fisher, C. (2023). Trauma-Informed Nature Therapy: A Case Study. *Ecopsychology*, 15(3), 214–221. DOI: 10.1089/eco.2022.0064

Freese, J. B. (2023). Towards Trauma-Informed Buddhist Spiritual Care: A Mutual Critical Correlation of Vipassana Meditation and Somatic Experiencing. *Pastoral Psychology*, 72(3), 447–464. DOI: 10.1007/s11089-023-01065-z

Fu, T. (2023). New Interventions for the Treatment of PTSD. *Journal of Education. Humanities and Social Sciences*, 8, 848–855.

Ha, A., Wilkins, S. S., Melrose, R. J., & Lee, C. C. (2023). Depression and PTSD as Predictors of Attrition in Older Adult Exercise Programs: A Systematic Review. *Topics in Geriatric Rehabilitation*, 39(1), 31–38. DOI: 10.1097/TGR.0000000000000383

Haller, H., Mitzinger, D., & Cramer, H. (2023). The integration of yoga breathing techniques in cognitive behavioral therapy for post-traumatic stress disorder: A pragmatic randomized controlled trial. *Frontiers in Psychiatry*, 14, 1101046. DOI: 10.3389/fpsyt.2023.1101046 PMID: 37139325

Jamil, A., Gutlapalli, S. D., Ali, M., Oble, M. J., Sonia, S. N., George, S., Shahi, S. R., Ali, Z., Abaza, A., & Mohammed, L. (2023). Meditation and its mental and physical health benefits in 2023. *Cureus*, 15(6). Advance online publication. DOI: 10.7759/cureus.40650 PMID: 37476142

Kaidesoja, M., Cooper, Z., & Fordham, B. (2023). Cognitive behavioral therapy for eating disorders: A map of the systematic review evidence base. *International Journal of Eating Disorders*, 56(2), 295–313. DOI: 10.1002/eat.23831 PMID: 36315392

Kerr, J. I., Weibel, R. P., Naegelin, M., Ferrario, A., Schinazi, V. R., La Marca, R., Hoelscher, C., Nater, U. M., & von Wangenheim, F. (2023). The effectiveness and user experience of a biofeedback intervention program for stress management supported by virtual reality and mobile technology: A randomized controlled study. *BMC Digital Health*, 1(1), 42. DOI: 10.1186/s44247-023-00042-z

Khwaja, K., Deban, M., Iqbal, S., Alowais, J., Al Bader, B., Deckelbaum, D., & Razek, T. (2023). The McGill simulation complexity Score (MSCS): A novel complexity scoring system for simulations in trauma. *Canadian Journal of Surgery*, 66(2), E206–E211. DOI: 10.1503/cjs.002220 PMID: 37085295

Laplaud, N., Perrochon, A., Gallou-Guyot, M., Moens, M., Goudman, L., David, R., Rigoard, P., & Billot, M. (2023). Management of post-traumatic stress disorder symptoms by yoga: An overview. *BMC Complementary Medicine and Therapies*, 23(1), 258. DOI: 10.1186/s12906-023-04074-w PMID: 37480017

Levesque, P., Desmeules, C., Béchard, L., Huot-Lavoie, M., Demers, M.-F., Roy, M.-A., & Deslauriers, J. (2023). Sex-specific immune mechanisms in PTSD symptomatology and risk: A translational overview and perspectives. *Brain Research Bulletin*, 195, 120–129. DOI: 10.1016/j.brainresbull.2023.02.013 PMID: 36822271

Li, N.-X., Hu, Y.-R., Chen, W.-N., & Zhang, B. (2022). Dose effect of psilocybin on primary and secondary depression: A preliminary systematic review and meta-analysis. *Journal of Affective Disorders*, 296, 26–34. DOI: 10.1016/j.jad.2021.09.041 PMID: 34587546

Li, T.-T., Wan, Q., Zhang, X., Xiao, Y., Sun, L.-Y., Zhang, Y.-R., Liu, X.-N., & Yang, W.-C. (2022). Stellate ganglion block reduces inflammation and improves neurological function in diabetic rats during ischemic stroke. *Neural Regeneration Research*, 17(9), 1991. DOI: 10.4103/1673-5374.335162 PMID: 35142688

Lowe, H., Toyang, N., Steele, B., Grant, J., Ali, A., Gordon, L., & Ngwa, W. (2022). Psychedelics: Alternative and potential therapeutic options for treating mood and anxiety disorders. *Molecules (Basel, Switzerland)*, 27(8), 2520. DOI: 10.3390/molecules27082520 PMID: 35458717

Magill, M., Kiluk, B. D., & Ray, L. A. (2023). Efficacy of Cognitive Behavioral Therapy for Alcohol and Other Drug Use Disorders: Is a One-Size-Fits-All Approach Appropriate? *Substance Abuse and Rehabilitation*, 14, 1–11. DOI: 10.2147/SAR.S362864 PMID: 36844999

Makhdoomi, S. M., Rakhra, M., Singh, D., & Singh, A. (2022). Artificial-Intelligence based Prediction of Post-Traumatic Stress Disorder (PTSD) using EEG reports. 2022 5th International Conference on Contemporary Computing and Informatics (IC3I)

Martínez, V., Iriondo De-Hond, A., Borrelli, F., Capasso, R., Del Castillo, M. D., & Abalo, R. (2020). Cannabidiol and other non-psychoactive cannabinoids for prevention and treatment of gastrointestinal disorders: Useful nutraceuticals? *International Journal of Molecular Sciences*, 21(9), 3067.

McGorrill, S. (2023). The Benefits of Sensory Exploration in Art Therapy with Children with Social, Emotional and Behavioral Difficulties Through a Trauma Informed Lens.

Merkley, T. L., Esopenko, C., Zizak, V. S., Bilder, R. M., Strutt, A. M., Tate, D. F., & Irimia, A. (2023). Challenges and opportunities for harmonization of cross-cultural neuropsychological data. *Neuropsychology*, 37(3), 237–246. DOI: 10.1037/neu0000818 PMID: 35549387

Metcalf, O., Finlayson-Short, L., Forbes, D., O'Donnell, M., & Varker, T. (2023). A systematic review of treatments for problem anger in veteran and military populations with PTSD. *Aggression and Violent Behavior*, 70, 101837. DOI: 10.1016/j.avb.2023.101837

Midyett, L. K. (2023). One Size Fits All Versus Individualized Medicine in Type 1 Diabetes Management. *Diabetes Technology & Therapeutics*, 25(S3), S-42–S-47. DOI: 10.1089/dia.2023.0109 PMID: 37306440

Morina, N., Kampmann, I., Emmelkamp, P., Barbui, C., & Hoppen, T. H. (2023). Meta-analysis of virtual reality exposure therapy for social anxiety disorder. *Psychological Medicine*, 53(5), 2176–2178. DOI: 10.1017/S0033291721001690 PMID: 34001293

Moser, D. A., Graf, S., Glaus, J., Urben, S., Jouabli, S., Perrizolo, V. P., Suardi, F., Robinson, J., Serpa, S. R., & Plessen, K. J. (2023). On the complex and dimensional relationship of maternal posttraumatic stress disorder during early childhood and child outcomes at school-age. *European Psychiatry*, 66(1), e20. DOI: 10.1192/j.eurpsy.2023.8 PMID: 36734250

Nacasch, N., Avni, C., & Toren, P. (2023). Medical cannabis for treatment-resistant combat PTSD. *Frontiers in Psychiatry*, 13, 1014630. DOI: 10.3389/fpsyt.2022.1014630 PMID: 36741572

Neuner, F. (2023). Physical and social trauma: Towards an integrative transdiagnostic perspective on psychological trauma that involves threats to status and belonging. *Clinical Psychology Review*, 99, 102219. DOI: 10.1016/j.cpr.2022.102219 PMID: 36395560

Nie, Y., Zhang, Y., Ren, R., Sanford, L. D., Vitiello, M. V., & Tang, X. (2023). Interventions for Trauma-Related Nightmare: Where Are We Now? *The International Journal of Neuropsychopharmacology*, 26(6), 412–414. DOI: 10.1093/ijnp/pyad022 PMID: 37226283

Niles, B., Lang, A., & Olff, M. (2023). *Complementary and integrative interventions for PTSD* (Vol. 14). Taylor & Francis.

Pacitto, R., Peters, C., Iadipaolo, A., & Rabinak, C. A. (2022). Cannabinoid modulation of brain activation during volitional regulation of negative affect in trauma-exposed adults. *Neuropharmacology*, 218, 109222. DOI: 10.1016/j.neuropharm.2022.109222 PMID: 35981598

Perez Alday, E. A., Da Poian, G., Levantsevych, O., Murrah, N., Shallenberger, L., Alkhalaf, M., Haffar, A., Kaseer, B., Ko, Y. A., Goldberg, J., Smith, N., Lampert, R., Bremner, J. D., Clifford, G. D., Vaccarino, V., & Shah, A. J. (2023). Association of Autonomic Activation with traumatic reminder challenges in posttraumatic stress disorder: A co-twin control study. *Psychophysiology*, 60(2), e14167. DOI: 10.1111/psyp.14167 PMID: 35959570

Pringle, G., Boddy, J., Slattery, M., & Harris, P. (2023). Adventure Therapy for Adolescents with Complex Trauma: A Scoping Review and Analysis. *Journal of Experiential Education*, 46(4), 433–454. DOI: 10.1177/10538259221147195

Punski-Hoogervorst, J. L., Avital, A., & Engel-Yeger, B. (2023). Challenges in basic and instrumental activities of daily living among adults with posttraumatic stress disorder: A scoping review. *Occupational Therapy in Mental Health*, 39(2), 184–210. DOI: 10.1080/0164212X.2022.2094523

Putri, V. S. I. S., Wijayanti, L. R., & Hidayati, I. N. (2023). The Positive Effect of The Forest Environment in The Ecotherapy Healing Forest Program on The Physical and Mental Health After COVID-19. BIO Web of Conferences

Salome, G., Vignaud, P., Galia, P., Prieto, N., & Chauliac, N. (2023). Determinants of care pathways for C-PTSD patients in French psychotrauma centers: A qualitative study. [PubMed]. *International Journal of Environmental Research and Public Health*, 20(13), 6278.

Sciarrino, N. A., & Myers, U. S. (2023). If it's offered, will they come? Practical considerations when offering intensive PTSD treatment in an outpatient Veterans Affairs PTSD clinic. *Bulletin of the Menninger Clinic*, 87(1), 46–62. DOI: 10.1521/bumc.2023.87.1.46 PMID: 36856477

Shafia, S., Ghadirzadeh, E., Fayyaz Shahandashti, A. S., & Ehsani Vostacolaee, S. (2023). Comparing the Effects of High and Moderate Intensity Exercise on Male and Female Rats with and without PTSD: A Behavioral and Biochemical Study. *Journal of Mazandaran University of Medical Sciences*, 32(216), 20–33.

Tedla, J. S., Sangadala, D. R., Reddy, R. S., Gular, K., & Dixit, S. (2023). High-definition trans cranial direct current stimulation and its effects on cognitive function: A systematic review. *Cerebral Cortex (New York, N.Y.)*, 33(10), 6077–6089. DOI: 10.1093/cercor/bhac485 PMID: 36533541

Vancampfort, D., De Soir, E., van Winkel, R., Louw, Q. A., McKeon, G., Rosenbaum, S., Seedat, S., & Pelayo Ramos-Sanchez, C. (2023). Physical activity, sedentary behaviour and mental health outcomes in firefighters: A cross-sectional study. *Journal of Workplace Behavioral Health*, •••, 1–18.

Vella, E. J., Lyman, T., & Lovering, T. (2023). Pilot Study: The Effects of a Mountain Wilderness Experience on Combat Veteran Psychosocial Wellness. *Military Behavioral Health*, 11(1-2), 1–12. DOI: 10.1080/21635781.2023.2221463

Wagner, C., & Cáceres-Melillo, R. (2023). Mindfulness-Based Cognitive Therapy (MBCT) and Mindfulness-Based Stress Reduction (MBSR) in the treatment of Post-Traumatic Stress Disorder (PTSD): A literature review. *Salud Mental*, 46(1), 35–42. DOI: 10.17711/SM.0185-3325.2023.005

Wahid, H., Ghazi, M., & Lashari, A. (2023). Impact of Meditation on the Level of Post-traumatic Stress in Flood Victims of Sindh. *Global Educational Studies Review, VIII*, 8(I), 272–278. DOI: 10.31703/gesr.2023(VIII-I).23

Wolfgang, A. S., & Hoge, C. W. (2023). Cannabis and cannabinoids for pain and posttraumatic stress disorder in military personnel and veterans. *JAMA Psychiatry*, 80(9), 869–870. DOI: 10.1001/jamapsychiatry.2023.1685 PMID: 37436761

Zabik, N., Iadipaolo, A., Peters, C., & Rabinak, C. A. (2022). P654. Varying Doses of THC Rescue Neural Fear Circuitry Dysfunction in Trauma-Exposed Adults. *Biological Psychiatry*, 91(9), S354–S355. DOI: 10.1016/j.biopsych.2022.02.891

Zaccari, B., Loftis, J. M., Haywood, T., Hubbard, K., Clark, J., & Kelly, U. A. (2022). Synchronous telehealth yoga and cognitive processing group therapies for women veterans with posttraumatic stress disorder: A multisite randomized controlled trial adapted for COVID-19. *Telemedicine Journal and e-Health*, 28(11), 1642–1650. DOI: 10.1089/tmj.2021.0612 PMID: 35357957

Zhang, L., Deng, L., Ma, C., Zhang, H., & Dang, Y. (2023). Brain-Derived Neurotrophic Factor Delivered Intranasally Relieves Post-Traumatic Stress Disorder Symptoms Caused by a Single Prolonged Stress in Rats. *Neuropsychobiology*, 82(1), 40–50. DOI: 10.1159/000528755 PMID: 36630922

Chapter 7

A Promising Mind-Body 4th Wave Approach to Treating Post-Traumatic Stress Disorder:

Clinical Emotional Freedom Techniques

Peta Stapleton
https://orcid.org/0000-0001-9916-7481
Bond University, Australia

ABSTRACT

This chapter presents Clinical Emotional Freedom Techniques (EFT) as a promising mind-body approach for treating post-traumatic stress disorder (PTSD). Through the compelling cases of Sarah and John, two individuals grappling with PTSD symptoms despite previous therapies, the chapter underscores the need for a more integrative treatment modality. It explores the foundations and principles of Clinical EFT, a technique that combines cognitive strategies with somatic acupressure point stimulation. The growing evidence base supporting EFT's efficacy is presented, and a detailed, step-by-step guide for clinicians is offered, including how clients can use at home, in and between sessions. Sarah and John's specific EFT protocol tailored to their cases is outlined, relating to repeated childhood trauma, and a single event military deployment trauma. With its emphasis on rapid symptom reduction, low dropout rates, and comparable efficacy to established therapies, Clinical EFT emerges as a valuable addition to the clinician's toolkit.

DOI: 10.4018/979-8-3693-2089-1.ch007

INTRODUCTION

As I meet with my patient, Sarah, I can see the effects of her childhood trauma. Her eyes have a distant, haunted look, reflecting the difficulties she has faced. Her body language is tense and guarded. She fidgets nervously, and her breathing is shallow. When I ask her about her recent experiences, she becomes visibly distressed, her hands trembling as she recounts intrusive memories and flashbacks that continue to plague her. Sarah is one of many individuals struggling with the debilitating impacts of posttraumatic stress disorder (PTSD), a complex and often treatment-resistant condition that can profoundly affect a person's well-being.

For years, Sarah has tried various evidence-based therapies, from cognitive-behavioral interventions to pharmacological treatments. While these approaches have provided some relief, the lingering symptoms of PTSD continue to impact her daily life. She is seeking a more holistic, mind-body solution that can address the root causes of her condition and empower her to reclaim her sense of self. Sarah has a history of childhood traumatic incidents such as physical and emotional abuse, and a chaotic family environment.

As a clinician, I have been intrigued by the emerging field of Clinical Emotional Freedom Techniques (Clinical EFT), a promising fourth wave mind-body approach that may hold the key to unlocking Sarah's path to healing and recovery. Through Sarah's journey and the experiences of other patients, this chapter outlines how this innovative technique can offer a transformative, integrative solution for clinicians dedicated to providing comprehensive, compassionate care for individuals struggling with the profound impact of trauma.

The Role of Mind Body Approaches in Trauma

While current trauma treatment approaches include medication (Schrader & Ross, 2021), side effects and relapse after treatment (Alexander, 2012) has resulted in clinical guidelines typically recommending that first-line treatments should be trauma-focused psychotherapies (American Psychological Association, 2017). These strategies for PTSD include trauma-focused therapies such as cognitive behavioral therapy (CBT), cognitive processing therapy (CPT), prolonged exposure therapy (PE), and eye movement desensitization and reprocessing (EMDR). These therapies have shown consistent reduction of PTSD symptoms and are considered effective treatments achieved in 12–16, 60-minute weekly sessions (Kar, 2011; Schrader & Ross, 2021).

However, it has been noted dropout rates from PE tend to be higher than that of other more cognitively-focused therapies such as CPT and EMDR, due to the difficulty in the verbal repeated retelling of the trauma (Schrader & Ross, 2021).

Nonresponse to CBT also been noted to be as high as 50% when comorbidity of other conditions is present (Kar, 2011), and studies show sufferers may still meet diagnosis of PTSD after CPT and PE (Steenkamp et al., 2015).

Reviews of PTSD treatments over the last 15 years has emphasized the importance of individual therapy and the potential benefits of incorporating mind-body approaches (Kim et al., 2013). Approaches that reduce stress in the body and restore balance to the autonomic nervous system are emerging as viable adjuncts to the treatment of PTSD (McEwen, 2000; Streeter et al., 2012). Research suggests these practices typically centering on breathing techniques, relaxation, imagery and hypnosis, may improve symptoms such as anxiety, depression, anger, fear and arousal (Kim et al., 2013). The US Department of Veteran Affairs now offers more than 80 percent of its specialized programs for PTSD as mind-body therapies, both as stand-alone and as complementary to other standard treatment (Niles et al., 2018). It appears the clinical advantages of including body-based or somatic elements into therapy may be crucial to not only target muscles and fascia, but the neurological connections in trauma (Stapleton et al., 2023). Integrating these into conventional psychotherapy approaches may enhance treatment outcomes and produce more rapid and durable effects.

Clinicians may want to consider incorporating a mind-body approach to PTSD treatment, in addition to traditional talk therapies, for several key reasons.

As with the case of Sarah above, many patients with PTSD continue to struggle with persistent symptoms despite undergoing evidence-based psychotherapies like cognitive-behavioral interventions. The mind-body connection is a crucial aspect of PTSD that is often not fully addressed through talk therapy alone. Mind-body practices such as yoga, meditation, and deep breathing can help regulate the autonomic nervous system, reduce physiological hyperarousal, and promote relaxation - all of which are central to alleviating the intrusive thoughts, avoidance, and hypervigilance that characterize PTSD.

Moreover, these approaches may enhance patients' engagement and adherence to treatment. Many individuals, like Sarah, are seeking more holistic, empowering solutions that go beyond just talking about their trauma. Incorporating mind-body techniques can provide patients with practical self-management skills that they can continue to utilize outside of the clinical setting, fostering a greater sense of control and self-efficacy in their recovery process. By addressing PTSD from both a psychological and physiological standpoint, clinicians can offer patients a more comprehensive, integrative treatment plan that optimizes their chances of achieving lasting symptom reduction and improved quality of life.

A Promising Mind-Body Approach: Clinical Emotional Freedom Techniques

As mentioned in the case of Sarah, an emerging evidence-based method that combines the somatic element of acupressure with components drawn from cognitive and exposure therapies, has been validated in more than 100 clinical trials, and 300 peer reviewed papers (Church et al., 2022; Feinstein, 2023; Stapleton et al., 2023). Emotional Freedom Techniques (EFT) is a psychophysiological mind-body intervention that combines techniques from CBT and PE including mindful awareness, imaginal exposure, cognitive reframing and systematic desensitization (Church et al., 2022; Stapleton et al., 2023). The somatic element of EFT includes self-stimulation of acupuncture points using a two-finger tapping process (Church et al., 2022; Stapleton et al., 2023). Clinical EFT is the term used to describe the manualized and standardized treatment protocol introduced in the 1990s (Church et al., 2018; Stapleton et al., 2023).

The integration of EFT into traditional talk therapy approaches has been proposed as a viable option to significantly enhance therapeutic outcomes. The dual ability of EFT to address both the physical (e.g., allostatic, stress load) and emotional aspects of psychological issues may lead to enhanced processing and resolution of underlying issues. Feinstein (2023) highlights another case study involving a client struggling with anxiety and panic attacks, and offers that the integration of EFT tapping alongside traditional cognitive therapy resulted in a substantial reduction in physiological anxiety symptoms and an increased sense of self-awareness and emotional control. Feinstein suggests the use of EFT can also strengthen the therapeutic alliance between the client and therapist. By incorporating EFT techniques, therapists can provide clients with additional tools for self-regulation and emotional processing outside of therapy sessions. This empowerment fosters a sense of agency and control in clients, ultimately enhancing the therapeutic relationship and promoting active engagement in recovery.

Given a common strategy in talk therapies is utilizing homework assignments as a mechanism to produce and strengthen beneficial treatment outcomes, then it is essential strategies be implemented outside therapy for beneficial outcomes (Mausbach et al., 2010). Meta-analyses indicate greater compliance with homework is associated with more beneficial treatment outcomes (Kazantaiz et al., 2000; Mausbach et al., 2010. However, one of the top cited reasons for therapy failure in CBT is homework noncompliance (Helbig, & Fehm, 2004). The implementation of a strategy such as Clinical EFT within session alleviates the need for the client to engage in homework activities, and is potentially a safer option when trauma is present.

Finally, EFT offers a complementary framework for therapists to work with clients who may not fully respond to traditional talk therapies alone. The process-oriented nature of EFT, and the ability to use it without the spoken word, allows for a holistic exploration of emotions and experiences, enabling therapists to delve deeper into unresolved issues contributing to psychological distress in a protected manner. For clients where trauma affects their ability to verbalise the content, mind-body approaches such as EFT may assist and provide a non-verbal avenue to processing. One key aspect of EFT is that past traumas can be revisited while the acupoint tapping reduces distress and allows for clients to remain in their window of tolerance, aiding the limbic system in processing unresolved emotional material *without speaking* (Feinstein, 2022a).

The Advantages of Clinical EFT for PTSD

Ultimately Clinical EFT offers several advantages over traditional talk therapies for the treatment of PTSD in clinical settings:

- Rapid symptom reduction in as few as 4-10 sessions;
- Low dropout rates: of less than 10% in PTSD populations;
- Comparable efficacy to well-established therapies such as EMDR and CBT; and
- A self-management tool that can be used outside of therapy sessions.

The Clinical EFT Protocol

Use of a manual for trauma therapy is the gold standard for treatment delivery (Schrader & Ross, 2021). Clinical EFT also adheres to a systematic approach that is manualized and structured. As a therapeutic modality that incorporates both cognitive and somatic elements, it is considered a psychophysiological intervention that aims to address psychological problems through this interaction. Acupressure points on the face and upper body are stimulated with a tapping technique with two fingers: usually the index and middle fingers. The strength of tapping is comfortable, and typically a person only uses tapping if they have a feeling or a thought they wish to change (usually negative or distressing). The approach emphasizes awareness and acceptance of the current state, and to this adds the somatic element of tapping on the acupressure points.

After acknowledging the emotional state one wishes to address, a subjective unit of distress (SUDS) rating is given (10=most distress, 0=no distress; Wolpe, 1969). A Setup Statement of acknowledgment is verbalized (typically three times) while an acupuncture point on the side of the hand is tapped upon (see Figure 1). The statement classically follows the format “Even though I am feeling (insert emotion, distress level), I accept myself anyway”. The remaining acupressure points (see Figure 2) are then tapped while the person verbalizes a reminder phrase or shortened version of the statement. This is usually the main emotion or distress (e.g., ‘angry’ or ‘sad’) and serves to encourage the person to remain present to the situation and thus acts as exposure. This constitutes a ‘round’ of CBT and at the end the person would re-rate the SUDS and continue tapping until there was a difference.

Figure 1. Side of the hand tapping point

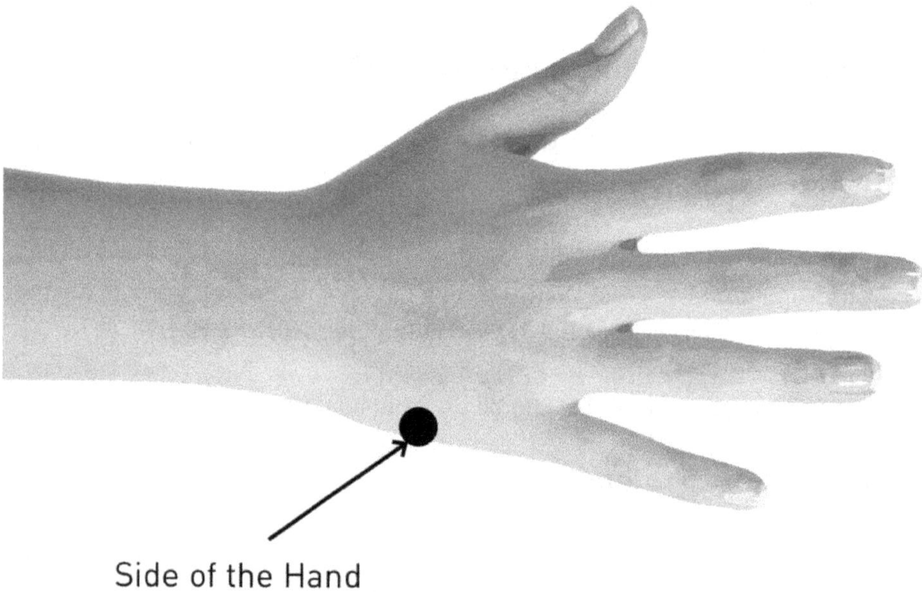

Figure 2. The tapping points

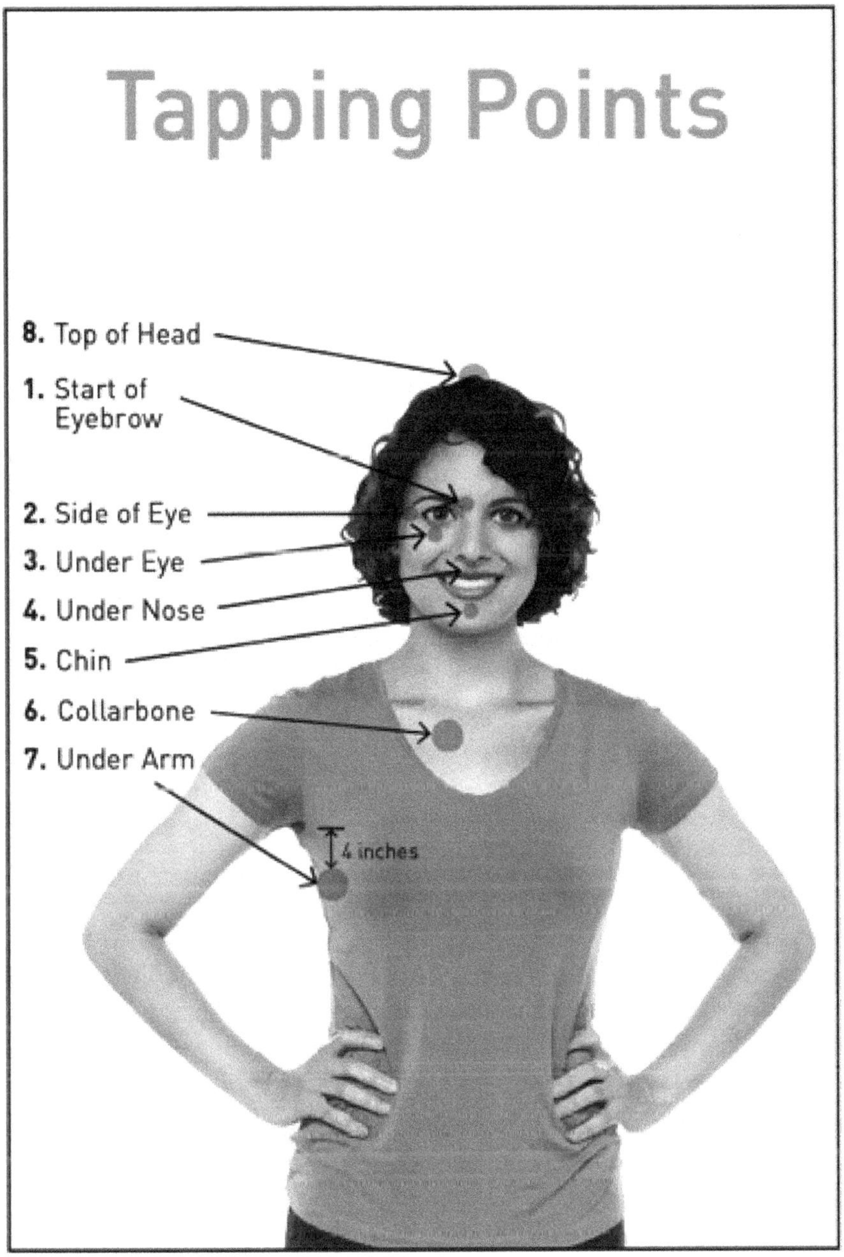

An Example

Imagine you feel angry about something that just happened at work and you rate it 9 out of 10. You would tap on the side of the hand while saying "Even though I feel really angry right now, and I feel sick, I accept I feel this way". You would state this three times while tapping on the side of the hand point. You would then begin tapping through the eight points in Figure 2 and say "so angry" or "I feel angry". If you felt the anger as a bodily sensation, that that area can be focused upon (e.g., this tight feeling in my chest). You would continue tapping until you felt a shift or difference, usually indicated by a low number out of 10.

Focusing on the Negative

It is common practice in the cognitive approaches to seek to reframe a person's issue, or simply learn to accept it. The EFT process appears to focus on the negative or distressing emotional state, however it is this present focused, mindful acknowledgement of one's state that allows for change. Just as cognitive therapies encourage confronting fears in order to integrate rational information in the fear memory (Kaczkurkin & Foa, 2015), Clinical EFT proposes to modify maladaptive emotional responses by first activating them through the spoken Setup Statement. To this it adds the somatic element of physically stimulating acupuncture points to regulate the autonomic nervous system, while the person remains exposed to the emotional state they are wanting to change.

A Simple 5-Step Process

In summary there are five steps for Clinical EFT:

1. Acknowledge there is something to change and rate distress/discomfort out of 10 (10=most distress, 0=no distress).
2. State problem in the setup statement while tapping on side of hand point in Figure 1 (3 times).
3. Tap through all 8 EFT points in Figure 2 while saying a short reminder phrase, which is usually the main feeling or body sensation, or thought. This is to stay engaged and not drift off in your thoughts.
4. Take a breath and re-rate the distress out of 10.
5. Tap again from the eyebrow point until the rating is 0. You only need to start again with the setup statement if you want to change the topic you are tapping on.

These steps represent the complete process; however, there is a way clients and patients can safely use it at home in between sessions.

EFT Emotional First Aid: Tap and Breathe

One of the key challenges in supporting patients is equipping them with practical, self-directed tools that they can utilize outside of the therapy setting to maintain emotional regulation and resilience. Clinical EFT can be used as a regulation activity, readily incorporated into a patient's daily routine to promote overall well-being and stress reduction. It is often called Tapping Emotional First Aid, and has clients just tap and breathe. Instead of speaking out loud, they just tap on each acupoint a few times, while taking a comfortable breath, before moving onto the next acupoint. Just a few rounds of tapping and breathing comfortably results in emotional regulation, and can be done as often as they need to throughout a day. This versatility and accessibility means patients can incorporate Clinical EFT into their daily routines, tapping for a few minutes whenever they feel the need to regain a sense of emotional control. This self-empowering approach encourages patients to take an active role in their own well-being, fostering a greater sense of control and self-efficacy. Moreover, the simplicity and non-invasive nature of Clinical EFT make it an appealing option for clinicians working with a diverse range of clients, from children to the elderly.

For Sarah in our case, who struggles with intrusive memories and hypervigilance related to her PTSD, learning to use EFT at home can be a powerful self-regulation tool. When she feels herself becoming overwhelmed by distressing thoughts or heightened anxiety, Sarah can take a few moments to tap through the EFT sequence while focusing on her breathing. She might start by tapping on the side of the hand point while silently acknowledging her current emotional state, such as "Even though I'm feeling anxious right now, I deeply and completely accept myself." Then, she can proceed to tap gently on the remaining acupoints, just taking slow, comfortable breaths with each tapping point.

By incorporating this simple tapping and breathing exercise into her daily routine, Sarah can take control of her emotional well-being without relying solely on external support.

A Typical Session of EFT for PTSD for Sarah

As I reflect on Sarah's case above, Clinical EFT offers a promising approach that could significantly benefit her PTSD journey to recovery. Sarah's persistent symptoms, including intrusive thoughts, hypervigilance, and difficulty regulating her emotions, despite her previous attempts at evidence-based therapies, suggest that a more integrative treatment plan may be warranted. The guidelines for using

Clinical EFT in the treatment of PTSD indicate that this approach can be effective in as little as 4-10 sessions, with significant reductions in symptom severity and, in many cases, the absence of a PTSD diagnosis altogether. Given the severity of Sarah's PTSD, and because she has numerous childhood incidents, they would be addressed in different sessions.

It is common practice for therapists to utilize standardized assessment measures and history taking to determine the appropriate approach for the EFT session. This may involve gathering information about Sarah's specific triggers, symptoms, risk assessment and the nature of her traumatic experiences. Sarah may also be taught additional stabilization and regulation activities prior to using Clinical EFT on traumatic experiences and memories. manual.

In a typical EFT session for Sarah, a therapist would guide her to tap (self-applied) while she focussed on a traumatic memory or feeling. The therapist would also tap with Sarah, which serves as a way for the therapist to remain regulated. This may involve Sarah speaking out loud about a memory, or not. The Clinical EFT manual specifies 48 techniques in the method, many of them specifically for the treatment of trauma in a gentle manner to enable her to remain in her window of distress tolerance, and includes imagining the past memories without verbalizing any details.

After a few rounds of tapping, the therapist would reassess Sarah's subjective distress level related to the memory or feeling and/or may utilize standardized assessment measures of distress, trauma or dysregulation, to determine its effectiveness. The process is repeated as needed until the Sarah's distress level related to the memory or feeling has significantly decreased.

The EFT process utilizes techniques such as verbalizing the trauma narrative and draws upon exposure therapy principles of CBT. The specific steps, wording of phrases and amount of tapping may vary based on the individual's needs, as will the number of required sessions. Some individuals may experience significant relief in just a few sessions, while others may require more extensive treatment.

The Clinical EFT approach, with its emphasis on eliciting the client's subjective experiences and utilizing exposure therapy principles, may provide Sarah with a more empowering and transformative path to healing. She can also stay safe during sessions but not *having* to retell the story of her trauma (which may potentially retraumatize her). The act of keeping her body calm while thinking (or speaking) of her trauma occurs through the actual tapping on acupoints, and then gives her brain and body a different experience.

Finally, the research indicates that Clinical EFT is a generally safe and well-tolerated intervention, with minimal adverse events reported. This, combined with the potential for rapid symptom reduction, makes it an attractive option for Sarah, who has struggled to find lasting relief through more traditional therapies.

Childhood trauma often involves prolonged, repeated exposure to traumatic events over many years during critical developmental periods. It can profoundly disrupt the development of secure attachment patterns and interpersonal relating capacities, and can shape core aspects of identity, self-concept, and worldview. Childhood trauma is also associated with a higher risk of complex trauma presentations, including comorbid conditions like personality disorders, dissociative disorders, and severe affective dysregulation. This may require additional care and pacing when using Clinical EFT.

A Typical Session of EFT for PTSD for Military

With military trauma however, EFT can be applied more directly to the specific traumatic deployment experiences (assuming these are single, time limited experiences), provided the individual has adequate emotional regulation capacities and existing relational resources. Here is a typical example.

John, a 35-year-old veteran who served in a combat zone, presents for a Clinical EFT session to address his PTSD symptoms stemming from a single traumatic event during his deployment. He struggles with intrusive memories, hypervigilance, and emotional numbness following an intense firefight where he witnessed the deaths of fellow soldiers.

For years, he has grappled with the debilitating effects of this trauma, including vivid flashbacks of the combat scene, exaggerated startle responses, and difficulties experiencing positive emotions or feeling connected to loved ones. Despite his best efforts, John has tried various evidence-based therapies, such as CBT and EMDR, with limited long-term success.

While these treatments provided some initial relief, he found that the benefits were often short-lived, and he continued to experience distressing intrusive memories, heightened arousal, and emotional constriction that significantly impacted his daily functioning and relationships. John's trauma response appears to be primarily focused on the single high-impact event during his deployment, rather than stemming from prolonged or repeated traumatic exposures.

Unlike individuals with complex trauma histories from childhood abuse or multiple deployments, John's relatively stable developmental background and sense of self prior to this event may allow for more focused trauma processing using an exposure-based approach like Clinical EFT. His existing attachment and relational capacities could also serve as resources in his recovery process.

Setup Statement. During the EFT session, the therapist guided John through a setup statement focusing on the specific traumatic incident he encountered during deployment. Based on the intake information and John's presenting concern, the therapist suggested he state:

"Even though I was in that firefight on that day in Iraq, and felt completely overwhelmed and helpless, I deeply and completely accept myself."

The emotions of feeling overwhelmed and helpless were rated by John as a 9 out of 10. At times, John did not want to speak out loud about the traumatic event, and he just thought about it, stayed present to it like he was watching the movie on a movie screen, while he kept tapping.

Reminder Phrases. For John's specific incident, reminder phrases for the rounds of tapping included:

"That firefight was terrifying."

"I felt overwhelmed and helpless."

"The memories of that moment haunt me still."

John engaged in 15 rounds of tapping in the first session, just focusing on the feelings of overwhelm and helplessness. He felt calmer and left the session. In between sessions John was asked to just use the tap and breathe process, to stay regulated without focussing on any specific events. When he returned the following week, the therapist enquired about any differences and asked him to retell the story of that incident (in order to check his reactions). John was calm as he retold the events of that day, but said he noticed himself thinking about a particular aspect of the event during the week. He started to feel guilty that he was alive, but that others had died that day. The guilt was as high as 8 out of 10 during the week.

The therapist suggested John tap with these words:

"Even though I now feel guilty that I am alive and my friends died that day, I accept this is how I feel."

John mentioned he had a lump in his throat and this was added to the setup statement: *"Even though I now feel guilty that I am alive, and I can feel a lump in my throat, when I think of my friends who died that day, I accept this is how I feel."*

Reminder Phrases included:

"This lump in my throat."

"I feel so guilty."

"This overwhelming guilt that I am alive."

While the guilt subsided related to this incident and notion that he was alive, and others were not, John started to think about feeling guilty during other times in life. The reported that was a common reaction he had throughout life., to many events and situations where he may not have done something he thought he should. The common thread here was the feeling of guilt, not the type of event, and the therapist systematically helped John tap on those events one at a time over the next few sessions, on the general theme of guilt.

After six sessions, John ceased his sessions, reporting a significant decrease in the frequency and intensity of intrusive memories related to the traumatic firefight. As well as feelings of guilt. He felt a greater sense of calm and relaxation in life generally (and his wife reported this too), and he was managing his feelings more effectively. Ultimately, John experienced a renewed sense of hope and optimism for the future.

When asked why he thought the six sessions of EFT may have assisted with his symptoms more effectively than the other therapies he tried, John shared:

"You know, after trying CBT and PE for my PTSD, I was really struggling to find lasting relief from the intrusive memories, hypervigilance, and emotional numbness I was experiencing. Those therapies helped a bit at first, but the benefits always seemed to fade over time.

When I started Clinical EFT, a few things really stood out to me. First off, the fact that it incorporates physical tapping along with the mental and emotional work was huge. By tapping on those acupressure points, it felt like I was addressing the physical stress and tension in my body that was so tied to my trauma. CBT and PE didn't really tackle that somatic side of things.

Secondly, the pace of progress with EFT was really rapid compared to the other therapies. In just six sessions, my symptom levels had dropped significantly.

Another big factor was learning the tapping techniques myself. Having that self-help tool to use whenever I needed it made me feel so much more in control and empowered to manage my symptoms on my own. The other therapies relied more heavily on the therapist guiding the process.

Overall, EFT just seemed to hit the nail on the head for me in a comprehensive way that CBT and PE couldn't quite manage. It gave me the lasting symptom relief I had been searching for."

The Research and Evidence

In order to make informed decisions about integrating new and emerging approaches such as Clinical EFT into their practice, clinicians often seek the research and evidence for several important reasons:

1. **Efficacy and Outcomes:** The primary concern for clinicians is whether a new therapy is effective in treating the targeted conditions or symptoms. Robust research evidence, particularly from randomized controlled trials (RCTs) and meta-analyses, provides valuable insights into the efficacy of new approaches.
2. **Comparison to Existing Therapies:** Clinicians need to understand how a new therapy like EFT compares to existing evidence-based treatments.
3. **Mechanisms of Action:** Understanding the underlying mechanisms of action may be important for clinicians to appreciate how a therapy works and its potential applications.

4. **Treatment Duration and Adherence:** Clinicians are interested in the time and resources required for a therapy to be effective, as well as patient adherence rates.
5. **Long-term Outcomes:** Clinicians need to know if the benefits of a therapy are sustainable over time.

The remaining section of this chapter is dedicated to a brief overview of these areas, but is not essential knowledge for the application of EFT.

Effectiveness of Clinical EFT for PTSD

The effectiveness of Clinical EFT for PTSD has been investigated in a variety of demographic groups including war veterans, victims of sexual violence, the spouses of PTSD sufferers, motor accident survivors, prisoners, hospital patients, adolescents, and survivors of natural and human-caused disasters (Feinstein, 2022b). Improvements in comorbid conditions such anxiety and depression, have been noted after treatment of PTSD (Church, 2013; Church et al., 2018), and adaptability to online and telemedicine applications have been successful (Sebastian & Nelms, 2017).

The research highlights significant physiological improvements after Clinical EFT interventions. A study by Bach et al. (2019) found decreases in subjective ratings of pain (-57%) and cravings (-74%), while happiness increased (+31%) after EFT training. Objective measures also showed improvements in resting heart rate (-8%), cortisol levels (-37%), blood pressure (systolic -6%, diastolic -8%), and salivary immunoglobulin A, a marker of immune function (+113%).

Several studies have examined the effects of EFT on gene expression, cortisol, and brain activity using functional MRI (fMRI). Differential expression of genes associated with processes like cancer suppression, immunity, neural plasticity, and oxidative stress reduction was observed after EFT (Church et al., 2018; Maharaj, 2016). EFT led to reduced cortisol levels compared to controls (Church et al., 2012; Stapleton et al., 2020), indicating its effectiveness in reducing stress.

fMRI studies showed decreased activation in brain areas related to cravings and hunger after EFT for obesity (Stapleton et al., 2019). In chronic pain patients, EFT decreased connectivity between brain regions involved in pain modulation and catastrophizing (Stapleton, 2022). Imagining tapping during fMRI led to downregulation of brain areas processing fear and disgust (Wittfoth et al., 2020, 2022).

Overall, the research suggests Clinical EFT can positively impact the autonomic nervous system.

Comparisons to Other Therapies

While many individual studies exist comparing Clinical EFT to other therapies, including gold standards, the focus here is on the meta-analyses.

Anxiety and Depression

One meta-analysis (Clond, 2016) focused on 14 RCTs using EFT for anxiety (n=658) and found a large effect size (Cohen's d = 1.23) compared to controls like progressive muscle relaxation, diaphragmatic breathing, and CBT. Notably, EFT produced superior treatment effects to these combined controls.

For depression, a meta-analysis of 20 studies (Nelms & Castel, 2016) indicated a large pre-post effect size (Cohen's d = 1.85) in RCTs (n=398) and outcome studies (n=461, d = 0.70). Follow-up effect sizes remained substantial at less than 90 days (d = 1.21) and 90 days or more (d = 1.11). EFT outperformed diaphragmatic breathing and supportive interviews and was comparable to EMDR. Importantly, the post-test effect size for EFT (d = 1.31) exceeded those reported in meta-analyses of antidepressant drug trials and traditional psychotherapy studies.

PTSD

Two meta-analyses have examined Clinical EFT for PTSD. The first (Sebastian & Nelms, 2017) analyzed seven studies and found a large pre-to-post treatment effect (d = 2.96) compared to usual care or waitlist controls. EFT outcomes were achieved in just 4-10 sessions, with a mean dropout rate below 10%. Notably, there were no significant differences in treatment effects when comparing EFT to other evidence-based therapies like EMDR and CBT.

The second meta-analysis (Stapleton et al., 2023) excluded two studies due to methodological issues and examined four trials comparing EFT to untreated controls and three trials comparing EFT to active treatment controls. Against untreated controls, EFT demonstrated large effect sizes (Hedge's g = 1.38 to 2.51), with highly statistically significant fixed and random effect summary estimates (g = 1.86 and 1.88, respectively). When compared to active controls like CBT, EMDR, and Narrative Exposure Therapy, effect sizes ranged from -0.15 to 0.79, indicating comparable treatment outcomes.

Adherence: Cost Effectiveness

The cost-effectiveness of a therapy is closely related to adherence for clients in several ways. Therapies that can produce significant improvements in fewer sessions are generally more cost-effective and have lower dropout rates. Clinical EFT has a mean dropout rate of less than 10% across PTSD studies, suggesting that clients are more likely to adhere to and complete the treatment (Libretto et al., 2015). In the case of John, his outcomes were achieved in 6 sessions, and for Sarah, she continued for 12 sessions to address multiple childhood traumatic events.

It is noted that the research indicates a six to 10 session protocol to treat PTSD with Clinical EFT, thus suggesting it is viable cost-effective treatment. A 2019 network meta-analysis of psychological and psychosocial interventions for children and young people with PTSD (Mavranezouli et al., 2019) examined 32 trials of 17 interventions (n=2260) that included trauma-focused CBT (TF-CBT), EMDR, and talk therapy. EFT was included in the combined somatic/cognitive therapies category, and was second most effective, to cognitive therapy for PTSD. The authors noted a large positive effect for EFT in particular, for these children and young people.

A second network meta-analysis for adults by the same team (Mavranezouli et al., 2020a) examined 90 trials and 22 interventions (n=6560). EMDR was the most effective at reducing symptoms and improving remission rates in adults with PTSD, but the combined somatic/cognitive therapies were second (with TF-CBT being third). Furthermore, a decision-analytic model comparing costs and quality-adjusted life-years indicated EMDR to be the most cost-effective intervention for adults with PTSD (with a probability of 0.34 amongst the 11 evaluated options at a cost-effectiveness threshold of £20,000/QALY), followed by combined somatic/cognitive therapies (Mavranezouli et al., 2020b). These independent reviews highlight the growing evidence and cost effectiveness of mind-body, somatic interventions treatments in addressing PTSD in children, young people and adults.

Proposed Physiological Mechanisms of Action

Emerging research provides insights into the potential physiological mechanisms underlying the effects of acupoint stimulation used in Clinical EFT. Studies using ultrasound and tracer dye injections suggest that acupuncture points and meridians may coincide with connective tissue planes and pathways in the body (de Vernejoul et al., 1992; Langevin & Yandow, 2002). The primo vascular system (PVS), a previously unknown system integrating features of the cardiovascular, nervous, immune, and hormonal systems, has been proposed as a physical substrate for acupuncture points and meridians (Stefanov et al., 2013).

Investigations into the electrical properties of acupoints have found differences in electrical resistance (Li et al., 2012), suggesting that mechanosensory transduction, where cells convert stimuli like tapping into electrical activity (Gillespie & Walker, 2001), may play a role. Collagen, highly concentrated in the body's interstitial tissue, has been proposed as a semi-conductor that allows rapid transmission of these electrical impulses, offering a potential anatomical explanation for the action of acupoint stimulation (Church et al., 2018).

Furthermore, a meta-analysis of six studies (n=403) comparing Clinical EFT protocols that included acupoint tapping with protocols using substitute activities (e.g., sham tapping or breathing exercises) found a large treatment effect for the full Clinical EFT protocol (Cohen's d = 1.28) and a moderate effect superior to controls (d = -0.47) (Church et al., 2018). These findings suggest that acupressure stimulation, or tapping, is an active ingredient in Clinical EFT, rather than solely attributable to placebo or non-specific therapy effects.

While more research is needed, these studies provide insights into the potential physiological mechanisms underlying the effects of Clinical EFT, including the involvement of connective tissue pathways, electrical signaling, and the specific contribution of acupoint stimulation.

Long Term Outcomes

Therapies that produce durable, long-lasting improvements are more cost-effective in the long run, as clients may not require additional treatment or incur further costs for managing their condition. nervous system, gene expression, cortisol levels, brain activity, and psychological symptoms. The effects of Clinical EFT appear durable, with follow-up periods ranging from one month to 2 years across various conditions (Feinstein, 2022a).

Acceptance as a PTSD Treatment

As an empirically validated, cost-effective therapy, Clinical EFT is recommended for clinicians treating PTSD, and is now included in conventional intervention programs, such as the *Warrior Combat Stress Reset Program* at Fort Hood, the largest US military base, using EFT and EMDR for the treatment of PTSD (Zhang, 2015). The BlueKnot Foundation included EFT in the 2019 Practice Guidelines for Clinical Treatment of Complex Trauma in Australia (Kezelman et al., 2019), and The National Institute for Health and Care Excellence in the United Kingdom has now indicated EFT is part of a "Combined Somatic and Cognitive Therapies" category that is a research priority for PTSD (Church et al., 2018).

While traditional sessions and many clinical trials focus on individual sessions, group applied EFT has been found to be effective in the treatment of PTSD and this is promising if cost and access necessitate group intervention (Bach et al., 2019). Group EFT has been applied where individual sessions are impractical (e.g., refugee camps, with earthquake survivors, education settings, hospital inpatient wards; Church & House, 2018) and still found to be effective. It appears the concept of borrowing benefits may be responsible for these significant outcomes from group EFT (Church & House, 2018). Borrowing benefits describes where participants in a group setting self-apply EFT while watching a demonstration or volunteer in front of the group who works with a therapist. It was first documented in an EFT 3-day workshop (n=102 people; Rowe, 2005). Participants completed a psychological symptom checklist one month prior to the workshop, immediately before starting, and 1- and 6-months afterwards. The 1- and 6-month follow-up indicated significant improvements in global psychological distress even though attendees only watched the EFT demonstrations on stage. Mirror neurons have been proposed as a possible explanation, and have been directly observed in primate species (Ramachandran, 1995).

Finally, while much of the research presented have been executed with universities, hospitals, and clinics, and published in English-language journals, there is a body of work published in non-English-language journals (Freedom et al., 2022). Many of these studies have been undertaken in primary care settings suggesting that EFT is available in many countries. This 2022 review identified 91 research studies on acupoint tapping not identified in standard Western databases (71% in Indonesia) and EFT was used in 47% of the studies. The remaining studies used "Spiritual EFT" (SEFT), a variation developed in Indonesia combining tapping with spiritual affirmations from the Quran.

7 Reasons Clinical EFT is Suitable for PTSD

A 2017 review (Church & Feinstein, 2017) of Clinical EFT for PTSD with a focus on veterans and service members indicated it is especially suitable for veterans and military for these seven reasons:

[Design: set as numbered list, 1–7]

- The depth and breadth of treatment effects
- The relatively brief time frames required for successful treatment
- The low risk of adverse events
- The minimal training time required for the approach to be applied effectively

- The simultaneous reduction of physical and psychological symptoms
- The utility and cost-effectiveness of Clinical EFT in a large-group format
- The method's adaptability to online and telemedicine applications

As a result of published research and clinical trials examining Clinical EFT for PTSD and a detailed practitioner survey, Clinical Guidelines have been published based on a stepped care approach (see Church et al., 2018) and the reader is courage to explore further.

The Final Stories

Sarah completed 12 EFT sessions, addressing multiple childhood events related to the emotional trauma and neglect she experienced growing up. Remarkably, due to a generalization effect - a phenomenon where resolving some specific traumatic events results in other events with a similar emotional signature also decreasing in intensity - Sarah did not need to process every single childhood incident.

As she worked through the most significant memories using EFT, she noticed a profound shift occurring. The overwhelming sense of fear, shame, and worthlessness that had permeated her entire being began to dissipate. Memories that were once paralyzing lost their intense emotional charge, allowing her to finally start shedding the weight of her past.

Empowered by this newfound emotional freedom, Sarah made the courageous decision to return to full-time study as a mature-aged adult, pursuing her long-held dream of becoming an architect. With a renewed sense of determination and self-belief, she immersed herself in her studies, excelling academically and ultimately achieving her degree.

Her personal life also blossomed in ways she had never imagined possible. Having worked through the deep-seated abandonment wounds from her childhood, Sarah found herself able to fully open her heart and enter into her second marriage - this time, with a profound sense of security and trust in herself and her partner. Upon graduating, Sarah secured employment at a prestigious local architecture firm, where her talents and passion for design quickly propelled her career. As she thrived in her professional life, she carried with her a deep sense of gratitude for the transformative power of EFT.

For John too, the intrusive memories from that fateful firefight, which had haunted him relentlessly since returning from deployment, began to lose their grip. Most significantly, John found himself rediscovering his ability to experience positive emotions and reconnect with loved ones on a deeper level. He celebrated 35 years of marriage with his wife, and found himself engaged at work as a cabinet maker, and handled the demands of his job with greater ease and resilience. He also found a deeper connection with his own parents and siblings, and was able to share about his deployment experiences.

FUTURE DIRECTIONS AND CONCLUSION

Future directions and examination of EFT will involve larger rigorous clinical trials, more comparative studies with established therapies such as CBT and EMDR, and replication attempts. It may be that the near future takes a personalized approach to psychological care, and combination approaches such as EFT being included in traditional talk therapy settings, become mainstream. The integration of mind-body practices in therapy may well become a pivotal aspect of trauma recovery in the future and more patients like Sarah and John will benefit. The research to date indicates EFT protocols are effective in treating various clinical conditions, indicate rapid results compared to conventional treatments, provide lasting benefits, induce changes in biological markers that align with clients' subjective assessments, and modulate arousal in specific brain regions. The research behind Clinical EFT supports effectiveness for PTSD, both at a psychological and also physiological level. Treatment outcomes are comparable to gold standard approaches, just achieved in half the time and therefore cost.

REFERENCES

American Psychological Association. (2017). *Clinical practice guideline for the treatment of Posttraumatic Stress Disorder (PTSD) in adults*. Retrieved December 30, 2023, from https://www.apa.org/ptsd-guideline

Bach, D., Groesbeck, G., Stapleton, P., Sims, R., Blickheuser, K., & Church, D. (2019). Clinical EFT (emotional freedom techniques) improves multiple physiological markers of health. *Journal of Evidence-Based Integrative Medicine, 24*, 2515690X18823691. DOI: 10.1177/2515690X18823691

Blevins, C. A., Weathers, F. W., Davis, M. T., Witte, T. K., & Domino, J. L. (2015). The Posttraumatic Stress Disorder Checklist for DSM-5 (PCL-5): Development and initial psychometric evaluation. *Journal of Traumatic Stress*, 28(6), 489–498. DOI: 10.1002/jts.22059 PMID: 26606250

Church, D. (2013). Clinical EFT as an evidence-based practice for the treatment of psychological and physiological conditions. *Psychology (Irvine, Calif.)*, 4(8), 645–654. DOI: 10.4236/psych.2013.48092

Church, D., & Feinstein, D. (2017). The manual stimulation of acupuncture points in the treatment of post-traumatic stress disorder: A review of clinical emotional freedom techniques. *Medical Acupuncture*, 29(4), 249–253. DOI: 10.1089/acu.2017.1213 PMID: 28874920

Church, D., & House, D. (2018). Borrowing benefits: Group treatment with clinical emotional freedom techniques is associated with simultaneous reductions in Posttraumatic Stress Disorder, anxiety, and depression symptoms. *Journal of Evidence-based Integrative Medicine*, 23, 2156587218756510. DOI: 10.1177/2156587218756510 PMID: 29468884

Church, D., Stapleton, P., Mollon, P., Feinstein, D., Boath, E., Mackay, D., & Sims, R. (2018). Guidelines for the treatment of PTSD using clinical EFT (emotional freedom techniques). *Healthcare (Basel)*, 6(4), 146. DOI: 10.3390/healthcare6040146 PMID: 30545069

Church, D., Stapleton, P., Vasudevan, A., & O'Keefe, T. (2022). Clinical EFT as an evidence-based practice for the treatment of psychological and physiological conditions: A systematic review. *Frontiers in Psychology*, 13, 951451. DOI: 10.3389/fpsyg.2022.951451 PMID: 36438382

Church, D., Stapleton, P., Yang, A., & Gallo, F. (2018). Is tapping on acupuncture points an active ingredient in emotional freedom techniques? A systematic review and meta-analysis of comparative studies. *The Journal of Nervous and Mental Disease*, 206(10), 783–793. DOI: 10.1097/NMD.0000000000000878 PMID: 30273275

Church, D., Stern, S., Boath, E., Stewart, A., Feinstein, D., & Clond, M. (2017). Emotional freedom techniques to treat Posttraumatic Stress Disorder in veterans: Review of the evidence, survey of practitioners, and proposed clinical guidelines. *The Permanente Journal*, 21(4), 16–100. DOI: 10.7812/TPP/16-100 PMID: 28678690

Church, D., Yount, G., & Brooks, A. J. (2012). The effect of emotional freedom techniques on stress biochemistry: A randomized controlled trial. *The Journal of Nervous and Mental Disease*, 200(10), 891–896. DOI: 10.1097/NMD.0b013e31826b-9fc1 PMID: 22986277

Church, D., Yount, G., Rachlin, K., Fox, L., & Nelms, J. (2018). Epigenetic effects of PTSD remediation in veterans using clinical emotional freedom techniques: A randomized controlled pilot study. *American Journal of Health Promotion*, 32(1), 112–122. DOI: 10.1177/0890117116661154 PMID: 27520015

Clond, M. (2016). Emotional freedom techniques for anxiety: A systematic review with meta-analysis. *The Journal of Nervous and Mental Disease*, 204(5), 388–395. DOI: 10.1097/NMD.0000000000000483 PMID: 26894319

de Vernejoul, P., Albarède, P., & Darras, J. C. (1992). Nuclear medicine and acupuncture message transmission. *Journal of Nuclear Medicine: Official publication, Society of Nuclear Medicine, 33*(3), 409–412.

Di Rienzo, F., Saruco, E., Church, D., Daligault, S., Delpuech, C., Gurret, J. M., & Guillot, A. (2019). Neuropsychological correlates of an energy psychology intervention on flight phobia: A MEG single-case study. *OSF Preprints,* https://doi.org/ DOI: 10.31234/osf.io/s3hce

Feinstein, D. (2022a). The energy of energy psychology. *OBM Integrative and Complimentary Medicine*, 7(2), 1–32. DOI: 10.21926/obm.icm.2202015 PMID: 35548526

Feinstein, D. (2022b). Uses of energy psychology following catastrophic events. *Frontiers in Psychology*, 13, 856209. DOI: 10.3389/fpsyg.2022.856209 PMID: 35548526

Feinstein, D. (2023). Integrating the manual stimulation of acupuncture points into psychotherapy: A systematic review with clinical recommendations. *Journal of Psychotherapy Integration*, 33(1), 47–67. Advance online publication. DOI: 10.1037/int0000283

Fournier, J. C., DeRubeis, R. J., Hollon, S. D., Dimidjian, S., Amsterdam, J. D., Shelton, R. C., & Fawcett, J. (2010). Antidepressant drug effects and depression severity: A patient-level meta-analysis. *Journal of the American Medical Association*, 303(1), 47–53. DOI: 10.1001/jama.2009.1943 PMID: 20051569

Freedom, J., Hux, M., & Warner, J. (2022). Research on acupoint tapping therapies proliferating around the world. *Energy Psychology*, 4(1), 22–37. Advance online publication. DOI: 10.9769/EPJ.2022.14.1.JF

Gillespie, P. G., & Walker, R. G. (2001). Molecular basis of mechanosensory transduction. *Nature*, 413(6852), 194–202. DOI: 10.1038/35093011 PMID: 11557988

Helbig, S., & Fehm, L. (2004). Problems with homework in CBT: Rare exception or rather frequent? *Behavioural and Cognitive Psychotherapy*, 32(3), 291–301. DOI: 10.1017/S1352465804001365

Hoskins, O. P., & Lewis, C. (2023). Post-traumatic stress disorder: Symptoms, diagnosis and treatment. *BMJ Best Practice*. Retrieved December 30, 2023, from https://bestpractice.bmj.com/topics/en-gb/430

Kaczkurkin, A. N., & Foa, E. B. (2015). Cognitive-behavioral therapy for anxiety disorders: An update on the empirical evidence. *Current Psychiatry Reports*, 17(3), 337–346. https://www.ncbi.nlm.nih.gov/pmc/articles/PMC4610618/ PMID: 26487814

Kar, N. (2011). Cognitive behavioral therapy for the treatment of post-traumatic stress disorder: A review. *Neuropsychiatric Disease and Treatment*, 7, 167–181. DOI: 10.2147/NDT.S10389 PMID: 21552319

Kazantzis, N., Deane, F. P., & Ronan, K. R. (2000). Homework assignments in cognitive and behavioral therapy: A meta-analysis. *Clinical Psychology : a Publication of the Division of Clinical Psychology of the American Psychological Association*, 7(2), 189–202. DOI: 10.1093/clipsy.7.2.189

Kezelman, C., & Stavropoulos, P. (Eds.). (2019). *Practice guidelines for clinical treatment of complex trauma*. Blue Knot Foundation. https://aztrauma.org/wp-content/uploads/2020/11/BlueKnot_Practice_Guidelines_2019.pdf

Kim, S. H., Schneider, S. M., Kravitz, L., Mermier, C., & Burge, M. R. (2013). Mind-body practices for posttraumatic stress disorder. *Journal of Investigative Medicine*, 61(5), 827–834. DOI: 10.2310/JIM.0b013e3182906862 PMID: 23609463

Langevin, H. M., & Yandow, J. A. (2002). Relationship of acupuncture points and meridians to connective tissue planes. *The Anatomical Record*, 269(6), 257–265. DOI: 10.1002/ar.10185 PMID: 12467083

Li, J., Wang, Q., Liang, H., Dong, H., Li, Y., Ng, E. H., & Wu, X. (2012). Biophysical characteristics of meridians and acupoints: A systematic review. *Evidence-Based Complementary and Alternative Medicine*, 793841, 1–6. Advance online publication. DOI: 10.1155/2012/793841 PMID: 23346214

Maharaj, M. (2016). Differential gene expression after Emotional Freedom Techniques (EFT) treatment: A novel pilot protocol for salivary mRNA assessment. *Energy Psychology*, 8(1), 17–32. DOI: 10.9769/EPJ.2016.8.1.MM

Mann, S. K., & Marwaha, R. (2023). Posttraumatic stress disorder. In *StatPearls*. StatPearls Publishing., https://www.ncbi.nlm.nih.gov/books/NBK559129/

Mausbach, B. T., Moore, R., Roesch, S., Cardenas, V., & Patterson, T. L. (2010). The relationship between homework compliance and therapy outcomes: An updated meta-analysis. *Cognitive Therapy and Research*, 34(5), 429–438. DOI: 10.1007/s10608-010-9297-z PMID: 20930925

Mavranezouli, I., Megnin-Viggars, O., Daly, C., Dias, S., Stockton, S., Meiser-Stedman, R., Trickey, D., & Pilling, S. (2019). Psychological and psychosocial treatments for children and young people with post-traumatic stress disorder: A network meta-analysis. *Journal of Child Psychology and Psychiatry, and Allied Disciplines*, 61(1), 18–29. DOI: 10.1111/jcpp.13094 PMID: 31313834

Mavranezouli, I., Megnin-Viggars, O., Daly, C., Dias, S., Welton, N. J., Stockton, S., Bhutani, G., Grey, N., Leach, J., Greenberg, N., Katona, C., El-Leithy, S., & Pilling, S. (2020). Psychological treatments for post-traumatic stress disorder in adults: A network meta-analysis. *Psychological Medicine*, 50(4), 542–555. DOI: 10.1017/S0033291720000070 PMID: 32063234

Mavranezouli, I., Megnin-Viggars, O., Grey, N., Bhutani, G., Leach, J., Daly, C., Dias, S., Welton, N. J., Katona, C., El-Leithy, S., Greenberg, N., Stockton, S., & Pilling, S. (2020). Cost-effectiveness of psychological treatments for post-traumatic stress disorder in adults. *PLoS One*, 15(4), e0232245. DOI: 10.1371/journal.pone.0232245 PMID: 32353011

McEwen, B. S. (2000). Allostasis and allostatic load: Implications for neuropsychopharmacology. *Neuropsychopharmacology*, 22(2), 108–124. DOI: 10.1016/S0893-133X(99)00129-3 PMID: 10649824

National Institutes of Health. (2021). *Post-traumatic stress disorder (PTSD) 2023.* Retrieved 23rd December 2023, https://hr.nih.gov/working-nih/civil/post-traumatic-stress-disorder-ptsd-2023

Nelms, J. A., & Castel, L. (2016). A systematic review and meta-analysis of randomized and nonrandomized trials of clinical emotional freedom techniques (EFT) for the treatment of depression. *Explore (New York, N.Y.)*, 12(6), 416–426. DOI: 10.1016/j.explore.2016.08.001 PMID: 27843054

Niles, B. L., Mori, D. L., Polizzi, C., Pless Kaiser, A., Weinstein, E. S., Gershkovich, M., & Wang, C. (2018). A systematic review of randomized trials of mind-body interventions for PTSD. *Journal of Clinical Psychology*, 74(9), 1485–1508. DOI: 10.1002/jclp.22634 PMID: 29745422

Ramachandran, V. (1995). Mirror neurons and imitation learning as the driving force behind the great leap forward in human evolution. Retrieved f2nd March 2024 from https://www.edge.org/conversation/vilayanur_ramachandran-mirror-neurons-and-imitation-learning-as-the-driving-force

Rowe, J. (2005). The effects of EFT on long-term psychological symptoms. *Counseling and Clinical Psychology Journal*, 2(3), 104.

Schrader, C., & Ross, A. (2021). A review of PTSD and current treatment strategies. *Annals of Clinical Psychiatry*, 33(6), 546–551. https://www.ncbi.nlm.nih.gov/pmc/articles/PMC8672952/ PMID: 34924624

Schulz, K. M. (2007). Integrating energy psychology into treatment for adult survivors of childhood sexual abuse: An exploratory clinical study from the therapist's perspective. *Dissertation Abstracts International. B, The Sciences and Engineering*, 68(1-B), 635.

Sebastian, B., & Nelms, J. (2017). The effectiveness of emotional freedom techniques in the treatment of posttraumatic stress disorder: A meta-analysis. *Explore (New York, N.Y.)*, 13(1), 16–25. DOI: 10.1016/j.explore.2016.10.001 PMID: 27889444

Stapleton, P., Baumann, O., O'Keefe, T., & Bhuta, S. (2022). Neural changes after emotional freedom techniques treatment for chronic pain sufferers. *Complementary Therapies in Clinical Practice*, 53, 101653. DOI: 10.1016/j.ctcp.2022.101653 PMID: 35933806

Stapleton, P., Buchan, C., Mitchell, I., McGrath, Y., Gorton, P., & Carter, B. (2019). An initial investigation of neural changes in overweight adults with food cravings after emotional freedom techniques. *OBM Integrative and Complementary Medicine, 4*(1), 010. DOI: 10.21926/obm.icm.1901010

Stapleton, P., Crighton, G., Sabot, D., & O'Neill, H. M. (2020). Reexamining the effect of emotional freedom techniques on stress biochemistry: A randomized controlled trial. *Traumatology*, 26(12), 869–877. DOI: 10.1037/tra0000563 PMID: 32162958

Stapleton, P., Kip, K., Church, D., Toussaint, L., Footman, J., Ballantyne, P., & O'Keefe, T. (2023). Emotional freedom techniques for treating posttraumatic stress disorder: An updated systematic review and meta-analysis. *Frontiers in Psychology*, 14, 1195286. DOI: 10.3389/fpsyg.2023.1195286 PMID: 37637920

Steenkamp, M. M., Litz, B. T., Hoge, C. W., & Marmar, C. R. (2015). Psychotherapy for military-related PTSD: A review of randomized clinical trials. *Journal of the American Medical Association*, 314(5), 489–500. DOI: 10.1001/jama.2015.8370 PMID: 26241600

Stefanov, M., Potroz, M., Kim, J., Lim, J., Cha, R., & Nam, M.-H. (2013). The primo vascular system as a new anatomical system. *Journal of Acupuncture and Meridian Studies*, 6(6), 331–338. DOI: 10.1016/j.jams.2013.10.001 PMID: 24290797

Streeter, C. C., Gerbarg, P. L., Saper, R. B., Ciraulo, D. A., & Brown, R. P. (2012). Effects of yoga on the autonomic nervous system, gamma-aminobutyric-acid, and allostasis in epilepsy, depression, and post-traumatic stress disorder. *Medical Hypotheses*, 78(5), 571–579. DOI: 10.1016/j.mehy.2012.01.021 PMID: 22365651

Veterans Affairs. (n.d.). Retrieved December 30, 2023, from https://www.ptsd.va.gov/understand/common/common_adults.asp

Wittfoth, D., Beise, J., Manuel, J., Bohne, M., & Wittfoth, M. (2022). Bifocal emotion regulation through acupoint tapping in fear of flying. *NeuroImage. Clinical*, 34, 102996. DOI: 10.1016/j.nicl.2022.102996 PMID: 35378497

Wittfoth, D., Pfeiffer, A., Bohne, M., Lanfermann, H., & Wittfoth, M. (2020). Emotion regulation through bifocal processing of fear-inducing and disgust-inducing stimuli. *BMC Neuroscience*, 21(1), 47. DOI: 10.1186/s12868-020-00597-x PMID: 33225884

Wolpe, J. (1969). *The practice of behavior therapy*. Pergamon Press.

Yount, G., Church, D., Rachlin, K., Blickheuser, K., & Cardonna, I. (2019). Do noncoding RNAs mediate the efficacy of energy psychology? *Global Advances in Health and Medicine : Improving Healthcare Outcomes Worldwide*, 8, 2164956119832500. DOI: 10.1177/2164956119832500 PMID: 30828482

Zhang, S. L., Hilton, L., & Gordon, W. (2015). Effects of integrative PTSD treatment in a military health setting. *Energy Psychology Journal*, 7(2). Advance online publication. DOI: 10.9769/EPJ.2015.11.1.SL

Chapter 8

The Search for the Sacred in a Traumatized Population:

An Investigation of the Impact of Spirituality on Posttraumatic Stress

Perella Perlstein
https://orcid.org/0009-0001-1063-3923
Perella Perlstein Therapeutic Services, USA

ABSTRACT

The chapter examines the role of spirituality and meaning in the aftermath of trauma. The chapter focuses on the variables that promote PTG and on the specific impact of spirituality and meaning. The chapter reviews PTG research results in multiple clinical settings, e.g., clinical psychotherapy centers and hospitals. The chapter conclude with a brief section on clinical applications. The goal of the chapter is to expand awareness of the necessity of spiritual resources into the assessment phase of treatment (e.g., assessment of client strengths and resources) and in the use of, whenever appropriate, a cognitive framework of spirituality in the treatment phase. Cognitive modification of posttraumatic expectations and infusion of meaning can support installation of hope in the face of trauma and tragedy.

DOI: 10.4018/979-8-3693-2089-1.ch008

INTRODUCTION

He who has a why to live can bear any how (Nietzsche, 1889).

In recent years, the ever-expansive body of posttraumatic stress disorder (PTSD) literature has evolved to accommodate the clinical needs of traumatized populations. Traditional treatment methods, e.g., Prolonged Exposure (PE; Foa et al., 2013) have been complimented by less traditional, but also promising methods, e.g., Transcranial Magnetic Stimulation (TMS; Harris & Reece, 2021) and equine-assisted therapy (Nelson et al., 2022). Similarly, whereas at the turn of the 21st century, the psychopathology model of human behavior largely dominated, the benefits of Positive Psychology gradually became recognized by practitioners (Lopez et al., 2018). The shift moved from a clinical model that emphasized human potential decay in the face of prolonged stress, to a model that supported human growth potential in the face of rising adversity.

The clinical application of the trend is best illustrated by the reorientation of the trauma research movement from a focus on posttraumatic stress, toward an interest in posttraumatic growth (PTG; Schubert et al., 2015). Tedeschi and Calhoun (1995) highlight the inherent need for trauma survivors to make their experience manageable, comprehensible, and therefore, *meaningful*. As such, spirituality and meaning, key players in the Positive Psychology arena, have emerged as significant moderators in the promotion of PTG.

Chapter Objectives and Goals

Cognitive modification of posttraumatic expectations and infusion of meaning can support installation of hope in the face of trauma and tragedy (Ehler & Clark, 2000). The goal of the chapter is to expand awareness of the necessity to incorporate spiritual resources into the assessment phase of treatment, and in the use, when deemed appropriate, of a cognitive framework for spirituality in the treatment phase. The chapter examines the role of spirituality and meaning in the aftermath of trauma and investigates their mediating contributions to PTG. The overall landscape of clinical theory and practice, predominately secular, has had limited use for spirituality and traditional metaphysical processes (Shafranske & Cummings, 2013). Clinical research has either ignored or oversimplified the role of spirituality and religion in daily living (Pargament, 1997), and has consequently limited their utility in clinical practice. For the significant segment of the population who regard religion and spirituality as significant sources of strength and coping, the omission of religion and spirituality is limiting at best, and negligent at worst (Pargament & Exline, 2022). As such, research results of PTG, as applied in multiple clinical settings, such as clinical psychotherapy centers and hospitals, are evaluated. The chapter concludes with a section on applied clinical practice.

The 'Meaning' of Spirituality

In his opening to the seminal work, *Man's Search for Meaning,* Victor Frankl (1963) presents his challenge to Maslow's (1943) hierarchy of needs and highlights the need for *meaning* as a protective life factor. Frankl's struggles, to both make sense of his existence in a post-Holocaust era, and his recognition of the limitations of the then traditional theory of motivation as exemplified by Freud's (1904) drive theory and Watson's (1913) theory of radical behaviorism, led to his development of logotherapy (1963). In tandem with the impact of life events on his psychotheoretical metamorphosis, Frankl progresses from a description of his experiences in a Nazi death camp in the first half of *Man's Search for Meaning,* to the evolution of his theory of human behavior in the second half. Frankel's transcendence from the traditional psychoanalytic model to one that emphasizes meaning, reflects the eventual, gradual shift of the broader psychotherapeutic community to integrate *meaning* and *spiritual needs* into the model of human behavior.

Interestingly, Frankl's (1963)*search for meaning* correlates with Pargament and Mahoney's (2017) definition of spirituality, that is, *the search for the sacred.* Spirituality is defined as "that which allows a person to experience transcendent meaning in life, often expressed as a relationship with God, but can also be about nature, art, music, family, or community—whatever beliefs and values give a person a sense of meaning and purpose in life" (Puchalski & Romer, 2000, p. 129). One could argue that the search for meaning, or *logos,* lies at the center of spirituality, that is, the expansion of self in the face of the material world. In a recent podcast interview, leading academics Peter Atia and Arthur Brooks (November 2023) discuss some of the neuroscientific literature referencing happiness and meaning. Meaning, Brooks explains, is a composite of three main variables: *coherence,* that everything has a reason, *direction*, the endpoint of one's life journey, and *significance,* something of deep value.

The beginning of the 21st century saw the birth of Positive Psychology, a school of thought which emphasizes a model of growth, rather than pathology (Lopez et al., 2018). Prior to the shift, psychological research predominantly either ignored spirituality or reduced spirituality to basic underlying psychological, social, or physiological components in order to meet the functional analytic standards of behaviors (Pargament & Mahoney, 2017). As such, little attention was given to the study and application of spirituality and growth in the lab or in the therapy room.

Fortunately, the third of wave of psychotherapy, namely Dialectical Behavior Therapy (DBT; Linehan, 1993) and Acceptance and Commitment Therapy (ACT; Hayes & Lillis, 2012) are influenced by spiritual elements. Marcia Linehan (2020) used her personal experiences with Zen Buddhism to shape the Core Mindfulness module of DBT. Similarly, the iconic hexaflex of ACT (Harris, 2009) emphasizes core values in multiple life domains, such as in the life domain of spirituality.

Assessment and intervention to correct the individual's dissatisfaction of life domains, such as work, leisure, social relationships, and spirituality, lie at the center of clinical treatment (Harris, 2009). Clinical case conceptualization requires the thorough evaluation of the client's problems of daily living and attempts to solve those problems through client resources (Fink, 2009). The discrepancy between client resources and environmental demands is the apex of client stress; the magnitude of discrepancy between resources and environmental demands is the climax of trauma.

At its best, the material world offers comfort and protection; at worst, the material world unleashes existential threat and nihilism. Stress is one of the most familiar challenges to the sustenance of emotional and psychological well-being (Fink, 2009). Stress represents a discrepancy between an individual's resources and expectations. When one encounters stressful life events, his or her resources are challenged. Consequently, the individual must increase his or her resources (problem-focused coping) or modify expectations (emotion-focused coping). Spiritual resources, which include accessing spiritual leadership, prayer, mediation, and acts of loving kindness, as well as modification of expectations by reframing the negative stressors in meaningful and expansive ways, expand coping mechanisms and promote adaptive well-being (Lopez, 2018). In the case where stressors increase to the point of threatening serious physical or psychological harm or death to self or a close other, *trauma,* the stressor is elevated and thus, the need for resourcing must rise to meet the demand.

Posttraumatic Stress Disorder

A traumatic event constitutes the direct experience or witness of an event or series of events involving actual or threatened death or severe injury to self or others (American Psychological Association [APA] 2013). The traumatic experience then elicits a response of intense fear, helplessness, or terror (APA, 2013). Traumatic events are episodic events posing imminent harm or even death (Type I Trauma), or an on-going series of events which erode physical or psychological safety (Type

II Trauma). Regardless of the nature of the trauma, the individual's safety is compromised, and available resources are devoted to survival.

PTSD was originally added to the DSM-III (APA, 1980) as an anxiety disorder. Interestingly, in the traditional anxiety model, cognitive appraisal is focused on an impending threat. In contrast, in the case of PTSD, the individual's cognitive appraisal is largely centered on a *memory* of an event which has already transpired (Ehler & Clark, 2000). In the case of PTSD, the individual processes the traumatic event in a way that produces and maintains a sense of serious and consistent threat. Ehler and Clark suggest the process is mediated by the traumatized individual's excess attachments to negative cognitive appraisals of the traumatized event, as well as modified autobiographical memory. The modified autobiographical memory is dominated by limited elaboration and contextualization in conjunction with significant associative memory of the trauma and perceptual priming from the current environment. The role of cognitive elaboration suggests that the potential clinical benefit for cognitive reframing processes like hope and meaning, be utilized as a means of altering the impacts of past memory and current cognitive process. Furthermore, cognitive reframing of past events highlights the opportunity for elaboration of past memories and reintegration into the context of current and future experiences.

Aligned with the adaptive mechanisms of survival, one strives to make sense of the events, whereas the subjective interpretation of events often adds an additional layer of distress (Courtois, 2015). Emergence of metacognitions such as guilt (DSM V; APA, 2013) and shame (López-Castro, et. al., 2019) deepen posttraumatic reactions and gradual decay of the self in the aftermath of trauma. Helen Block Lewis's (1971) distinction between guilt (the attribution of a transgression or a perceived transgression *to a behavior*) and shame (the attribution of a transgression or a perceived transgression *to the self*) represent clinical application of cognitive interventions for PTSD sufferers.

A further clinical focus must concern the capacity for, or exploration of the failure to, derive meaning from one's experiences. Deficits in finding meaning from one's traumatic experiences have shown to exacerbate the development of PTSD (Cann et al., 2011). In addition to managing symptoms, treatment must also address the client's modification of reality. In some cases, the meaning placed on the trauma creates a transformative experience and the trauma survivor undergoes a period of unanticipated growth (Schubert et al., 2015).

Posttraumatic Stress Growth (PTG)

Some fortunate trauma survivors find meaning in the aftermath of trauma, and in so doing, can experience a period of growth which transcends their pre-trauma psychological state (Schubert et al., 2015). PTG, also referred to in the literature as thriving (Carver, 1998; O'Leary & Ickovics, 1995), stress-related growth (Park et al, 1996), and adversarial growth (Linley & Joseph, 2004), has shown to positively impact worldview (Butler et al., 2005), posttraumatic coping, and positive relationships with others (Tedeschi & Calhoun, 2004). Calhoun and Tedeschi (2000) define PTG as "positive change that an individual experiences as a result of the struggle with a traumatic event" (p. 135). Cann and colleagues (2013) note the presence of challenge to core beliefs as a significant predictor of posttraumatic growth. Resilient individuals return to baseline functioning following exposure to a traumatic event (O'Leary & Ickovics 1995; Morland et al, 2008); individuals who experience *PTG* benefit from posttraumatic adaptation that exceeds pre-event levels. In elevated terms, PTG offers greater psychological currency compared to resilience. Tedeschi and Calhoun (2004) highlight five life domains that may be positively impacted by PTG. These domains are enhancements in relationships, a renewed appreciation for life, broadened life opportunities, a greater sense of personal strength, and spiritual development. Once again, spirituality occupies a central position in moderating the development of PTG and is a cornerstone of resourcing for the posttraumatic survivor.

Similar to the development of PTSD, PTG outcomes are mediated by types of trauma and demographic variables of the post-traumatized survivors. Specifically, PTG is found to effect Type I PTSD (episodic), rather than Type II PTSD (prolonged), suggesting that it is easier reconstruct a one-time negative experience, rather than prolonged, unrelented exposure to stressful life events (Kira e t al., 2013). Furthermore, religiosity has been shown to mediate the occurrence of PTG, a factor that may explain the increase in PTG in African American and Hispanic populations, compared to Caucasian samples (Bellizzi et al., 2019). Notably, there has been an expansion of the PTG literature in recent years to include the role of spirituality as a potential protective factor for the development of PTG (see Butler et al., 2005).

Butler and colleagues (2005) conducted a longitudinal, Internet study of changes in cognitions, posttraumatic coping, and posttraumatic growth, following the 9/11 terrorist attacks in New York City (n = 1,505). PTSD symptoms were assessed via the PTSD Checklist – Specific (PCL-S; Weathers & Ford, 1996). Positive and negative changes in existential outlook or worldview were measured by the Changes in Outlook Questionnaire (CIO; Joseph et al., 1993; Joseph et al., 2005), a measure that asks respondents to indicate the degree to which they agree with statements, such as "I don't take life for granted anymore" (positive change) and "My life has no meaning anymore" (negative change). Posttraumatic coping was assessed by the Brief COPE (Carver, 1997), a measure of 14 categories of coping, i.e., active coping, use of emotional supports, use of instrumental supports, positive reframing, planning, humor, acceptance, religion, distraction, denial, behavioral disengagement, substance use, and self-blame. Posttraumatic growth was assessed via the Posttraumatic Growth Inventory (PTGI; Tedeschi & Calhoun, 1995, 1996), a measure of growth-related changes experienced by traumatized individuals in five domains:0new possibilities, relating to others, personal strength, spiritual change, and appreciation of life.

Initial results (mean nine weeks post-9/11) showed that those who indicated post-9/11 trauma responses also showed high rates of PTG, positive changes in worldview, post-trauma coping skills of denial, and less behavioral disengagement (Butler et al., 2005). Interestingly, PTG showed a curvilinear relationship with level of trauma symptoms, for instance those reporting symptoms at intermediate levels reported the highest levels of growth. Most noteworthy, 6.5 months follow-up PTG results showed a significant decline across all PTG subscales, with the exception of spiritual change. The sustained positive impact of spirituality highlights the inextricable relationship between spirituality and PTG and reinforces its use in the assessment and treatment phases of PTSD.

PTG and Spirituality

Growth occupies the simultaneous position of a roadmap and destination (Pargament & Exline, 2022). Moreover, growth represents characterological change, the individual's regard toward one's world, and relationship with spirituality. For example, spiritual and religious adaptive and creative benefits have been found among children and grandchildren of Holocaust Survivors (Jacobs, 2022), in Germans soldiers in the aftermath of World War I (Croutelhand, 2021), in cancer patients (Namisango et al., 2022), in trauma clinicians (Muehlhausen, 2021), in adult survivors of childhood abuse (Kosarkova et al., 2020), and in suffers of chronic and acute anxiety (Tolentino et al., 2022).

Notably, the initial impacts of posttraumatic growth appear to lay firm roots which upon follow-up study, produce sustainable and positive change. For example, McMilen and colleagues (1997) interviewed survivors of three community-based disasters, these disasters included a tornado that resulted in the significant destruction and loss of life in a northern Florida town, a plane crash into a hotel that killed nine of the hotel's inhabitants, and a mass shooting in a cafeteria in Texas. In two separate follow-up interviews, three months, and three years posttraumatic event respectively, most individuals surveyed reported sustained positive posttraumatic benefits. In another study, Tsai and colleagues, (2015) analyzed data from the National Health and Resilience in Veterans Study *(n* = 3,157). Data included the Posttraumatic Growth Inventory-Short Form (PTGI-SF; Cann et al., 2010). Results indicate a moderate presence of PTG in 50.1% of all veterans and 72% of veterans who met criteria for PTDS. Tsai and colleagues point to an inverted u-shaped relationship between veteran symptoms of PTSD and the presence of PTG. Veterans with PTSD and PTG reported enhanced levels of mental functioning and greater general health outcomes, compared with their non-PTG counterparts. Moreover, increased connectedness, intrinsic religiosity, and stated life purpose, were positively associated with greater PTG.

There is an accumulating body of evidence suggesting the intrinsic value (e.g., positive state of mind) and extrinsic benefits (e.g., personal resources) of PTG on overall well-being (Park & Fenster, 2004). In particular, PTG was shown to correlate with increased optimism, social support, and positive affect (Park et al., 1996). Haugen (2011) further extended the link between PTG and spirituality. Posttraumatic spiritual growth was shown to correlate with changes in spirituality and religiosity, mainly, silence, integration, and belief-behavior congruence in the spiritual domain.

Spirituality and Religion

Spirituality is far from a straightforward construct. Some researchers debate whether or not PTG represents actual growth or something else, e.g., a cognitive mechanism to bolster self-worth via emphasis of post-stressor progress (McFarland & Alvaro, 2000), Freudian denialism of real pain and reidentification of it via a growth lens (Maercker & Zoellner, 2004), a logotherapeutic interpretation of traumatic events (Jayawickrene & Blackie, 2014), or the results of a sociocultural script that assures a positive outgrowth of pain (Linley & Joseph, 2004). Perhaps the central feature underlying the challenges to the veracity of spirituality lies in the debaters' limited experience with the topic itself. For example, spirituality is positively related to religion (Pargament, 1997). Unfortunately, psychologists are largely unacquainted with religion (Pargament, 1997). The nature of religion to elicit strong positive and negative feelings in clinicians and their clients, along with psychologists' discomfort with its meta-physic and nonmetric-orientation, results in a significant reduction of the religious domain as a medium for therapeutic use. It is limiting, as "religion is often present in the most remarkable times of life….Any understanding of the human response to extraordinary moments remain incomplete without an appreciation for religion (Pargament, 1997, p. 4)." Finally, crises are often pivotal points of existence that lead to choice crossroads of posttraumatic stress and posttraumatic growth.

For example, Lazar Research surveyed the spiritual impact of the October 7th terrorist attacks on an Israeli sample (Klein, 2024). Results reveal a strengthened faith in God in 33% of the sample, compared to a decline in faith (8%), or no change in impact (59%). Faith reinforcement was particularly deepened for those with traditional leanings (44%), compared to those with secular leanings (16%).

Religion, according to Leuba (1912), is a way of "dismissing the worrying complications of this world, of escaping a dreaded sense of isolation, of entering into a circle of solacing and elevating thoughts and feelings, and forgetting and of surmounting evil (p. 8)." To the religious mind, the social scientist's relegation of religion to its specific elements and psychological benefits, strips it of its core essence, *the spiritual,* that is, the expansion of self (Pargament, 1997).The expansion of self in the face of adversity allows for complete coping and added adaptation to posttraumatic events.

Evidence of Religious Coping

Coping rejects the notion of psychic and contextual determinism; rather, it represents a *choice point,* in which one is able to rebound from stress and loss (Pargament, 1997).

Yalom (1980) declares,

"All of face natural adversities that influence our lives….but that does not mean that we have no responsibility (or choice) in the situation….When all else fails, when the coefficient of adversity is formidable, still one is responsible for the attitude one adopts toward the adversity – whether to live a life of bitter regret or to find a way to transcend the handicap and to fashion a meaningful life despite it (p. 272)."

Moreover, Meninger (1963) regards coping as a means of regulating everyday emergencies. Similarly, Chodoff and colleagues (1963) describe coping as "mechanisms, utilized by an individual to meet a significant threat to his psychological stability and to enable him to function effectively (p. 616)."

For example, religion has been found to be a significant source of coping among veterans and their spouses (Stouffer et al., 1965), in patients with a medical illness (David et al., 1992) and victims of violence (Horton et al., 1988), in World War II veterans (Stouffer et al., 1965), in pre-op cardiac patients (Saudia et al., 1991), in parents of children with physical disabilities (Barsch, 1968), in women with breast cancer (David et al., 1992), in wives of Vietnam war POWs (Hunter et al., 1974), and in physically abused spouses (Horton et al., 1988). Once again, the widespread impact of spirituality in PTG further underscores the clinical obligation for its inclusion in clinical treatment protocols.

Clinical Considerations

Most recently, researchers have determined that some sufferers of psychiatric disorders suffer from a "meaning crisis" and recommend that mental health professional assess the spiritual and religious (S/R) domain and expand their referral resources to include spiritual and religious resources (Berzengi et al., 2017). Smith and colleagues (2012) examine the relationship between spirituality, resilience, and positive emotions, to create a trifecta worth applying to trauma survivors. Similarly, Koenig (2021) examines the general pathway of S/R in a Mental Health model, an area that must be applied to the treatment of the traumatized. In particular, Cist and Choi (2017) highlight the need to accommodate religious rituals and spiritual intervention on Intensive Care Units and for nurses (Swinton & Vanderpot, 2017).

The rise of alternative treatment methods to treat PTSD highlights the benefits of perspective broadening. A broadened treatment view must therefore include the role of spirituality and meaning in the treatment of the traumatized. Spirituality has been currently recognized by the APA as an aspect of "cultural diversity." Thus, the benefits of spirituality shown by researchers (see Cist & Choi, 2017), coupled with the practitioner's ethical obligation to attend to the dimension of spirituality as a matter of diversity (see Ethical Principles of Psychologists and Code of Conduct of APA, 1992), necessitates the consideration of including spirituality to the growing body of scientific research and clinical application. Treatment structures which include spirituality present an elevated potential for client growth. Consequentially, *meaning* is elevated to *meaningful* and the suffering client experiences a transformation from helpless victim of life circumstance, to that of an active agent of life's potential.

It has been said that the mental health field is suffering from a "professional dissociation disorder" concerning spirituality and client spiritual struggles (Pargament & Exline, 2022). An understanding of human response to extraordinary life events is incomplete without consideration of spiritual and religious processes (Pargament, 1997). Crises are pivotal points that call for new solutions; religion offers guidelines toward new solutions. Moreover, psychology and religion are both concerned with the areas of personal control. As exemplified by the Health Belief Model (Rosenstock, 1974), psychologists argue that one is not as powerless as one imagines oneself to be, and can, through self-actualization of untapped potential, override the system's limits. As demonstrated by the Twelve Step program of Alcoholics Anonymous, religious figures proclaim that one *is* in fact powerless, and that one must look past himself alone for answers to life's important questions (Pargament, 1997). The willing clinician can help her client extend areas of control (personal control) *and* accept personal limitations and look elsewhere for solutions to those limitations (spiritual resources).

Posttraumatic stress sufferers seek treatment because their life story has either been disrupted or challenged in seemingly irredeemable ways. The role of psychotherapy is, in part, to help sufferers reconstruct the fragmented narrative to one of meaning and hope (Pargament & Exline, 2022). The case has been made for the integration of spiritual processes in the assessment phase, and, when deemed clinically appropriate, the incorporation into the treatment phase of therapy; the final sections offer several avenues of integration.

Clinical Practice

The barriers of integration of spirituality and spiritual struggles into clinical practice may begin at the outset of therapy. The client may wonder whether it is even appropriate to raise the concern of spiritual struggle, or whether the mental health professional, often secular, is a qualified and suitable resource. As such, the clinician must approach the assessment of spirituality and spiritual struggles, particularly in the traumatized population, with sensitivity and care. At times, assessment of spiritual resources and spiritual struggles for posttraumatic sufferers are compounded by several factors. First, the metaphysical nature of spirituality may make it difficult for the suffering individual to articulate intrapsychic growth and struggle with the supernatural. Second, as is the general case of posttraumatic stress, post event spiritual struggles may elicit personal feelings of shame and guilt (López-Castro et al., 2019), and fears of disappointment of others and disapproval of God (Exline et al., 2012).

Assessment of spirituality in the general assessment of posttraumatic stress serves two functions; the first objective is to assess for potential areas of posttraumatic stress vs. posttraumatic growth and the second objective is to assess the appropriateness of incorporating spirituality in treatment. To do so, the clinician must approach the assessment of the client's spiritual life and struggles with general curiosity and openness. Questions such as "That is really interesting; can you tell me more?" are more effective than rejoinders such as, "God does not give us more than we can handle." As part of the general assessment phase, the clinician can assess for: spiritual salience ("Do you see yourself as a religious or spiritual person?"); salience of spirituality to the problem ("Has your struggles effected your religious or spiritual domain?"); and, salience of spirituality to the solution ("Has your religion or spirituality helped you cope with your struggles?"). When the initial assessment reveals client spiritual struggles, it may be necessary for broader assessment (see Pargament & Exline, 2022, for a review). The assessment phase concludes with a collaborative process of treatment goal-setting. Spiritual goals may include: the processing of spiritual struggles, the broadening of understanding of pain and suffering, acceptance of spiritual pain, harnessing of spirituality to promote coping, greater self-awareness, and the development of a sustainable life-vison (Pargament & Exline, 2022).

The strength of a collaborative working relationship predicts therapeutic outcomes over the specific therapeutic modality used (Horwath Del Re et al., 2011). As such, it is not necessary for the clinician to be an active member of a religious group to promote spiritual growth in her clients. Clinicals who are present and oriented to their client's spirituality and spiritual struggles intervene by naming and normalizing the spiritual struggles. Naming the struggle places it in a normative, developmental context. Clinicians can apply cognitive modification of traumatic events to promote client PTG. For example, when appropriate, practitioners can reframe the client's stressful life experiences as opportunities for growth. The practitioner can emphasize the cycle nature of life; endings are beginnings, loss breeds growth. At times, the practitioner may be unwilling to use the reframe out of fear of appearing dismissive of her client's suffering. On the contrary, when successfully applied, the reframe of traumatic events in spiritual terms offers client hope, renewal, and growth. Thus, meaning is added to trauma; the process is transformative, and the client is freed from the bonds of pain.

CONCLUSIONS

Trauma and tragedy are inevitable parts of life's journey; crises are crossroads for posttraumatic stress and posttraumatic growth. The impact of spiritual process in the promotion of PTG has been well documented. Though mental health professionals are considerably less religious than those they serve (Shafranske & Cummings, 2013), the integration of spirituality and meaning in the treatment of the traumatized offers opportunities of expansion and growth for both client and clinician.

It is our prayer that spiritual treatment strategies, strengthened by applied research findings, will offer relief from the human suffering that comes from pain without meaning.

REFERENCES

American Psychiatric Association. (2000). *Diagnostic and statistical manual of mental disorders* (4th ed., text rev.). Author.

American Psychiatric Association. (2013). *Diagnostic and statistical manual of mental disorders* (5th ed.)., DOI: 10.1176/appi.books.9780890425596

American Psychological Association. (2017). Ethical principles of psychologists and code of conduct (2002, amended effective June 1, 2010, and January 1, 2017). https://www.apa.org/ethics/code/

Barsch, R. H. (1968). *The parent of the handicapped child: The study of child-raring practices.* Charlse C. Thomas. `Bellizzi, K.M., Smith, A.W., Reeve, B.B., Alfano, C.M., Bernstein, L, Meeske, K. et al. (2010). Posttraumatic growth and health-related quality of life in a racially diverse cohort of breast cancer survivors. *Health Psychology,* 15(4). 615–626.

Berzengi, A., Berzenji, L., Kadim, A., Mustafa, F., & Jobson, L. (2017). Role of Role of Islamic appraisals, trauma-related appraisals, and religious coping in the posttraumatic adjustment of Muslim trauma survivors. *Psychological Trauma: Theory, Research, Practice, and Policy*, 9(2), 189–197. DOI: 10.1037/tra0000179 PMID: 27504962

Brookls, A. (Nov. 2023). On cultivating happiness, emotional self-management, and more. *On the Peter Atia Drive*. Episode 280.

Butler, L. D., Blasey, C. M., Garlan, R. W., McCaslin, S. E., Azarow, J., Chen, X. H., Desjardins, J. C., DiMiceli, S., Seagraves, D. A., Hastings, T. A., Kraemer, H. A., & Spiegel, D. (2005). Posttraumatic growth following the terrorist attacks of September 11, 2001: Cognitive, coping, and trauma symptom predictors in an Internet convenience sample. *Traumatology*, 11(4), 247–267. DOI: 10.1177/153476560501100405

Calhoun, L. G., & Tedeschi, R. G. (2000). Early posttraumatic intervention: Facilitating possibilities for growth. In Patton, D., & Dunning, C. (Eds.), *Posttraumatic Stress Intervention: Challenges, Issues, and Perspectives* (pp. 135–152). Charles C. Thomas.

Cann, A., Calhoun, L. G., Tedeschi, R. G., Taku, K., Vishnevsky, T., Triplett, K. N., & Danhauer, S. C. (2010). *Posttraumatic Growth Inventory—Short Form (PTGI-SF)* [Database record]. APA PsycTests.

Cann, A., Calhoun, L. G., Tedeschi, R. G., Triplett, K. N., Vishnevsky, T., & Lindstrom, C. M. (2011). Assessing posttraumatic cognitive processes: The event related rumination inventory. *Anxiety, Stress, and Coping*, 24(2), 137–156. DOI: 10.1080/10615806.2010.529901 PMID: 21082446

Carver, C. S. (1997). You want to measure coping but your protocol's too long: Consider the Brief COPE. *International Journal of Behavioral Medicine*, 4(1), 92–100. DOI: 10.1207/s15327558ijbm0401_6 PMID: 16250744

Cist, A., & Choi, P. (2017). Religion and spirituality in the Intensive Care Unit. In Balboni, M., & Peteet, J. J. (Eds.), *Spirituality and Religion Within the Culture of Medicine: From Evidence to Practice*.

Courtois, C. A. (2015). First, do no more harm: Ethics of attending to spiritual issues in trauma treatment. In Walker, D. F., Courtois, C. A., & Aten, J. D. (Eds.), *Spiritually oriented psychotherapy for trauma* (pp. 55–75). American Psychological Association. DOI: 10.1037/14500-004

Crouthamel, J. (2001). *Trauma, Religion, and Spirituality in Germany during the First World War*. Bloomsbury Academic.

David, J. P., Ladd, K., & Spilka, B. (1992). *The multidimensionality of prayer and its roles as a source of secondary control.* Paper presented at the meeting of the American Psychological Association, Washington, DC.

Ehlers, A., & Clark, D. (2000). A cognitive model of posttraumatic stress disorder. *Behaviour Research and Therapy*, 38(4), 319–345. DOI: 10.1016/S0005-7967(99)00123-0 PMID: 10761279

Exline, J. J., Kaplan, K. J., & Grubbs, J. B. (2012). Anger, exit, and assertion: Do people see protest toward God as morally acceptable? *Psychology of Religion and Spirituality*, 4(4), 264–277. DOI: 10.1037/a0027667

Fink, G. (2009). Stress: definition and history. *Encyclopedia ofNeuroscience*. 549-555.

Foa, E., Carmen, P., Capaldi, S., & Rosenfield, D. (2013). Prolonged exposure vs supportive counseling for sexual abuse–related PTSD in adolescent girls. A randomized clinical trial. *Journal of the American Medical Association*, 310(24), 650–2657. DOI: 10.1001/jama.2013.282829 PMID: 24368465

Frankl, V. E. (1963). *Man's search for meaning*. Simon and Schuster.

Freud, S. (2002). *The Psychopathology of Everyday Life* (Bell, A. L., Trans.). Penguin Modern Classics. Penguin Classics.

Friedman, S. B., Chodoff, P., Mason, J. W., & Hamburg, D. A. (1963). Behavioral observations on parents anticipating the death of a child. *Pediatrics*, 32(4), 610–625. DOI: 10.1542/peds.32.4.610 PMID: 14069103

Harris, A., & Reece, J. (2021). Transcranial magnetic stimulation as a treatment for posttraumatic stress disorder: A meta-analysis. *Journal of Affective Disorders*, 289(15), 55–65. DOI: 10.1016/j.jad.2021.04.003 PMID: 33940319

Harris, R. (2009). *ACT Made Simple: An Easy-To-Read Primer on Acceptance and Commitment Therapy*. New Harbinger Publications.

Haugen, M. R. G. (2011). *Does trauma lead to religiousness? A longitudinal study of the effects of traumatic events on religiousness and spirituality during the first three years at university.* (Unpublished doctoral dissertation). Bowling Green State University.

Hayes, S. C., & Lillis, J. (2012). *Acceptance and commitment therapy*. American Psychological Association. DOI: 10.1037/17335-000

Horton, A. L., Wilkins, M. M., & Wright, W. (1988). Women who ended abuse: What religious leaders and religion did for these victims. In Horton, A. L., & Williamson, J. A. (Eds.), *Abuse and religion: When praying isn't enough* (pp. 235–246). Lexington Books.

Horwath, A. O., Del Re, A. C., Fluckiger, C., & Symonds, D. (2011). Alliance in individual psychotherapy. *Psychotherapy (Chicago, Ill.)*, 48(1), 9–16. DOI: 10.1037/a0022186 PMID: 21401269

Hunter, E. J., McCubbin, H. I., & Metres, P. J.Jr. (1974). Religion and POW/MIA wife. In McCubbin, H. I., Dahl, B. B., Metres, P. J.Jr, Hunter, E. J., & Plag, J. A. (Eds.), *Family separation and reunion: Families of prisoners of war and servicemen missing in action* (pp. 85–93). US Government Printing Office.

Jacobs, J. (2022). The Intergenerational Transmission of Trauma: Religion, Spirituality, and Ritual among Children and Grandchildren of Holocaust Survivors. In *Interpreting Religion*. Bristol University Press., DOI: 10.2307/j.ctv2m7c5ks.8

Jayawickrene, E., & Blackie, L. E. R. (2014). Posttraumatic growth as positive personality change: Evidence, controversies, and future directions. *European Journal of Personality*, 28(4), 312–331. DOI: 10.1002/per.1963

Joseph, S., Linley, P. A., Andrews, L., Harris, G., Howle, B., Woodward, C., & Shevlin, M. (2005). Assessing positive and negative changes in the aftermath of adversity: Psychometric evaluation of the Changes in Outlook Questionnaire. *Psychological Assessment*, 17(2), 70–80. DOI: 10.1037/1040-3590.17.1.70 PMID: 15769229

Joseph, S., Williams, R., & Yule, W. (1993). Changes in outlook following disaster: The preliminary development of a measure to assess positive and negative responses. *Journal of Traumatic Stress*, 6(2), 271–279. DOI: 10.1002/jts.2490060209

Kira, I. A., Aboumediene, S., Ashby, J. S., Odenat, L., Mohanesh, J., & Alamia, H. (2013). The dynamics of posttraumatic growth across different trauma types in a Palestinian sample. *Journal of Loss and Trauma*, 18(2), 120–139. DOI: 10.1080/15325024.2012.679129

Klein, T. (2024). Editor's Note: War with Hamas pushes Israelis closer to God. The Jerusalem Post.

Koenig, H. G. (2021). Mechanisms: religion's impact on mental health. In Moreira-Almeida, A. (Ed.), *Spirituality and Mental Health Across Cultures*. Oxford University Press.

Kosarkova, A., Malinakova, K., Koncalova, Z., Tavel, P., & van Dijk, J. P. (2020). Childhood Trauma is associated with the spirituality of non-religious respondents. *International Journal of Environmental Research and Public Health*, 17(4), 1268. DOI: 10.3390/ijerph17041268 PMID: 32079153

Leuba, J. H. (1912). *A psychological study of religion*. Macmillan.

Lewis, H. B. (1971). *Shame and guilt in neurosis*. International Universities.

Linehan, M. M. (1993). *Cognitive-behavioral treatment of borderline personality disorder*. Guilford Press.

Linehan, M. M. (2020). *Building a life worth living: a memoire*. Random House.

Linley, P. A., & Joseph, S. (2004). Positive change following trauma and adversity: A review. *Journal of Traumatic Stress*, 17(1), 11–21. DOI: 10.1023/B:JOTS.0000014671.27856.7e PMID: 15027788

Lopez, S. J., Pedrotti, J. T., & Snyder, C. R. (2018). *Positive psychology: the scientific practical explorations of human strengths* (4th ed.). Sage Publications.

López-Castro, T., Saraiya, T., Zumberg-Smith, K., & Dambreville, N. (2019). Association between shame and posttraumatic stress disorder: A meta-analysis. *Journal of Traumatic Stress*, 32(4), 484–495. DOI: 10.1002/jts.22411 PMID: 31291483

Maercker, A., & Zoellner, T. (2004). The Janus face of self-perceived growth: Toward a two-component model of posttraumatic growth. *Psychological Inquiry*, 15(1), 41–48.

Maslow, A. H. (1943). A theory of human motivation. *Psychological Review*, 50(4), 370–396. DOI: 10.1037/h0054346

McFarland, C., & Alvaro, C. (2000). The impact of motivation of temporal comparisons: Coping with traumatic events by perceiving personal growth. *Journal of Personality and Social Psychology*, 79(3), 327–343. DOI: 10.1037/0022-3514.79.3.327 PMID: 10981837

McMillen, J. C., Smith, E. M., & Fisher, R. H. (1997). Perceived benefit and mental health after three types of disaster. *Journal of Consulting and Clinical Psychology*, 65(5), 733–739. DOI: 10.1037/0022-006X.65.5.733 PMID: 9337492

Menninger, K. (1963). *The vital balance: The life process in mental health and illness*. Viking.

Morland, L. A., Butler, L. D., & Leskin, G. A. (2008). Resilience and thriving in a time of terrorism. In Joseph, S., & Linley, P. A. (Eds.), *Trauma, Recovery, and Growth: Positive Psychological Perspectives on Posttraumatic Stress* (pp. 39–61). John Wiley & Sons, Inc. DOI: 10.1002/9781118269718.ch3

Muehlhausen, B. L. (2020). Spirituality and vicarious trauma among trauma clinicians: A qualitative study. [Published online.]. *International Journal of Environmental Research and Public Health*, 17(4), 1268. PMID: 32079153

Namisango, E., Matovu, L., Harding, R., & Berger, A. (2022). Existentialism and spirituality in the healing processes of cancer patients. In (Ed.). in *Global Perspectives in Cancer Care: Religion, Spirituality, and Cultural Diversity in Health and Healing*. Oxford University Press.

Nelson, C., Dossett, K., & Walker, D. L. (2022). Equine-assisted therapy for post-traumatic stress disorder among first responders. *Psychological Reports*. Advance online publication. DOI: 10.1177/00332941221146707 PMID: 36542680

Nietzsche, F. (1889). *Twilight of the idols*. Penguin Classics.

O'Leary, V. E., & Ickovics, J. R. (1995). Resilience and thriving in response to challenge: An opportunity for a paradigm shift in women's health. *Women's Health: Research on Gender, Behavior, and Policy*, 1(2), 121–142. PMID: 9373376

Pargament, K. I., & Exline, J. J. (2022). *Working with spiritual struggles in psychotherapy: From research to practice*. The Guilford Press.

Pargament, K. I. (1997). *The Psychology of Religion and Coping Theory, Research, Practice*. The Guildford Press.

Pargament, K. J., & Mahoney, A. (2017). Spirituality: the search for the sacred. In C. R. Snyder, S. J. Lopez, L. Edwards, & S. C. Marques (Eds), *Oxford handbook of positive psychology* (3rd ed.) (pp. 1-27), Oxford University Press.

Park, C. L., Cohen, L. H., & Murch, R. L. (1996). Assessment and prediction of stress-related growth. *Journal of Personality*, 6(1), 71–105. DOI: 10.1111/j.1467-6494.1996.tb00815.x PMID: 8656319

Park, C. L., & Fenster, J. R. (2004). Stress-related growth: Predictors of occurrence and correlates with psychological adjustment. *Journal of Social and Clinical Psychology*, 23(2), 195–215. DOI: 10.1521/jscp.23.2.195.31019

Puchalski, C., & Romer, A. L. (2000). Taking a spiritual history allows clinicians to understand patients more fully. *Journal of Palliative Medicine*, 3(1), 129–137. DOI: 10.1089/jpm.2000.3.129 PMID: 15859737

Rosenstock, I. M. (1974). Historical origins of the Health Belief Model. *Health Education Monographs*, 2(4), 328–335. DOI: 10.1177/109019817400200403

Saudia, T. L., Kinney, M. R., Brown, K. C., & Yong-Ward, L. (1991). Health locus of control and helpfulness of prayer. *Heart & Lung*, 20, 60–65. PMID: 1988394

Schubert, C. F., Schmidt, U., & Rosner, R. (2015). PTSD growth in populations with posttraumatic stress disorder-a systematic review on growth-related psychological constructs and biological variables. *Clinical Psychology & Psychotherapy*, •••, 1985. PMID: 26514236

Shafranske, E. P., & Cummings, J. P. (2013). Religious and spiritual beliefs, affirmations, and practices of psychologist. In Pargament, K. I., Mahoney, A., & Shafranske, E. P. (Eds.), APA handbook of psychology, religion, and spirituality: Vol. 2. *An applied psychology of religion and spirituality. (* (pp. 23–42). American Psychological Association.

Smith, B. W., Oritz, J. A., Wiggins, K. T., Bernard, J. F., & Dalen, J. (2012). Spirituality, resilience, and positive emotions. In Miller, A. (Ed.), *The Oxford Handbook of Psychology and Spirituality*. Oxford University Press.

Stouffer, S. A., Consadaine, A. A., Consadaine, M. H., Willians, R. W., Jr., & Smith, M. B., Janis, J. L., Star, S. A., & Cottrell, L. S., Jr. (1963). *The American soldier: Combat and its aftermath* (Vol. 2). Wiley.

Swinton, J., & Vanderport, L. (2017). The unforeseen relationship between spirituality and psychiatric medication: A hermeneutic phenomenological study. *Journal of Spirituality in Mental Health*. Advance online publication. DOI: 10.1080/19349637.2017.1297692

Tedeschi, R. G., & Calhoun, L. G. (1995). Trauma and Transformation: Growing in the Aftermath of Suffering. *Sage (Atlanta, Ga.)*. Advance online publication. DOI: 10.4135/9781483326931

Tedeschi, R. G., & Calhoun, L. G. (1996). The Posttraumatic Growth Inventory: Measuring the positive legacy of trauma. *Journal of Traumatic Stress*, 9(3), 455–472. DOI: 10.1002/jts.2490090305 PMID: 8827649

Tedeschi, R. G., & Calhoun, L. G. (2004). Posttraumatic growth: Conceptual foundations and empirical evidence. *Psychological Inquiry*, 15(1), 1–18. DOI: 10.1207/s15327965pli1501_01

Tolentino, J. C., Gjorup, A. L. T., Mello, C. R., de Assis, S. G., Marques, A., Filho, A. C., Salazar, H. R. M., van Duinkerken, E., & Schmidt, S. L. (2022). Spirituality as a protective factor for chronic and acute anxiety in Brazilian healthcare workers during the COVID-19 outbreak. *PLoS One*, 17(5), e0267556. DOI: 10.1371/journal.pone.0267556 PMID: 35503766

Tsai, J., El-Gabalawy, R., Sledge, W. H., Southwick, S. M., & Pietrzak, R. H. (2015). Post-traumatic growth among veterans in the USA: Results from the National Health and Resilience in Veterans Study. *Psychological Medicine*, 45(1), 165–179. DOI: 10.1017/S0033291714001202 PMID: 25065450

Watson, J. B. (1913). Psychology as the behaviorist views it. *Psychological Review*, 20(2), 158–177. DOI: 10.1037/h0074428

Weathers, F. W., & Ford, J. (1996). Psychometric review of PTSD Checklist (PCL-C, PCL-S, PCL-M, PCL-PR). In Stamm, B. H. (Ed.), *measurement of stress, trauma, and adaptation* (pp. 250–251). Sidran Press.

Yalom, L. D. (1980). *Existential psychotherapy*. Basic Books.

Chapter 9
Social Media as a Conduit for Secondary Trauma

Sanam Hafeez
https://orcid.org/0000-0001-7428-0103
Comprehensive Consultation Corp, USA

ABSTRACT

Secondary trauma, once limited to therapists and first responders, is part of our everyday lives. Anyone with a phone and an account can talk about harrowing experiences sharing with the world at large. This creates social and psychological awareness but also trauma, inherited. We watched the murder of George Floyd, because it was filmed on several phones. No one really thinks of the trauma of a Black man or a Black mother, watching that clip. The carnage in Gaza, unrelenting for over four months, has been the most traumatizing experience I have had, and that is the reality of millions if not billions of people in the world. This chapter gives that reality a voice as a Psychologist who is one of the masses. The impact on the brain is indelible when it is readily available on the little screen that is your constant companion. This chapter talks about the very personal experience of watching a war unfold on my instagram and how we are all unwittingly witnessing some of the most graphic violence via social media.

INTRODUCTION

Twenty-two years ago, I defended my doctoral dissertation, "Degree of exposure to violence related trauma and PTSD on EMS personnel," under the guidance of Robert Motta, PhD. Having been under the tutelage of Dr. Motta my entire academic career at Hofstra University, you could say studying PTSD was not a choice. During my time, I had also worked on developing a secondary trauma questionnaire with

DOI: 10.4018/979-8-3693-2089-1.ch009

him (Motta et al., 2001; Motta et al., 1999), and yet had to discover what it was to experience it. Secondary Traumatic Stress (STS, also called Vicarious Trauma or Compassion Fatigue) is the behaviors and emotions that result from knowing about a traumatizing event experienced by a significant other, though it has also been observed in more general populations like individuals consuming news media. Those who come into close contact with trauma victims can experience symptoms similar to those of the victims, including anxiety, anger, intrusive thoughts, nightmares, sleep disturbances, and emotional numbing (Bercier & Maynard, 2015; Lamba et al., 2023).

While developing my dissertation study on the EMS personnel, through the FDNY, I became familiar with fire stations where the EMS ambulances were housed. This was before iPhones or mobile internet, so while I waited for more EMS personnel to return to their firehouses, there was time to chat. In speaking to these first responders, I came to understand trauma through their eyes. I imagined some of the graphic imagery they would describe. I remember a paramedic telling me how he "cleaned the brains off the sidewalk of a baby that had fallen six stories". Some of these tales stuck with me, but not for too long, as they were passing verbal exchanges, and the brain cannot hold onto images it conjures up for too long.

Then 9/11 happened. 9/11, or as we Americans refer to it, is the date in 2001, that terrorists flew planes into the World Trade Center in New York City, my backyard, my hometown, causing unimaginable devastation and a profound, senseless loss of innocent lives. I recalled seeing names on TV that I had come to know, people I had sought permission from for my research for my dissertation. I was glued to the TV when I was home, even listening to the AM radio in my car, needing more information about survivors or heroes. I wept, a lot. On a nightly basis, I dreamt of planes and wreckage. I had developed a traumatic response to the events of 9/11. As the data collection part of my study fell squarely during this time, I had to integrate 9/11 and its impact on first responders carefully into my research without losing focus of the daily violence I was studying. My study examining differences between the Bronx, Brooklyn, and Queens correctly hypothesized that the greater the violence EMTs experienced, the greater the PTSD would be (Hafeez, 2002).

9/11 was the first time I had seen a war-like state and right in my own backyard. I had worked near the Twin Towers and had it not been for a new class I had started teaching that semester as a graduate student, I might have been on the E train at that very moment. The collective buzzing and pinging of beepers started going off in my lecture hall class, and many people just laughed it off. Even when I called to see what had happened, I could not actually fathom the massacre. There was no iPhone, Twitter, or Instagram. There is a difference between hearing something and seeing it; the brain's ability to visualize images in the absence of a frame of reference is actually quite unsophisticated (Pearson et al., 2015). When I got home, the same video kept playing on all the channels showing the planes flying into the buildings. I was eventually able to turn off the TV and sleep, only to dream of more planes. The nightmares and the hypervigilance lasted a couple of weeks, though not long enough to become PTSD. It was Acute Stress Disorder, its little, less anxious sibling.

To this day, I still feel the hairs on my neck stand up when I watch footage from 9/11. I feel queasy, sad, anxious, and angry, all at once. Even as someone so impacted emotionally, I can only think of a handful of stories I saw on the news. A father who would show up looking for his daughter with a photo of her will sometimes play in my mind, as he would often talk tearfully to reporters. The image of a man jumping out of the north tower published on the front page of the New York Times, infamously called "The Falling Man" still haunts me to this day (Drew, 2001).

Looking back, it was such an innocent time. You watched the news when it was on, and then went about your day. You spoke to people about it briefly and went back to doing whatever it was you were doing. You read the paper as time went on, shook your head, and went back to your coffee. Every now and then, the History Channel would broadcast a documentary, and slowly, we even stopped watching those. The harrowing images on TV were eventually replaced by depictions of the invasions of Iraq and Afghanistan in the following years. Slowly, those of us who wanted to get "those sons of bitches" started to see that we were sending troops in and killing scores of people who had nothing to do with it. Jon Stewart became a leader to those of us who dared question the administration's motivations through his skeptical reporting of the Iraq War (Blake, 2015). The images of war, dust, shelling, and even explosions, were curated and predetermined for our consumption by mainstream media, not only for visual gore, but also for political reasons. As we now know, big news networks have owners and stockholders who decide which war is important, how much to show us, which angle, which people, whose pain and suffering, and to what extent they deserve attention.

Enter social media.

In today's world, social media is no longer merely something to pass the time– it is where we all come together in the form of a digital space called the online community of news, fashion, gossip and finding common ground through the algorithm created for us, by us (Ashar, 2024). We share glimpses into what we are doing in our lives and forge connections through networks, having conversations that stretch thousands of miles between friends, and those we have never met. But there is also an underside to these online communities, which are increasingly difficult to ignore: there is online bullying and interpersonal violence in comments and posts. There is violent content that slips through on our feeds, to test if we'll pause for more than a few seconds to watch. We're scrolling through posts of puppies, recipes, and celebrity news, and suddenly, there is a harrowing scene you didn't ask for, but you are glued. It's not just disturbing— it can really do damage to our emotional state by altering it, but also leaves you craving for more. When you are constantly being shown images that depict the worst of humanity, you can walk around with a pit in your stomach all day and not remember why. People may feel more anxious, a kind of nagging discomfort that just won't go away, only to return to the trigger unknowingly. Though findings on specific groups differ, the literature largely supports the effects that social media can have on mental health, particularly in increasing anxiety and depression in susceptible populations (Barman et al., 2018; Karim et al., 2020; Lai et al., 2023).

As the 21st century got under way, some questions were strongly raised about social media and sociopolitical changes. This has been where Twitter, Facebook, Reddit, Instagram, and TikTok have garnered the power to overturn things entirely. We saw this with the now forgotten Arab Spring of the early 2010s, often pointed to as an example of the socio-political reach of social media (Emmanouilidou, 2020). It mobilized and organized one of the earliest political movements and brought it to America. This was in its time a novel concept but such is the power of connecting continents. Social media has facilitated and sped-up long-distance communication, bringing together different groups that have shared objectives. Social media has also become an influential method of raising public awareness about sociopolitical issues. Hashtag activism, where a particular phrase or word preceded by '#' is employed to group together conversations about a given subject, is common (Goswami, 2018). It can lead to issues coming into sharper focus than they might under conventional media coverage.

In recent years, the proliferation of violent imagery on social media platforms has been called into question and is of great concern to both the public and academic researchers going beyond traditional media (Bostic, 2014). Social media makes possible instant and at times malicious dissemination and consumption of graphic material, often without filtering or warnings, such as the livestreamed Christchurch mass shootings in New Zealand (Mulholland, 2019). While most people did not return to see that, (and if you did, please see a Psychologist), most people cannot always control what they'll scroll to next, in a post, a story, even a direct message from your sister, whom you trust. In that moment of grief, she shared a post that will haunt you till lunch.

Studies have well-documented the impact of violent imagery on mental health, collectively. Holman et al, (2019) explored the mass trauma experienced by those consuming news on social media. Media-based stories of traumatic events expand the events' boundaries from geographically constrained to virtually boundless experiences, transforming local events into widespread collective traumas, according to the authors. Although access to media stories about these events may appropriately inform us about events in our world, prolonged exposure to media coverage also may serve to amplify and heighten public anxiety and fear. A growing body of literature suggests that with the 24-hr news cycle and ubiquitous digital news platforms, media coverage following disasters and mass violence events may have a more complex, unintended, injurious impact, they stated. The study further clarifies that witnessing intrusive and traumatic images, such as car accident victims, can produce flashbacks by activating areas of the brain that are linked to fear and threat processing. They cite research showing that children exposed to media images of war injuries and death reported more severe posttraumatic stress symptoms after the first Gulf War, and subsequent studies of 9/11 and the Iraq War some images, particularly those depicting severe injury or death, are more likely to cause distress, and longer-term studies showed that these images can have a prolonged effect even 2-3 years later (Holman, 2019; Silver, 2013). The brain sees and emotionally processes actual footage differently than the carnage wreaked by the Avengers in a Marvel movie.

Even as recent as pre-pandemic, social media did not stream news like it does now. With individuals using their handles as news accounts, they have gained legitimacy. A large majority of Americans now prefer getting their news through digital devices (i.e., phones, laptops, tablets), and at least half get news through social media (Forman-Katz & Matsa, 2023). Slowly, even I started turning to these accounts for what I was not being shown on mainstream media. As a long-time reader of the New York Times, I found myself disillusioned with their trite headlines pandering to the West's agenda, and instead turned to Instagram pages that would repost these headlines crossed out, saying "there, I fixed it for you" as they countered the manufactured mainstream narratives.

During the pandemic, Instagram became a haven for me and many others. Mothers, like me, found something to do in between remote classes, work, cooking, cleaning, and ordering abnormally expensive eggs from Amazon Fresh. I could immediately see horrors unfolding at Elmhurst Hospital where bodies of Covid-19 deaths were piling up just a few miles from my home (Carrington, 2021), but also find a recipe on BuzzFeed to cook that evening. It became a portal to a world I was too scared to breathe in, for a period that seemed like eternity.

Donald Trump became an entertainment, and sometimes the scariest thing for some on social media, especially if you were a woman or a minority, or just well-informed (Graham et al., 2019; Prasad, 2019). You would find out what he said in an obscure fundraiser from a video someone had made at Mar-a-Lago. We learned about his dealings behind the scenes and watched countless videos of the January 6 insurrection on our phones. Black Lives Matter, a movement originating in 2013 online communities, was newly invigorated during his presidency and expanded its reach to educate younger people through social media (Bestvater et al., 2023). Social media discussion allowed people to understand concepts such as 'critical race theory', and 'systemic racism', as if they were always part of the public discourse (Cineas, 2021).

Then came the Ukraine war. We initially showed concern and quickly realized that the president of Ukraine was on the cover of Vogue and doing better than you. Not to mention the pandering to Congress for our taxpayer money. Zelensky's speeches wedged between Oscar winners and every mainstream media showcasing him, saturation which made social media lose interest in Ukraine and Zelensky, fast (Mitrovica, 2023). We can tell if the mainstream newspapers or primetime channels are showing you, you probably don't need our attention. People are obsessed with social media because it shows us what is really happening while giving a break by following it with an empowering quote, a celebrity without makeup, and how to organize your sock drawer. We now turn to social media because it is unfiltered. It does not insult your intelligence unless you want it to. You see, social media is authentically tailored to you, reading your thoughts like a little best friend.

Matthew Price in his PTSD Bytes podcast addresses a term coined during the pandemic; 'doomscrolling'. Researchers found an increase in negative emotions people felt after looking through endless negative social media stories. Doomscrolling may make you feel anxious or worried without offering a particular solution or helping you address some of the challenges you're facing (Buchanan et al., 2021). Doomscrolling exposes us to a lot of emotionally charged information, and that can be especially challenging for individuals with PTSD to handle (Kartol et al., 2023).

Social media truly came to collect souls on October 7th, 2023, and the days and months following it. People who had never heard of Palestine and Gaza had questions about this "middle east" situation they had heard about for so long. Optics and headlines that had been around and floated as fact for decades were destroyed in a matter of hours, let alone days, on social media. CNN journalist Sara Sidner spurred news of "40 headless babies", and social media demanded proof (Sara Sidner, 2023). When there was none, social media turned on mainstream media for allowing such inflammatory lies to be presented as truth. Mainstream media lost most if not all its virtue. I was invited to be a guest on a CBS news show a couple of days after the attacks. I told the producer that people were getting their news without them, and if they wanted to remain in the news business, they were going to have to change their scripts. To my surprise, they agreed, and stated that they were aware of what their viewers wanted to see. As a Psychologist, I spoke about the impact of the violence on social media, on the young minds, and how parents can protect them.

The 1200 Israeli deaths and the 250 hostages taken at the hand of Hamas remained a focus of mainstream media, and the White House, but on social media where the majority of the world was getting its news, images of thousands of Palestinian burnt babies and shredded children, at the hands of the Israeli army, flooded our screens. Social media algorithms and content production favored pro-Palestine content, likely indicating that it receives more engagement from users (Scott, 2023). Calls for ceasefire and to stop funding Israel became a staple on social media, especially

Instagram and Tik-Tok. History lessons abound, everyone became an expert on the Middle East, Israel and Palestine. For several months, the trauma of gory images became the trauma of feeling betrayed and silenced by the powers that be. People became disillusioned with the mainstream media's exclusive focus on Israeli victims while ignoring the Palestinian victims, even though estimates of Palestinian deaths directly related to the conflict are around 35,000 (and combined with indirect deaths could be up to 186,000, or nearly 9% of the Palestinian population) (Khatib et al., 2024). The Onion, a satirical newspaper, which has been around since I was in college, stated that they "stand with Israel, because it seems you get in far less trouble for that" (The Onion Editorial Board, 2023).

People's emotions, raw vulnerability, empathy, and ancestral connections suddenly seemed at the forefront. We are a tribal people, we need to find affiliation and connection, and the long history of antisemitism, the Holocaust, and the Muslim experience in the West, all played into the tragedies we selectively saw. Every post was littered with insults being hurled with expletives or genuine reasoning, with emojis, the Israeli and Palestinian flags. People started to lose sight of reality feeling so tied into their blood lines, and religious affiliations, not having been to a mosque or observing sabbath, maybe ever. It awoke humanity, and many were heartened to see people of all backgrounds come together for humanity. One example of this is the survivors of the Holocaust or children of the survivors of the Holocaust making the most noise, "not in our name" (Le Masurier, 2023). Others are powerful groups such as 'Jewish Voices for Peace', and scholars such as Gabor Mate, a powerhouse in his own right in the field of neuropsychological advances, have been vocal about this violence even prior to the October 7th attacks (Mate & Hollington-Sawyer, 2014). However, many were unwilling to notice the disparity between the numbers, facts, and there were those who negated the Hamas attacks on October 7th. Trauma is multi-layered and there is no better global or collective example than of this very moment in history.

Secondary trauma occurs when anyone who bears witness to someone else's tragedy and trauma, may feel the after-effect as the primary victim (Brecier & Maynard, 2015). Douglas Yeung wrote for the USA Today, as an Opinion Contributor, "Secondary trauma was, for a long time, largely confined to people involved in the initial event, like first responders. Thanks to technology, however, it can now afflict anyone with a smartphone" (Yeung, 2023). Malaka Gharib writes for NPR News "I've noticed that something strange is happening to me. Even when I am not watching the news, I feel irritable and anxious, like I am on high alert. Whenever I am with my own 8-month-old child, I get flashbacks of posts I've seen, especially of children and infants killed, and I worry for his safety. What is going on? How can I pull myself out of this nightmare loop?" (Gharib, 2023). Once you get hooked on these images, as unpleasant as they may be, the brain starts to crave them, as the balance of dopamine in the brain is continually upset by the intentionally addictive design of digital devices and social media sites (e.g., quick bursts of dopamine produced by consuming content followed by desire to consume more from withdrawals from the dopamine imbalance) that encourage continuous use even when the content is not pleasurable for users (Gross, 2021). The cry may feel like relief, or an awareness of how blessed you are or how small your problems may be, but they are all dopamine hits that keep you scrolling for more gore.

The stark difference in mainstream news, the politics, and the trauma scrolling on our screens was undeniable. Social media with its global power created awareness leading to unprecedented marches in major cities across the world, including London, Madrid, Istanbul, Jerusalem, Tel Aviv, Tokyo, and Sydney (Al Jazeera News Agencies, 2024; "Pro-Palestine student protests," 2024). What really held the world captive, was the horrific imagery, often uploaded by Palestinian journalists, and disseminated by social media activists. We could not stop watching them, and relating to people most people knew nothing about. Meta and Facebook started shadow banning these accounts if not completely deleting them. The uproar over free speech became yet another battle for the disillusioned. There is a trauma attached to one's own sense of safety that the war in Gaza took away from those following it on social media. It went beyond just the pileup of dead children or wailing mothers. It was a reminder that human life did not matter equally. It triggered insecurities, moral and morality discussions, and just like with American politics a few years ago, divided people.

I started to analyze my own reactions. In the early months, I found myself crying openly into my coffee, or welling up at the most inopportune moments. I wept at my desk, and at least once a day, would have a patient who would start talking about the genocide in Gaza. How could this be happening in real time? How could we stand by and let it? This wasn't the 1940s where Hitler got away with mass murdering millions of Jews. We could see these horrors on the little screen in our palms before we brush our teeth in the morning. Each scene filmed by another on the ground, shared by several accounts, triggered the viewers. There was a steady rise in anti-Semitic and anti-Islamic hate. Celebrities were too quiet; people looked at them with disdain and disgust for not saying anything. Some deleted their posts after being told that the photo they had posted was not of Israeli children or wreckage, but of Gaza's. Washington Post published an article about this phenomenon about Jamie Lee Curtis, and Justin Bieber, and how they had been victims of this social media verification (Chery, 2023). There was a strange feeling of seeing what had been behind the curtain most of our lives, sheltered by the usual newspapers and TV news channels like CNN. An award-winning Anthony Bourdain episode about Gaza garnered attention as did a movie called 'Israelism', that campuses tried to ban, without success. Social media won every battle against a mainstream outlet on its small scale, but the movement continued to gain momentum.

My mood was non celebratory, anxious and depressed. I hadn't felt like this even when my father had died a few years ago. I found it hard to enjoy things and wanted to hold on to my children at drop off to school. I started to see people I knew on social media with disdain for posting a photo of their coffee, or dog. I started to notice a lack of empathy and compassion in my then-husband, perhaps not for the first time, but it stuck. I filed for divorce only two months later, disillusioned and disconnected from him. True story.

Some days, I was grateful that I had been protected from these grotesque images in my younger years. They were unnerving. I am not just an adult, but one trained to understand PTSD and trauma, even more than many of my peers. I consider myself well-adjusted, and fortunately, largely free of major traumas that others have endured. What was this doing to those who had previous trauma? Those that had been in an accident? Those that had lost a loved one to violence? Or simply a first responder or counselor who had numbed himself over the year as "this is just part of the job". How did that woman, who had escaped from a war-torn country of her own, react? A new mother, who was nursing her baby, while seeing a Palestinian woman rock hers in a white shroud. Media exposure of traumatic events has been shown to increase the risk of Post-Traumatic Stress Disorder (PTSD) and Secondary Traumatic Stress (STS) as well as reduce people's trust in media reliability, which begs the question of how this barrage of traumatic events displayed on social media is doubly affecting those with existing trauma and how they further engage with content (Abdalla et al., 2021; Lamba et al., 2023). It is even of concern for those who help these individuals process their experiences, as even therapists can experience secondary trauma stemming from interactions with patients (Johansen et al., 2019).

The definition of PTSD describes witnessing or experiencing a traumatic or abnormal event, with symptoms including recurrent memories and flashbacks of the events causing distress, sleep disturbances, and avoidant behaviors, among others (Taylor-Desir, 2022). There was nothing normal about this real-life horror show. People's colonial and generational traumas were being triggered. Researchers looking into the responses of Jordanian teenagers, more than half of whom have shared ancestry with Palestinians, found increased stress levels from witnessing the violence in the Gaza Strip. A respondent said "What can I do for Gaza? I am just one person. . .I feel hopeless," and another explained how nightmares kept them up at night and they had difficulty concentrating on their studies, showing the deep emotional response experienced by those witnessing these traumatic events from a secondary perspective (Al-Maghaireh et al., 2024).

This feeling of hopelessness and helplessness has not been limited to those with Palestinian ancestry or those across the border from the West Bank and Gaza Strip, however. I started to get private messages from men and women from different backgrounds and cultures looking to find more answers. I was just like them, albeit with a longer standing knowledge of both the region and the role of mainstream news. They spoke to me about their mental health crises, and forged friendships with merely an account on Instagram. This is also an example of collective trauma, or psychological reactions to a traumatic event affecting an entire society, in the new, virtual world (Hirschberger, 2018).

While this chapter is dedicated to the impact of unfettered social media on mental health, and particularly as a conduit to secondary trauma, I would be remiss if I did not mention the incredible impact of social media on political movements, even compelling South Africa to bring a case of genocide against Israel to the International Court of Justice (ICJ) ("'Chilling evidence'," 2024). It brought worldwide attention to a long-standing occupation and apartheid conditions, long kept under wraps by mainstream Western media. In response, the US government, which took decades to put a warning label on cigarette cartons, banned TikTok, a social media platform instrumental in showing real time images and livestreams of Palestine's destruction and the atrocities committed by Israel, to the extent that these images and videos were presented as evidence in the International Court of Justice, such was their mark (Fatafta, 2024). The US government cited concerns that the Chinese government could access sensitive user data in banning a very popular social media platform, despite the fact that sites like Facebook, Instagram, and Twitter were infiltrated by Russian interference with the 2016 election and were not held accountable by the government (Mak, 2019).

The continued movement on social media and the lack of action by our own politicians led to rampant, undeterred college encampments across the US in 2024, nation-wide protests demanding divestment from Israel, and that the Western world stop treating the rest of us like imbeciles.

Clearly, social media is here to stay and is giving rise to scholars, activists, and even playing a major role in bringing awareness to mental health issues. How can we find a way to live with it?

Let's talk neuropsychology for a minute;

How does trauma embed itself into the brain?

After the brain receives violent image, a series of complex psychological and physiological events are set in motion:

Step 1: Visual Processing. The primary visual cortex and other parts of the brain process image's simplest features like shape and color.

Step 2: Emotional Reaction. The amygdala, a part of the brain which processes emotions and fearful stimuli's most sensitive site, immediately issues some kind of emotional response - such as fear, disgust, or anger. The brain attaches this emotion to the visual imagery it has just seen.

Step 3: Cognitive Appraisal. The prefrontal cortex--which governs higher-order cognitive activities--evaluates the image. It mediates emotional response by evaluating context and relevance to decide whether this is or is not a real threat. Even when it is not deemed a real or viable threat to oneself, the brain recognizes that this is not a movie, that the image or a short clip seen is real. If it came from a reliable source or forwarded by a friend or sibling, it raises in value and authenticity.

Step 4: Physical Response. Through the hypothalamus, the brain communicates with the rest of your body and may activate a "fight or flight" reaction. Such activation of the body can mean an elevated heart rate, spiked blood pressure, and increased respiration rate--readying oneself for potential threats. This happens when we are on a roller coaster, watching a movie, readying for an argument with a partner, because the human brain is designed to protect the body at all costs.

Step 5: Desensitization. As the brain has been repeatedly exposed to violent images, it can gradually become less responsive to such stimuli. This is called desensitization and helps reduce the emotional impact of violent images over time. However, this repeated trauma can damage the brain, its ability to trust its environment, and others. Children who have been exposed to violence at a younger age have a much greater likelihood of developing depression, anxiety, and violent tendencies.

Step 6: Formation of memories. Because the hippocampus is involved in forming memories and calling them back up again for use later, repeated exposures to violent images can make these thoughts more easily remembered. It may even bring on delusions about part of what one has experienced. Regurgitation of memories, involuntarily, retraumatizes the brain.

7: Reaction to stress. If the body releases stress hormones such as cortisol (and for long periods), then mood and stress states will alter.

8: Activation of mirror neurons. In a person's mind, mirror neurons might simulate or even literally "mirror" the observed actions—so that when someone else is being aggressive the viewer might feel empathy or distress for them. As if he were actually doing it himself.

9. Long-term effects. People who see too much violence over time will suffer more aggression later, be more scared, see their minds insensibly turned away from real-life violence until it has no effect at all, and in certain cases develop post-traumatic stress disorder (PTSD) especially if they have a personal history with trauma or have been victimized themselves.

10: Different people's coping strategies are probably crucial to how the mind reacts over time to violent images: some people will become more vigilant; others may actively shun them or like a stone learn not to feel.

While many posts or stories on social media started carrying trigger warnings before going to graphic content, it was either disregarded or even created more suspense. There is much discussion as to how this sort of media should be regulated.

What are some possible solutions? As technology and various social media platforms evolve, there are several possibilities and solutions on the horizon to protect the human mind and race;

1. Content tailoring: Platforms could adjust their algorithms to do a better job of personalizing news content. This way they might eliminate triggering posts that could upset certain users, such as those with mental health problems, or provide contextual suggestions like talking to a trusted adult (McHugh et al., 2018). This helps safeguard the most vulnerable, yet at the same time it raises questions about echo chambers and the balance between mental well-being and informed citizenship. Even worse, if people start censoring information in order to make sensitive issues "politically correct" for others' comfort (either intentionally or by unconsciously turning a blind eye), then there will also be challenges for public discourse and education.
2. Digital well-being handles: As increasing numbers of people become concerned about the impact of social media on mental health, platforms are likely to offer users more tools and tricks to manage their consumption and exposure to news. These could include screen-time limits, reminders to take breaks, stops for keywords that evoke strong feelings or addictions (McHugh et al., 2018).
3. Mental Health Education: Social media is increasingly being used as a tool for raising public consciousness and teaching people what mental health resources exist on the Internet, providing information about how they work. It could become more common for mental health organizations and social media platforms to join forces in joint efforts.
4. AI and Emotional Analysis: Artificial intelligence is set to play a larger role in reading the emotional tenor of news stories and reactions to those stories. Suggestions could come in the form of real-time mental health support, like a link to a virtual counselor, using a deep breathing app or tool, or even a prompt to call one of your favorites.
5. Privacy and Data Ethics: The ethical uses of data for predicting mental-health problems or crafting user experiences will continue to be much debated, as they should. As these technologies grow more complex in their capabilities, ensuring privacy and standards of ethical conduct--will become increasingly important.

6. Empowerment of the users: Users could receive more control over what sorts of news they see, with possibilities for even finer-grained content preferences. This might help people engage with the news in a way healthier for their mental health.
7. Peer Support Networks: Social media could see the growth of peer support networks, where people can discuss their reactions to news events under a safe and moderated environment of people promoting mental well-being. To some degree, this is already available but there is no way to filter abusive language, bots, and those looking to disrupt.
8. Oversight: There might be increased pressure on social media companies to adhere to directives aimed at safeguarding mental health, demands like requiring them give transparency about their news algorithms and conduct service impact evaluations on well-being.
9. Collaboration between mental health and technology companies: As more and more research data is accumulating about the junction of social media, news consumption and mental health, collaborative research and solutions will likely allow us to generate more sophisticated risk-mitigation strategies--including cooperation between tech companies and mental health experts.
10. Traditional mental health interventions: Both traditional and more modern, holistic psychotherapeutic approaches such as interpersonal psychotherapy (ITP) and Trauma-Focused Cognitive-Behavioral Therapy (TF-CBT), as well as art and recreational programs like aerobic laughter therapy and drumming group therapy, have been shown to have positive outcomes in reducing symptoms of PTSD and secondary trauma, which could be helpful for those experiencing secondary stress from social media exposure (Bercier & Maynard, 2015; Kim et al., 2022; Ramirez de Arellano et al., 2014). Teaching patients mindfulness strategies and implementing mindfulness interventions, particularly smartphone-based trainings, can also help reduce trauma and stress symptoms, even in group settings (Kim et al., 2022; Wylde et al., 2017)

It is thus undisputed, given the biology of visual imagery of a violent, graphic nature, and its impact on the brain that repeated and extended contact can lead to more chronic psychological problems such as symptoms consistent with post-traumatic stress disorder (PTSD), especially in individuals who predispose themselves to or have a history of psychological trauma.

Here is the big question; is it too late? Can we quit social media? Can we quit our need for not just news but news from various sources, all at the same time? The other big movement across all races and nations is striving for better mental health while we plunge our brains into darkness the minute we wake up. We know that brain volume, experiences of happiness, and future psychopathology, least of which is PTSD, is all greatly impacted by the continuous stream of consumption of real-life violence.

In the meantime, my next dating profile will emphasize the value of an empathetic, emotionally and politically intelligent partner, because I need some compassion to combat the PTSD, at the end of a tiring day of doomscrolling.

REFERENCES

Abdalla, S. M., Cohen, G. H., Tamrakar, S., Koya, S. F., & Galea, S. (2021). Media Exposure and the Risk of Post-Traumatic Stress Disorder Following a Mass traumatic Event: An In-silico Experiment. *Frontiers in Psychiatry*, 12, 674263. Advance online publication. DOI: 10.3389/fpsyt.2021.674263 PMID: 34899406

Ashar, L. C. (2024, May 2). Social Media Impact: How Social Media Sites Affect Society. https://www.apu.apus.edu/area-of-study/business-and-management/resources/how-social-media-sites-affect-society/

Barman, L., Mukhopadhyay, D. K., & Bandyopadhyay, G. K. (2018). Use of Social Networking Site and Mental Disorders among Medical Students in Kolkata, West Bengal. *Indian Journal of Psychiatry*, 60(3), 340–345. DOI: 10.4103/psychiatry.IndianJPsychiatry_210_18 PMID: 30405262

Bercier, M. L., & Maynard, B. R. (2015). Interventions for Secondary Traumatic Stress With Mental Health Workers: A Systematic Review. *Research on Social Work Practice*, 25(1), 81–89. DOI: 10.1177/1049731513517142

Bestvater, S., Gelles-Watnick, R., Odabas, M., Anderson, M., & Smith, A. (2023, June 29). #BlackLivesMatter Turns 10. Pew Research Center. https://www.pewresearch.org/internet/2023/06/29/blacklivesmatter-turns-10/

Blake, M. (2015, August 6). Nine times Jon Stewart proved he was more than just a comedian. Los Angeles Times. https://www.latimes.com/entertainment/tv/showtracker/la-et-st-jon-stewart-definitive-moments-the-daily-show-20150805-html-htmlstory.html

Bostic, B. (2014, February 20). Does Social Media Perpetuate Youth Violence? Michigan Youth Violence Prevention Center. https://yvpc.sph.umich.edu/social-media-perpetuate-youth-violence/

Buchanan, K., Aknin, L. B., Lotun, S., & Sandstrom, G. M. (2021). Brief exposure to social media during the COVID-19 pandemic: Doom-scrolling has negative emotional consequences, but kindness-scrolling does not. *PLoS One*, 16(10), e0257728. DOI: 10.1371/journal.pone.0257728 PMID: 34644310

Carrington, A. E. (2021, March 28). How NY hospital faced COVID devastation and came back from the brink. ABC News. https://abcnews.go.com/Health/ny-hospital-faced-covid-devastation-back-brink/story?id=76638912

Chery, S. (2023, October 25). Where celebrities went wrong opining on the Israel-Gaza war. Washington Post. https://www.washingtonpost.com/entertainment/2023/10/25/celebrities-react-israel-gaza-war-palestinian-hamas/

'Chilling' evidence: ICJ hears South Africa's genocide case against Israel. (2024, January 11). Al Jazeera. https://www.aljazeera.com/news/2024/1/11/icj-hears-south-africas-genocide-case-against-israel-over-gaza-war

Cineas, F. (2021, June 24). What the hysteria over critical race theory is really all about. Vox. https://www.vox.com/22443822/critical-race-theory-controversy

Drew, R. (2001, September 20). A Day of Terror. https://archive.nytimes.com/www.nytimes.com/slideshow/2001/09/20/12DEST.9.slideshow_4.html

Emmanouilidou, L. (2020, December 17). Arab uprisings: What role did social media really play? The World from PRX. https://theworld.org/stories/2020/12/17/arab-uprisings-what-role-did-social-media-really-play

Fatafta, M. (2024, March 20). Genocide in the digital age: What role do social media companies play? Association for Progressive Communications. https://www.apc.org/en/blog/genocide-digital-age-what-role-do-social-media-companies-play

Gharib, M. (2023, November 24). Watching war unfold is distressing—Here's how to protect your mental health. NPR. https://www.npr.org/sections/health-shots/2023/11/24/1214534579/images-war-gaza-israel-vicarious-trauma-stress

Goswami, M. (2018). Social Media and Hashtag Activism. In Liberty, Dignity, and Change in Journalism (pp. 252–262). Kanishka.

Graham, D. A., Green, A., Murphy, C., & Richards, P. (2019, May 13). An Oral History of Trump's Bigotry. The Atlantic. https://www.theatlantic.com/magazine/archive/2019/06/trump-racism-comments/588067/

Gross, T. (2021, August 25). In "Dopamine Nation," Overabundance Keeps Us Craving More. NPR. https://www.npr.org/sections/health-shots/2021/08/25/1030930259/in-dopamine-nation-overabundance-keeps-u-s-craving-more

Hafeez, S. (2002). The relationship between violence-related trauma and length of exposure to PTSD in emergency medical technicians [Unpublished doctoral dissertation]. Hofstra University.

Hirschberger, G. (2018). Collective Trauma and the Social Construction of Meaning. *Frontiers in Psychology*, 9, 1441. DOI: 10.3389/fpsyg.2018.01441 PMID: 30147669

Holman, E. A., Garfin, D. R., Lubens, P., & Silver, R. C. (2020). Media Exposure to Collective Trauma, Mental Health, and Functioning: Does It Matter What You See? *Clinical Psychological Science*, 8(1), 111–124. DOI: 10.1177/2167702619858300

Johansen, A. B., Kristiansen, E., Bjelland, I., & Tavakoli, S. (2019). Secondary traumatic stress in Norwegian SUD-therapists: Symptoms and related factors. Nordisk Alkohol- & Narkotikatidskrift. *Nordisk Alkohol- & Narkotikatidskrift*, 36(6), 522–531. DOI: 10.1177/1455072519847014 PMID: 32934585

Karim, F., Oyewande, A. A., Abdalla, L. F., Chaudhry Ehsanullah, R., & Khan, S. (2020). Social Media Use and Its Connection to Mental Health: A Systematic Review. *Cureus*, 12(6), e8627. DOI: 10.7759/cureus.8627 PMID: 32685296

Kartol, A., Üztemur, S., & Yaşar, P. (2023). 'I cannot see ahead': Psychological distress, doomscrolling and dark future among adult survivors following Mw 7.7. and 7.6 earthquakes in Türkiye. *BMC Public Health*, 23(1), 2513. DOI: 10.1186/s12889-023-17460-3 PMID: 38102569

Khatib, R., McKee, M., & Yusuf, S. (2024). Counting the dead in Gaza: Difficult but essential. *Lancet*, 0(0), 237–238. Advance online publication. DOI: 10.1016/S0140-6736(24)01169-3 PMID: 38976995

Kim, J., Chesworth, B., Franchino-Olsen, H., & Macy, R. J. (2022). A scoping review of vicarious trauma interventions for service providers working with people who have experienced traumatic events. *Trauma, Violence & Abuse*, 23(5), 152483802199131. DOI: 10.1177/1524838021991310 PMID: 33685294

Lai, F., Wang, L., Zhang, J., Shan, S., Chen, J., & Tian, L. (2023). Relationship between Social Media Use and Social Anxiety in College Students: Mediation Effect of Communication Capacity. *International Journal of Environmental Research and Public Health*, 20(4), 3657. DOI: 10.3390/ijerph20043657 PMID: 36834357

Lamba, N., Khokhlova, O., Bhatia, A., & McHugh, C. (2023). Mental health hygiene during a health crisis: Exploring factors associated with media-induced secondary trauma in relation to the COVID-19 pandemic. *Health Psychology Open*, 10(2), 20551029231199578. Advance online publication. DOI: 10.1177/20551029231199578 PMID: 37746585

Mak, T. (2019, October 8). Senate Report: Russians Used Social Media Mostly To Target Race In 2016. NPR. https://www.npr.org/2019/10/08/768319934/senate-report-russians-used-used-social-media-mostly-to-target-race-in-2016

Mate, G., & Hollington-Sawyer, S. (2014, July 28). Israel: The Beautiful Dream has become a Nightmare. https://drgabormate.com/beautiful-dream-israel-become-nightmare/

McHugh, B. C., Wisniewski, P., Rosson, M. B., & Carroll, J. M. (2018). When social media traumatizes teens: The roles of online risk exposure, coping, and post-traumatic stress. *Internet Research*, 28(5), 1169–1188. DOI: 10.1108/IntR-02-2017-0077

Mitrovica, A. (2023, December 7). Volodymyr Zelenskyy: The forgotten man. Al Jazeera. https://www.aljazeera.com/opinions/2023/12/7/volodymyr-zelenskyy-the-forgotten-man

Motta, R., Hafeez, S., Sciancalepore, R., & Diaz, A. (2001). Discriminant Validation of the Modified Secondary Trauma Questionnaire. *Journal of Psychotherapy in Independent Practice*, 24(4), 17–25. DOI: 10.1300/J288v02n04_02

Motta, R. W., Kefer, J. M., Hertz, M. D., & Hafeez, S. (1999). Initial evaluation of the Secondary Trauma Questionnaire. *Psychological Reports*, 85(3 Pt 1), 997–1002. DOI: 10.2466/pr0.1999.85.3.997 PMID: 10672764

Mulholland, J. M. Tara. (2019, March 15). How the Christchurch terrorist attack was made for social media | CNN Business. CNN. https://www.cnn.com/2019/03/15/tech/christchurch-internet-radicalization-intl/index.html

Prasad, R. (2019, November 29). How Trump talks about women—And does it matter? https://www.bbc.com/news/world-us-canada-50563106

Pro-Palestine student protests spread to Japan. (2024, May 3). Middle East Monitor. https://www.middleeastmonitor.com/20240503-pro-palestine-student-protests-spread-to-japan/

Ramirez de Arellano, M. A., Lyman, D. R., Jobe-Shields, L., George, P., Dougherty, R. H., Daniels, A. S., Ghose, S. S., Huang, L., & Delphin-Rittmon, M. E. (2014). Trauma-Focused Cognitive-Behavioral Therapy for Children and Adolescents: Assessing the Evidence. *Psychiatric Services (Washington, D.C.)*, 65(5), 591–602. DOI: 10.1176/appi.ps.201300255 PMID: 24638076

Scott, M. (2023, December 14). Does social media favor Palestine over Israel? POLITICO. https://www.politico.eu/newsletter/digital-bridge/does-social-media-favor-palestine-over-israel/

Taylor-Desir, M. (2022, November). What is post-traumatic stress disorder (PTSD)? Psychiatry.org; American Psychiatric Association. https://www.psychiatry.org/patients-families/ptsd/what-is-ptsd

The Onion Editorial Board. (2023, October 13). 'The Onion' Stands With Israel Because It Seems Like You Get In Less Trouble For That. The Onion. https://www.theonion.com/the-onion-stands-with-israel-because-it-seems-like-yo-1850922505

Wylde, M. C., Mahrer, E. N., Meyer, M. L. R., & Gold, I. J. (2017). Mindfulness for Novice Pediatric Nurses: Smartphone Application Versus Traditional Intervention. *Journal of Pediatric Nursing*, 36, 205–212. DOI: 10.1016/j.pedn.2017.06.008 PMID: 28888505

Yeung, D. (2023, November 3). I can't help but follow graphic images from Israel-Hamas war. I should know better. USA TODAY. https://www.usatoday.com/story/opinion/voices/2023/11/03/israel-hamas-war-images-trauma-mental-health/71334176007/

Compilation of References

Abdalla, S. M., Cohen, G. H., Tamrakar, S., Koya, S. F., & Galea, S. (2021). Media Exposure and the Risk of Post-Traumatic Stress Disorder Following a Mass traumatic Event: An In-silico Experiment. *Frontiers in Psychiatry*, 12, 674263. Advance online publication. DOI: 10.3389/fpsyt.2021.674263 PMID: 34899406

Abd-Alrazaq, A. A., Alajlani, M., Ali, N., Denecke, K., Bewick, B. M., & Househ, M. (2021). Perceptions and Opinions of Patients About Mental Health Chatbots: Scoping Review. *Journal of Medical Internet Research*, 23(1), e17828. DOI: 10.2196/17828 PMID: 33439133

Acheson, D. T., Gresack, J. E., & Risbrough, V. B. (2012). Hippocampal dysfunction effects on context memory: Possible etiology for post-traumatic stress disorder. *Neuropharmacology*, 62(2), 674–685. DOI: 10.1016/j.neuropharm.2011.04.029 PMID: 21596050

Adamowska, S., Adamowski, T., Frydecka, D., & Kiejna, A. (2014). Diagnostic validity polish language version of the questionnaire MINI-KID (Mini international neuropsychiatry interview for children and adolescent). *Comprehensive Psychiatry*, 55(7), 1744–1750. DOI: 10.1016/j.comppsych.2014.05.019 PMID: 25023384

Aerni, A., Traber, R., Hock, C., Roozendaal, B., Schelling, G., Papassotiropoulos, A., Nitsch, R. M., Schnyder, U., & de Quervain, D. J.-F. (2004). Low-dose cortisol for symptoms of posttraumatic stress disorder. *The American Journal of Psychiatry*, 161(8), 1488–1490. DOI: 10.1176/appi.ajp.161.8.1488 PMID: 15285979

Agustini, E. N., & Matsuo, H. (2012). Children and Adolescents-Survivors of the 2004 Indian Ocean Tsunami: Prevalence of Long-Term PTSD and Coping Strategies. In Lopez, G. I. (Ed.), *Tsunami-Analysis of a Hazard-From Physical Interpretation to Human Impact*. IntechOpen Limited.

Ahmedani, B. K. (2011). Mental health stigma: society, individuals, and the profession. J Soc Work Values Ethics, 8(2), 4-1–4-16.

Aimone, J. B., Li, Y., Lee, S. W., Clemenson, G. D., Deng, W., & Gage, F. H. (2014). Regulation and function of adult neurogenesis: From genes to cognition.*Physiological Reviews*, 94(4), 991–1026. DOI: 10.1152/physrev.00004.2014 PMID: 25287858

Al Jowf, G. I., Ahmed, Z. T., Reijnders, R. A., de Nijs, L., & Eijssen, L. M. T. (2023). To Predict, Prevent, and Manage Post-Traumatic Stress Disorder (PTSD): A Review of Pathophysiology, Treatment, and Biomarkers.*International Journal of Molecular Sciences*, 24(6), 6. Advance online publication. DOI: 10.3390/ijms24065238 PMID: 36982313

Aliev, G., Beeraka, N. M., Nikolenko, V. N., Svistunov, A. A., Rozhnova, T., Kostyuk, S., Cherkesov, I., Gavryushova, L. V., Chekhonatsky, A. A., Mikhaleva, L. M., Somasundaram, S. G., Avila-Rodriguez, M. F., & Kirkland, C. E. (2020). Neurophysiology and psychopathology underlying PTSD and recent insights into the PTSD therapies—A comprehensive review.*Journal of Clinical Medicine*, 9(9), 1–19. DOI: 10.3390/jcm9092951 PMID: 32932645

Alneyadi, M., Drissi, N., Almeqbaali, M., & Ouhbi, S. (2021). Biofeedback-based connected mental health interventions for anxiety: Systematic literature review. *JMIR mHealth and uHealth*, 9(4), e26038. DOI: 10.2196/26038 PMID: 33792548

Altman, J. (1969). Autoradiographic and histological studies of postnatal neurogenesis. IV. Cell proliferation and migration in the anterior forebrain, with special reference to persisting neurogenesis in the olfactory bulb.*The Journal of Comparative Neurology*, 137(4), 433–457. DOI: 10.1002/cne.901370404 PMID: 5361244

Altman, J., & Das, G. D. (1965). Autoradiographic and histological evidence of postnatal hippocampal neurogenesis in rats.*The Journal of Comparative Neurology*, 124(3), 319–335. DOI: 10.1002/cne.901240303 PMID: 5861717

Ambrosini, P. J. (2000). Historical development and present status of the schedule for affective disorders and schizophrenia for school-age children (K-SADS).*Journal of the American Academy of Child and Adolescent Psychiatry*, 39(1), 49–58. DOI: 10.1097/00004583-200001000-00016 PMID: 10638067

American Psychiatric Association. (1980). *Diagnostic and statistical manual of mental disorders* (3rd ed.). Author.

American Psychiatric Association. (1994). *Diagnostic and Statistical Manual of Mental Disorders* (4th ed.).

American Psychiatric Association. (2004). *Practice guideline for the treatment of patient with acute stress disorder and posttraumatic stress disorder*. American Psychiatric Association.

American Psychiatric Association. (2009). *Practice guideline for the treatment of patients with acute stress disorder and posttraumatic stress disorder: guideline watch*. American Psychiatric Association.

American Psychiatric Association. A. P., & Association, A. P. (1994). *Diagnostic and statistical manual of mental disorders: DSM-IV* (Vol. 4). American psychiatric association Washington, DC.

American Psychological Association. (2017). *Clinical practice guideline for the treatment of Posttraumatic Stress Disorder (PTSD) in adults*. Retrieved December 30, 2023, from https://www.apa.org/ptsd-guideline

American Psychological Association. (2017). Ethical principles of psychologists and code of conduct (2002, amended effective June 1, 2010, and January 1, 2017). https://www.apa.org/ethics/code/

American Psychological Association. (2017). Guideline Development Panel for the Treatment of PTSD in Adults. Clinical practice guideline for the treatment of Posttraumatic Stress Disorder (PTSD) in adults [Internet]. Available from: https://www.apa.org/ptsdguidelines/

Andreassen, O. A., Hindley, G. F. L., Frei, O., & Smeland, O. B. (2023). New insights from the last decade of research in psychiatric genetics: Discoveries, challenges and clinical implications.*World Psychiatry; Official Journal of the World Psychiatric Association (WPA)*, 22(1), 4–24. DOI: 10.1002/wps.21034 PMID: 36640404

Annerstedt, M., & Wahrborg, P. (2011). Nature-assisted therapy: Systematic review of controlled and observational studies.*Scandinavian Journal of Public Health*, 39(4), 371–388. DOI: 10.1177/1403494810396400 PMID: 21273226

Aoki, S., & Nozawa, E. (2024). Pilot Study on Classification of Sensory Symptoms in PTSD.*Journal of Child & Adolescent Trauma*, 17(2), 283–293. Advance online publication. DOI: 10.1007/s40653-023-00602-5 PMID: 38938954

APA Presidential Task Force on Evidence-Based Practice. (2006). Evidence-based Practice in psychology.*The American Psychologist*, 61(4), 271–285. DOI: 10.1037/0003-066X.61.4.271 PMID: 16719673

Apfel, B. A., Ross, J., Hlavin, J., Meyerhoff, D. J., Metzler, T. J., Marmar, C. R., Weiner, M. W., Schuff, N., & Neylan, T. C. (2011). Hippocampal volume differences in Gulf War veterans with current versus lifetime posttraumatic stress disorder symptoms.*Biological Psychiatry*, 69(6), 541–548. DOI: 10.1016/j.biopsych.2010.09.044 PMID: 21094937

Arakawa, R., Stenkrona, P., Takano, A., Svensson, J., Andersson, M., Nag, S., Asami, Y., Hirano, Y., Halldin, C., & Lundberg, J. (2019). Venlafaxine ER Blocks the Norepinephrine Transporter in the Brain of Patients with Major Depressive Disorder: A PET Study Using [18F]FMeNER-D2.*The International Journal of Neuropsychopharmacology*, 22(4), 278–285. DOI: 10.1093/ijnp/pyz003 PMID: 30649319

Arango, V., Ernsberger, P., Marzuk, P. M., Chen, J.-S., Tierney, H., Stanley, M., Reis, D. J., & Mann, J. J. (1990). Autoradiographic demonstration of increased serotonin 5-HT2 and β-adrenergic receptor binding sites in the brain of suicide victims.*Archives of General Psychiatry*, 47(11), 1038–1047. DOI: 10.1001/archpsyc.1990.01810230054009 PMID: 2173513

Armour, C., Greene, T., Contractor, A. A., Weiss, N., Dixon-Gordon, K., & Ross, J. (2020). Posttraumatic Stress Disorder Symptoms and Reckless Behaviors: A Network Analysis Approach.*Journal of Traumatic Stress*, 33(1), 29–40. DOI: 10.1002/jts.22487 PMID: 32086982

Arnon, S., Fisher, P. W., Pickover, A., Lowell, A., Turner, J. B., Hilburn, A., Jacob-McVey, J., Malajian, B. E., Farber, D. G., Hamilton, J. F., Hamilton, A., Markowitz, J. C., & Neria, Y. (2020). Equine-Assisted Therapy for Veterans with PTSD: Manual Development and Preliminary Findings.*Military Medicine*, 185(5-6), e557–e564. DOI: 10.1093/milmed/usz444 PMID: 32034416

Asalgoo, S., Jahromi, G. P., Meftahi, G. H., & Sahraei, H. (2015). Posttraumatic stress disorder (ptsd): Mechanisms and possible treatments.*Neurophysiology*, 47(6), 482–489. DOI: 10.1007/s11062-016-9559-9

Ashar, L. C. (2024, May 2). Social Media Impact: How Social Media Sites Affect Society. https://www.apu.apus.edu/area-of-study/business-and-management/resources/how-social-media-sites-affect-society/

Asmundson, G. J., & Taylor, S. (2009). PTSD diagnostic criteria: Understanding etiology and treatment.*The American Journal of Psychiatry*, 166(Suppl. 6), 726. DOI: 10.1176/appi.ajp.2009.08121799 PMID: 19487404

Australian Centre for Posttraumatic Mental Health. (2013).*Australian guidelines for the treatment of acute stress disorder and posttraumatic stress disorder*. Australian Centre for Posttraumatic Mental Health.

Averill, L. A., Purohit, P., Averill, C. L., Boesl, M. A., Krystal, J. H., & Abdallah, C. G. (2017). Glutamate dysregulation and glutamatergic therapeutics for PTSD: Evidence from human studies.*Neuroscience Letters*, 649, 147–155. DOI: 10.1016/j.neulet.2016.11.064 PMID: 27916636

Bach, D., Groesbeck, G., Stapleton, P., Sims, R., Blickheuser, K., & Church, D. (2019). Clinical EFT (emotional freedom techniques) improves multiple physiological markers of health. *Journal of Evidence-Based Integrative Medicine, 24*, 2515690X18823691. DOI: 10.1177/2515690X18823691

Baik, J.-H. (2020). Stress and the dopaminergic reward system.*Experimental & Molecular Medicine*, 52(12), 1879–1890. DOI: 10.1038/s12276-020-00532-4 PMID: 33257725

Baldwin, D. S., Anderson, I. M., Nutt, D. J., Allgulander, C., Bandelow, B., den Boer, J. A., Christmas, D. M., Davies, S., Fineberg, N., Lidbetter, N., Malizia, A., McCrone, P., Nabarro, D., O'Neill, C., Scott, J., van der Wee, N., & Wittchen, H. U. (2014). Evidence-based pharmacological treatment of anxiety disorders, post-traumatic stress disorder and obsessive-compulsive disorder. A revision of the 2005 guidelines from the British Association for Psychopharmacology.*Journal of Psychopharmacology (Oxford, England)*, 28(5), 403–439. DOI: 10.1177/0269881114525674 PMID: 24713617

Bale, T. L., & Vale, W. W. (2004). CRF and CRF receptors: Role in stress responsivity and other behaviors.*Annual Review of Pharmacology and Toxicology*, 44(1), 525–557. DOI: 10.1146/annurev.pharmtox.44.101802.121410 PMID: 14744257

Bandelow, B., Baldwin, D., Abelli, M., Bolea-Alamanac, B., Bourin, M., Chamberlain, S. R., Cinosi, E., Davies, S., Domschke, K., Fineberg, N., Grünblatt, E., Jarema, M., Kim, Y.-K., Maron, E., Masdrakis, V., Mikova, O., Nutt, D., Pallanti, S., Pini, S., & Riederer, P. (2017). Biological markers for anxiety disorders, OCD and PTSD: A consensus statement. Part II: Neurochemistry, neurophysiology and neurocognition.*The World Journal of Biological Psychiatry*, 18(3), 162–214. DOI: 10.1080/15622975.2016.1190867 PMID: 27419272

Banzi, R., Cusi, C., Randazzo, C., Sterzi, R., Tedesco, D., & Moja, L. (2015). Selective serotonin reuptake inhibitors (SSRIs) and serotonin-norepinephrine reuptake inhibitors (SNRIs) for the prevention of migraine in adults.*Cochrane Database of Systematic Reviews*, 4(4), CD002919. Advance online publication. DOI: 10.1002/14651858.CD002919.pub3 PMID: 25829028

Barbui, C., Purgato, M., Abdulmalik, J., Acarturk, C., Eaton, J., Gastaldon, C., Gureje, O., Hanlon, C., Jordans, M., Lund, C., Nose, M., Ostuzzi, G., Papola, D., Tedeschi, F., Tol, W., Turrini, G., Patel, V., & Thornicroft, G. (2020). Efficacy of psychosocial interventions for mental health outcomes in low income and middle-income countries: An umbrella review.*The Lancet. Psychiatry*, 7(2), 162–172. DOI: 10.1016/S2215-0366(19)30511-5 PMID: 31948935

Bar-Haim, Y., Stein, M. B., Bryant, R. A., Bliese, P. D., Ben Yehuda, A., Kringelbach, M. L., Jain, S., Dan, O., Lazarov, A., Wald, I., Levi, O., Neria, Y., & Pine, D. S. (2021). Intrusive Traumatic Reexperiencing: Pathognomonic of the Psychological Response to Traumatic Stress.*The American Journal of Psychiatry*, 178(2), 119–122. DOI: 10.1176/appi.ajp.2020.19121231 PMID: 33517759

Barman, L., Mukhopadhyay, D. K., & Bandyopadhyay, G. K. (2018). Use of Social Networking Site and Mental Disorders among Medical Students in Kolkata, West Bengal.*Indian Journal of Psychiatry*, 60(3), 340–345. DOI: 10.4103/psychiatry.IndianJPsychiatry_210_18 PMID: 30405262

Barsch, R. H. (1968). *The parent of the handicapped child: The study of child-raring practices.* Charlse C. Thomas. `Bellizzi, K.M., Smith, A.W., Reeve, B.B., Alfano, C.M., Bernstein, L, Meeske, K. et al. (2010). Posttraumatic growth and health-related quality of life in a racially diverse cohort of breast cancer survivors. *Health Psychology,*15(4). 615–626.

Barua, R. (2024). An In-Depth Exploration of AI and Humanoid Robotics' Role in Contemporary Healthcare. In V. Grover, B. Balusamy, N. M.K., V. Anand, & M. Milanova (Eds.), *Approaches to Human-Centered AI in Healthcare* (pp. 42-61). IGI Global. https://doi.org/DOI: 10.4018/979-8-3693-2238-3.ch003

Barua, R., Das, D., & Biswas, N. (2024). Revolutionizing Drug Discovery With Artificial Intelligence: Enhancing Efficiency, Addressing Ethical Concerns, and Overcoming Limitations. In V. Grover, B. Balusamy, N. M.K., V. Anand, & M. Milanova (Eds.), *Approaches to Human-Centered AI in Healthcare* (pp. 62-85). IGI Global. https://doi.org/DOI: 10.4018/979-8-3693-2238-3.ch004

Barua, R., Datta, S., & Bardhan, N. (2021). Impact of Social Media on Pandemic COVID-19 Outbreak. In G. Sarı (Ed.), *Handbook of Research on Representing Health and Medicine in Modern Media* (pp. 422-435). IGI Global. https://doi.org/DOI: 10.4018/978-1-7998-6825-5.ch025

Barua, R. (2024). An Investigation of AI Techniques for Detecting Kidney Stones in CT Scan Images Through Advanced Image Processing. In Sharma, A., Chanderwal, N., Tyagi, S., Upadhyay, P., & Tyagi, A. (Eds.), *Enhancing Medical Imaging with Emerging Technologies* (pp. 133–150). IGI Global., DOI: 10.4018/979-8-3693-5261-8.ch008

Barua, R., & Bardhan, N. (2021). Downfall of the Sports Industry Due to the Pandemic of COVID-19. In Faganel, A., Rižnar, I., & Baruca, A. (Eds.), *Impacts and Implications for the Sports Industry in the Post-COVID-19 Era* (pp. 60–72). IGI Global., DOI: 10.4018/978-1-7998-6780-7.ch004

Barua, R., & Das, S. (2022). Improvements of Virtual and Augmented Reality for Advanced Treatments in Urology. In Coelho, L., Queirós, R., & Reis, S. (Eds.), *Emerging Advancements for Virtual and Augmented Reality in Healthcare* (pp. 117–131). IGI Global., DOI: 10.4018/978-1-7998-8371-5.ch008

Barua, R., Datta, P., & Chowdhury, A. R. (2022). The Impact of 3D Printing Technology on the COVID-19 Pandemic. In Moumtzoglou, A. (Ed.), *Quality of Healthcare in the Aftermath of the COVID-19 Pandemic* (pp. 135–154). IGI Global., DOI: 10.4018/978-1-7998-9198-7.ch008

Barua, R., & Datta, S. (2023). Artificial Intelligence in Modern Medical Science: A Promising Practice. In Rajest, S., Singh, B., Obaid, A. J., Regin, R., & Chinnusamy, K. (Eds.), *Recent Developments in Machine and Human Intelligence* (pp. 1–12). IGI Global., DOI: 10.4018/978-1-6684-9189-8.ch001

Barua, R., & Datta, S. (2024). An Extensive Evaluation of New Federated Learning Approaches for COVID-19 Identification. In Hassan, A., Prasad, V., Bhattacharya, P., Dutta, P., & Damaševičius, R. (Eds.), *Pioneering Smart Healthcare 5.0 with IoT, Federated Learning, and Cloud Security* (pp. 246–257). IGI Global., DOI: 10.4018/979-8-3693-2639-8.ch014

Barua, R., Datta, S., Datta, P., & Chowdhury, A. R. (2022). The Study of Traditional Medicine for the Treatment of COVID-19. In El Hiba, O., Radhakrishnan, J., Balzano, T., & Isbaine, F. (Eds.), *Handbook of Research on Pathophysiology and Strategies for the Management of COVID-19* (pp. 221–241). IGI Global., DOI: 10.4018/978-1-7998-8225-1.ch014

Barua, R., Datta, S., & Sarkar, A. (2023). Artificial Intelligence and Robotics-Based Minimally Invasive Surgery: Innovations and Future Perceptions. In Karthick, G., & Karupusamy, S. (Eds.), *Contemporary Applications of Data Fusion for Advanced Healthcare Informatics* (pp. 350–368). IGI Global., DOI: 10.4018/978-1-6684-8913-0.ch015

Bell, S. L., Hickman, C., & Houghton, F. (2023). From therapeutic landscape to therapeutic 'sensescape' experiences with nature? A scoping review. *Wellbeing, Space and Society*, 4, 100126. DOI: 10.1016/j.wss.2022.100126

Benedek, D. M., & Wynn, G. H. (2016). *Complementary and alternative medicine for PTSD*. DOI: 10.1093/med/9780190205959.001.0001

Ben-Zion, Z., Zeevi, Y., Keynan, N. J., Admon, R., Kozlovski, T., Sharon, H., Halpern, P., Liberzon, I., Shalev, A. Y., Benjamini, Y., & Hendler, T. (2020). Multi-domain potential biomarkers for post-traumatic stress disorder (PTSD) severity in recent trauma survivors.*Translational Psychiatry*, 10(1), 208. DOI: 10.1038/s41398-020-00898-z PMID: 32594097

Bercier, M. L., & Maynard, B. R. (2015). Interventions for Secondary Traumatic Stress With Mental Health Workers: A Systematic Review.*Research on Social Work Practice*, 25(1), 81–89. DOI: 10.1177/1049731513517142

Berzengi, A., Berzenji, L., Kadim, A., Mustafa, F., & Jobson, L. (2017). Role of Role of Islamic appraisals, trauma-related appraisals, and religious coping in the posttraumatic adjustment of Muslim trauma survivors.*Psychological Trauma: Theory, Research, Practice, and Policy*, 9(2), 189–197. DOI: 10.1037/tra0000179 PMID: 27504962

Besnard, A., & Sahay, A. (2016). Adult hippocampal neurogenesis, fear generalization, and stress.*Neuropsychopharmacology*, 41(1), 24–44. DOI: 10.1038/npp.2015.167 PMID: 26068726

Bestvater, S., Gelles-Watnick, R., Odabas, M., Anderson, M., & Smith, A. (2023, June 29). #BlackLivesMatter Turns 10. Pew Research Center. https://www.pewresearch.org/internet/2023/06/29/blacklivesmatter-turns-10/

Bijanki, K. R., Van Rooij, S. J. H., Ely, T. D., Stevens, J. S., Inman, C. S., Fasano, R. E., Carter, S. E., Winters, S. J., Baman, J. R., Drane, D. L., Jovanovic, T., & Willie, J. T. (2020). Case series: Unilateral amygdala ablation ameliorates post-traumatic stress disorder symptoms and biomarkers.*Neurosurgery*, 87(4), 796–802. DOI: 10.1093/neuros/nyaa051 PMID: 32259241

Bismark, M., Scurrah, K., Pascoe, A., Willis, K., Jain, R., & Smallwood, N. (2022). Thoughts of suicide or self-harm among Australian healthcare workers during the COVID-19 pandemic.*The Australian and New Zealand Journal of Psychiatry*, 56(12), 1555–1565. DOI: 10.1177/00048674221075540 PMID: 35128948

Bisson, J. I., Roberts, N. P., Andrew, M., Cooper, R., & Lewis, C. (2013). Psychological therapies for chronic post-traumatic stress disorder (PTSD) in adults. *Cochrane Database of Systematic Reviews*, 2015(8), 12. DOI: 10.1002/14651858.CD003388.pub4 PMID: 24338345

Blake, M. (2015, August 6). Nine times Jon Stewart proved he was more than just a comedian. Los Angeles Times. https://www.latimes.com/entertainment/tv/showtracker/la-et-st-jon-stewart-definitive-moments-the-daily-show-20150805-html-htmlstory.html

Blanchard, E. B., Kolb, L. C., Pallmeyer, T. P., & Gerardi, R. J. (1982). A psychophysiological study of post traumatic stress disorder in Vietnam veterans.*The Psychiatric Quarterly*, 54(4), 220–229. DOI: 10.1007/BF01064817 PMID: 7187510

Blanchard, E. B., Kolb, L. C., Prins, A., Gates, S., & McCOY, G. C. (1991). Changes in plasma norepinephrine to combat-related stimuli among Vietnam veterans with posttraumatic stress disorder.*The Journal of Nervous and Mental Disease*, 179(6), 371–373. DOI: 10.1097/00005053-199106000-00012 PMID: 2051153

Blank, A. A. (1985). The unconscious flashback to the war in Vietnam veterans: clinical mystery, legal defense, and community problem. In Sonnenberg, S. M., & Talbot, J. A. (Eds.), *The Trauma of War: Stress and Recovery in Vietnam Veterans* (pp. 293–308). American Psychiatric Association.

Blevins, C. A., Weathers, F. W., Davis, M. T., Witte, T. K., & Domino, J. L. (2015). The Posttraumatic Stress Disorder Checklist for DSM-5 (PCL-5): Development and initial psychometric evaluation.*Journal of Traumatic Stress*, 28(6), 489–498. DOI: 10.1002/jts.22059 PMID: 26606250

Bomyea, J., Risbrough, V., & Lang, A. J. (2012). A consideration of select pre-trauma factors as key vulnerabilities in PTSD.*Clinical Psychology Review*, 32(7), 630–641. DOI: 10.1016/j.cpr.2012.06.008 PMID: 22917742

Bonne, O., Vythilingam, M., Inagaki, M., Wood, S., Neumeister, A., Nugent, A. C., Snow, J., Luckenbaugh, D. A., Bain, E. E., Drevets, W. C., & Charney, D. S. (2008). Reduced posterior hippocampal volume in posttraumatic stress disorder.*The Journal of Clinical Psychiatry*, 69(7), 1087–1091. DOI: 10.4088/JCP.v69n0707 PMID: 18572983

Bostic, B. (2014, February 20). Does Social Media Perpetuate Youth Violence? Michigan Youth Violence Prevention Center. https://yvpc.sph.umich.edu/social-media-perpetuate-youth-violence/

Bourassa, K. J., Smolenski, D. J., Edwards-Stewart, A., Campbell, S. B., Reger, G. M., & Norr, A. M. (2020). The impact of prolonged exposure therapy on social support and PTSD symptoms.*Journal of Affective Disorders*, 260, 410–417. DOI: 10.1016/j.jad.2019.09.036 PMID: 31539674

Bourla, A., Mouchabac, S., Hage, W. E., & Ferreri, F. (2018). e-PTSD: an overview on how new technologies can improve prediction and assessment of posttraumatic stress disorder (PTSD). Eur J Psychotraumatol, 9(sup1), 1424448.

Bowen, D. J., & Neill, J. T. (2013). A meta-analysis of adventure therapy outcomes and moderators.*The Open Psychology Journal*, 6(1), 28–53. DOI: 10.2174/1874350120130802001

Bowers, M. E., & Yehuda, R. (2016). Intergenerational Effects of PTSD on Offspring Glucocorticoid Receptor Methylation. In Spengler, D., & Binder, E. (Eds.), *Epigenetics and Neuroendocrinology: Clinical Focus on Psychiatry* (Vol. 2, pp. 141–155). Springer International Publishing., DOI: 10.1007/978-3-319-29901-3_6

Boyd, J. E., Lanius, R. A., & McKinnon, M. C. (2018). Mindfulness-based treatments for posttraumatic stress disorder: A review of the treatment literature and neurobiological evidence.*Journal of Psychiatry & Neuroscience*, 43(1), 7–25. DOI: 10.1503/jpn.170021 PMID: 29252162

Bradley, R., Greene, J., Russ, E., Dutra, L., & Westen, D. (2005). A multidimensional meta-analysis of psychotherapy for PTSD.*The American Journal of Psychiatry*, 162(2), 214–227. DOI: 10.1176/appi.ajp.162.2.214 PMID: 15677582

Bremner, J. D., & Pearce, B. (2016). Neurotransmitter, neurohormonal, and neuropeptidal function in stress and PTSD. *Posttraumatic Stress Disorder*, 179–232.

Bremner, J. D., Charney, D. S., Stein, D. J., Hollander, E., & Rothbaum, B. O. (2010). *Neural circuits in fear and anxiety.*

Bremner, J. D., Southwick, S. M., & Charney, D. S. (1999). *The neurobiology of posttraumatic stress disorder: an integration of animal and human research.*

Bremner, J. D. (2002). *Does stress damage the brain?: Understanding trauma-related disorders from a mind-body perspective*. WW Norton & Company.

Bremner, J. D. (2003). Functional neuroanatomical correlates of traumatic stress revisited 7 years later, this time with data.*Psychopharmacology Bulletin*, 37(2), 6–25. PMID: 14566211

Bremner, J. D. (2006). Traumatic stress: Effects on the brain.*Dialogues in Clinical Neuroscience*, 8(4), 445–461. DOI: 10.31887/DCNS.2006.8.4/jbremner PMID: 17290802

Bremner, J. D., Elzinga, B., Schmahl, C., & Vermetten, E. (2007). Structural and functional plasticity of the human brain in posttraumatic stress disorder.*Progress in Brain Research*, 167, 171–186. DOI: 10.1016/S0079-6123(07)67012-5 PMID: 18037014

Bremner, J. D., Narayan, M., Staib, L. H., Southwick, S. M., McGlashan, T., & Charney, D. S. (1999). Neural correlates of memories of childhood sexual abuse in women with and without posttraumatic stress disorder.*The American Journal of Psychiatry*, 156(11), 1787–1795. DOI: 10.1176/ajp.156.11.1787 PMID: 10553744

Bremner, J. D., Vythilingam, M., Vermetten, E., Southwick, S. M., McGlashan, T., Staib, L. H., Soufer, R., & Charney, D. S. (2003). Neural correlates of declarative memory for emotionally valenced words in women with posttraumatic stress disorder related to early childhood sexual abuse.*Biological Psychiatry*, 53(10), 879–889. DOI: 10.1016/S0006-3223(02)01891-7 PMID: 12742675

Breslau, N. (2009). The epidemiology of trauma. PTSD and other posttrauma disorders.*Trauma, Violence & Abuse*, 10(3), 198–210. DOI: 10.1177/1524838009334448 PMID: 19406860

Brewin, C. R. (2015). Re-experiencing traumatic events in PTSD: New avenues in research on intrusive memories and flashbacks.*European Journal of Psychotraumatology*, 6(1), 27180. DOI: 10.3402/ejpt.v6.27180 PMID: 25994019

Britton, J. C., Phan, K. L., Taylor, S. F., Fig, L. M., & Liberzon, I. (2005). Corticolimbic blood flow in posttraumatic stress disorder during script-driven imagery. *Biological Psychiatry*, 57(8), 832–840. DOI: 10.1016/j.biopsych.2004.12.025 PMID: 15820703

Brookls, A. (Nov. 2023). On cultivating happiness, emotional self-management, and more. *On the Peter Atia Drive*. Episode 280.

Brown, G. L., & Linnoila, M. I. (1990). CSF serotonin metabolite (5-HIAA) studies in depression, impulsivity, and violence.*The Journal of Clinical Psychiatry*, 51, 31–41. PMID: 1691169

Brown, S. L., Wanamaker, K. A., Greiner, L., Scott, T., & Skilling, T. A. (2021). Complex Trauma and Criminogenic Needs in a Youth Justice Sample: A Gender-Informed Latent Profile Analysis.*Criminal Justice and Behavior*, 48(2), 175–194. DOI: 10.1177/0093854820964513

Bryant, R. A. (2019). Post-traumatic stress disorder: A state-of-the-art review of evidence and challenges.*World Psychiatry; Official Journal of the World Psychiatric Association (WPA)*, 18(3), 259–269. DOI: 10.1002/wps.20656 PMID: 31496089

Bryant, R. A. (2022). The nature of posttraumatic stress disorder in treatment-seeking first responders.*European Journal of Psychotraumatology*, 13(1), 2011602. DOI: 10.1080/20008198.2021.2011602 PMID: 35096284

Bryant, R. A., Dawson, K. S., Azevedo, S., Yadav, S., Cahill, C., Kenny, L., Maccallum, F., Tran, J., Rawson, N., Tockar, J., Garber, B., & Keyan, D. (2023). Augmenting trauma-focused psychotherapy for post-traumatic stress disorder with brief aerobic exercise in Australia: A randomised clinical trial.*The Lancet. Psychiatry*, 10(1), 21–29. DOI: 10.1016/S2215-0366(22)00368-6 PMID: 36436532

Buchanan, K., Aknin, L. B., Lotun, S., & Sandstrom, G. M. (2021). Brief exposure to social media during the COVID-19 pandemic: Doom-scrolling has negative emotional consequences, but kindness-scrolling does not.*PLoS One*, 16(10), e0257728. DOI: 10.1371/journal.pone.0257728 PMID: 34644310

Burback, L., Brult-Phillips, S., Nijdam, M. J., McFarlane, A., & Vermetten, E. (2024). Treatment of Posttraumatic Stress Disorder: A State-of-the-art Review. *Current Neuropharmacology*, 22(4), 557–635. DOI: 10.2174/1570159X21666230428091433 PMID: 37132142

Burghardt, N. S., Bush, D. E. A., McEwen, B. S., & LeDoux, J. E. (2007). Acute selective serotonin reuptake inhibitors increase conditioned fear expression: Blockade with a 5-HT2C receptor antagonist.*Biological Psychiatry*, 62(10), 1111–1118. DOI: 10.1016/j.biopsych.2006.11.023 PMID: 17524369

Butler, L. D., Blasey, C. M., Garlan, R. W., McCaslin, S. E., Azarow, J., Chen, X. H., Desjardins, J. C., DiMiceli, S., Seagraves, D. A., Hastings, T. A., Kraemer, H. A., & Spiegel, D. (2005). Posttraumatic growth following the terrorist attacks of September 11, 2001: Cognitive, coping, and trauma symptom predictors in an Internet convenience sample.*Traumatology*, 11(4), 247–267. DOI: 10.1177/153476560501100405

Cabib, S., Ventura, R., & Puglisi-Allegra, S. (2002). Opposite imbalances between mesocortical and mesoaccumbens dopamine responses to stress by the same genotype depending on living conditions.*Behavioural Brain Research*, 129(1–2), 179–185. DOI: 10.1016/S0166-4328(01)00339-4 PMID: 11809509

Cacabelos, R., Torrellas, C., Fernandez-Novoa, L., & Aliev, G. (2016). Neuroimmune crosstalk in CNS disorders: The histamine connection.*Current Pharmaceutical Design*, 22(7), 819–848. DOI: 10.2174/1381612822666151209150954 PMID: 26648474

Cahill, S. P., Rothbaum, B. O., Resick, P. A., & Follette, V. M. (2009). *Cognitive-behavioral therapy for adults.*

Calcerano, D., & Ciurlia, G. (2023). *Neurofeedback in Virtual Reality Naturalistic Scenarios for Enhancing Relaxation: Visual and Auditory Stimulation to Promote Brain Entrainment.* Politecnico di Torino.

Calhoun, L. G., & Tedeschi, R. G. (2000). Early posttraumatic intervention: Facilitating possibilities for growth. In Patton, D., & Dunning, C. (Eds.), *Posttraumatic Stress Intervention: Challenges, Issues, and Perspectives* (pp. 135–152). Charles C. Thomas.

Calinescu, A. (2023). The Many Worlds of Trauma: An Interdisciplinary Perspective. *Border Crossing*, 13(2), 2. Advance online publication. DOI: 10.33182/bc.v13i2.2843

Callahan, R. (1997). Thought field therapy: The case of Mary.*Traumatology*, 3(1), 30–37. DOI: 10.1177/153476569700300105

Cameron, R. P., & Gusman, D. (2003). The primary care PTSD screen (PC-PTSD): Development and operating characteristics.*Primary Care Psychiatry*, 9(1), 9–14.

Cann, A., Calhoun, L. G., Tedeschi, R. G., Taku, K., Vishnevsky, T., Triplett, K. N., & Danhauer, S. C. (2010). *Posttraumatic Growth Inventory—Short Form (PTGI-SF)* [Database record]. APA PsycTests.

Cann, A., Calhoun, L. G., Tedeschi, R. G., Triplett, K. N., Vishnevsky, T., & Lindstrom, C. M. (2011). Assessing posttraumatic cognitive processes: The event related rumination inventory.*Anxiety, Stress, and Coping*, 24(2), 137–156. DOI: 10.1080/10615806.2010.529901 PMID: 21082446

Carlini, S. V., Osborne, L. M., & Deligiannidis, K. M. (2023). Current pharmacotherapy approaches and novel GABAergic antidepressant development in postpartum depression.*Dialogues in Clinical Neuroscience*, 25(1), 92–100. DOI: 10.1080/19585969.2023.2262464 PMID: 37796239

Carmi, L., Zohar, J., Juven-Wetzler, A., Desarnaud, F., Makotkine, L., Bierer, L. M., Cohen, H., & Yehuda, R. (2023). Promoter methylation of the glucocorticoid receptor following trauma may be associated with subsequent development of PTSD.*The World Journal of Biological Psychiatry*, 24(7), 578–586. DOI: 10.1080/15622975.2023.2177342 PMID: 36748398

Carrington, A. E. (2021, March 28). How NY hospital faced COVID devastation and came back from the brink. ABC News. https://abcnews.go.com/Health/ny-hospital-faced-covid-devastation-back-brink/story?id=76638912

Carrion, V. G., Garrett, A., Menon, V., Weems, C. F., & Reiss, A. L. (2008). Posttraumatic stress symptoms and brain function during a response-inhibition task: An fMRI study in youth.*Depression and Anxiety*, 25(6), 514–526. DOI: 10.1002/da.20346 PMID: 17598145

Carver, C. S. (1997). You want to measure coping but your protocol's too long: Consider the Brief COPE.*International Journal of Behavioral Medicine*, 4(1), 92–100. DOI: 10.1207/s15327558ijbm0401_6 PMID: 16250744

Castro-Vale, I., van Rossum, E. F. C., Machado, J. C., Mota-Cardoso, R., & Carvalho, D. (2016). Genetics of glucocorticoid regulation and posttraumatic stress disorder—What do we know?*Neuroscience and Biobehavioral Reviews*, 63, 143–157. DOI: 10.1016/j.neubiorev.2016.02.005 PMID: 26872620

Catlow, B. J., Song, S., Paredes, D. A., Kirstein, C. L., & Sanchez-Ramos, J. (2013). Effects of psilocybin on hippocampal neurogenesis and extinction of trace fear conditioning.*Experimental Brain Research*, 228(4), 481–491. DOI: 10.1007/s00221-013-3579-0 PMID: 23727882

Chalquist, C. (2009). A look at the ecotherapy research evidence.*Ecopsychology*, 1(2), 64–74. DOI: 10.1089/eco.2009.0003

Charuvastra, A., & Cloitre, M. (2008). Social Bonds and Posttraumatic Stress Disorder.*Annual Review of Psychology*, 59(1), 301–328. DOI: 10.1146/annurev.psych.58.110405.085650 PMID: 17883334

Chauhan, N., Soni, S., & Jain, U. (2021). Optimizing testing regimes for the detection of COVID-19 in children and older adults.*Expert Review of Molecular Diagnostics*, 21(10), 999–1016. DOI: 10.1080/14737159.2021.1962708 PMID: 34324823

Chen, C. R., Hung, C. F., Lee, Y. W., Tseng, W. T., Chen, M. L., & Chen, T. T. (2022). Functional Outcomes in a Randomized Controlled Trial of Animal-Assisted Therapy on Middle-Aged and Older Adults with Schizophrenia.*International Journal of Environmental Research and Public Health*, 19(10), 6270. DOI: 10.3390/ijerph19106270 PMID: 35627807

Cheng, C., & Ebrahimi, O. V. (2023). Gamification: A Novel Approach to Mental Health Promotion.*Current Psychiatry Reports*, 25(11), 577–586. DOI: 10.1007/s11920-023-01453-5 PMID: 37801212

Chery, S. (2023, October 25). Where celebrities went wrong opining on the Israel-Gaza war. Washington Post. https://www.washingtonpost.com/entertainment/2023/10/25/celebrities-react-israel-gaza-war-palestinian-hamas/

Chiba, T., Kanazawa, T., Koizumi, A., Ide, K., Taschereau-Dumouchel, V., Boku, S., Hishimoto, A., Shirakawa, M., Sora, I., Yoneda, H., & Kawato, M. (2019). Current status of neurofeedback for post-traumatic stress disorder: A systematic review and the possibility of decoded neurofeedback.*Frontiers in Human Neuroscience*, 13, 233. DOI: 10.3389/fnhum.2019.00233 PMID: 31379538

Choi, Y.-J., Choi, E.-J., & Ko, E. (2023). Neurofeedback Effect on Symptoms of Posttraumatic Stress Disorder: A Systematic Review and Meta-Analysis.*Applied Psychophysiology and Biofeedback*, 48(3), 1–16. DOI: 10.1007/s10484-023-09593-3 PMID: 37314616

Christiansen, D. M., & Hansen, M. (2015). Accounting for sex differences in PTSD: A multi-variable mediation model.*European Journal of Psychotraumatology*, 6(1), 26068. DOI: 10.3402/ejpt.v6.26068 PMID: 25604705

Church, D., & Feinstein, D. (2013). Energy psychology in the treatment of PTSD: Psychobiology and clinical principles. In T, Van Leeuwen & T. Van Brouwer (Eds.). *Psychology of trauma* (pp. 211-224). Hauppauge, N.Y: Nova Science

Church, D. (2013). Clinical EFT as an evidence-based practice for the treatment of psychological and physiological conditions.*Psychology (Irvine, Calif.)*, 4(8), 645–654. DOI: 10.4236/psych.2013.48092

Church, D., & Feinstein, D. (2017). The manual stimulation of acupuncture points in the treatment of post-traumatic stress disorder: A review of clinical emotional freedom techniques.*Medical Acupuncture*, 29(4), 249–253. DOI: 10.1089/acu.2017.1213 PMID: 28874920

Church, D., & House, D. (2018). Borrowing benefits: Group treatment with clinical emotional freedom techniques is associated with simultaneous reductions in Posttraumatic Stress Disorder, anxiety, and depression symptoms.*Journal of Evidence-based Integrative Medicine*, 23, 2156587218756510. DOI: 10.1177/2156587218756510 PMID: 29468884

Church, D., Stapleton, P., Mollon, P., Feinstein, D., Boath, E., Mackay, D., & Sims, R. (2018). Guidelines for the treatment of PTSD using clinical EFT (emotional freedom techniques).*Healthcare (Basel)*, 6(4), 146. DOI: 10.3390/healthcare6040146 PMID: 30545069

Church, D., Stapleton, P., Vasudevan, A., & O'Keefe, T. (2022). Clinical EFT as an evidence-based practice for the treatment of psychological and physiological conditions: A systematic review.*Frontiers in Psychology*, 13, 951451. DOI: 10.3389/fpsyg.2022.951451 PMID: 36438382

Church, D., Stapleton, P., Yang, A., & Gallo, F. (2018). Is tapping on acupuncture points an active ingredient in emotional freedom techniques? A systematic review and meta-analysis of comparative studies.*The Journal of Nervous and Mental Disease*, 206(10), 783–793. DOI: 10.1097/NMD.0000000000000878 PMID: 30273275

Church, D., Stern, S., Boath, E., Stewart, A., Feinstein, D., & Clond, M. (2017). Emotional freedom techniques to treat Posttraumatic Stress Disorder in veterans: Review of the evidence, survey of practitioners, and proposed clinical guidelines.*The Permanente Journal*, 21(4), 16–100. DOI: 10.7812/TPP/16-100 PMID: 28678690

Church, D., Yount, G., & Brooks, A. J. (2012). The effect of emotional freedom techniques on stress biochemistry: A randomized controlled trial.*The Journal of Nervous and Mental Disease*, 200(10), 891–896. DOI: 10.1097/NMD.0b013e31826b9fc1 PMID: 22986277

Church, D., Yount, G., Rachlin, K., Fox, L., & Nelms, J. (2018). Epigenetic effects of PTSD remediation in veterans using clinical emotional freedom techniques: A randomized controlled pilot study.*American Journal of Health Promotion*, 32(1), 112–122. DOI: 10.1177/0890117116661154 PMID: 27520015

Cineas, F. (2021, June 24). What the hysteria over critical race theory is really all about. Vox. https://www.vox.com/22443822/critical-race-theory-controversy

Cist, A., & Choi, P. (2017). Religion and spirituality in the Intensive Care Unit. In Balboni, M., & Peteet, J. J. (Eds.), *Spirituality and Religion Within the Culture of Medicine: From Evidence to Practice.*

Clark, C. R., McFarlane, A. C., Morris, P., Weber, D. L., Sonkkilla, C., Shaw, M., Marcina, J., Tochon-Danguy, H. J., & Egan, G. F. (2003). Cerebral function in posttraumatic stress disorder during verbal working memory updating: A positron emission tomography study.*Biological Psychiatry*, 53(6), 474–481. DOI: 10.1016/S0006-3223(02)01505-6 PMID: 12644352

Clark, T. J., Conrad, C. G., Cummings, A. D. P., & Johnson, A. D. (2022). Trauma-Informed Policing: The Impact of Adult and Childhood Trauma on Law Enforcement Officers.*Case Western Reserve Law Review*, 73, 843. https://heinonline.org/HOL/Page?handle=hein.journals/cwrlrv73&id=880&div=&collection=

Cloitre, M., Garvert, D. W., & Weiss, B. J. (2017). Depression as a moderator of STAIR Narrative Therapy for women with post-traumatic stress disorder related to childhood abuse.*European Journal of Psychotraumatology*, 8(1), 1377028. DOI: 10.1080/20008198.2017.1377028 PMID: 29038682

Clond, M. (2016). Emotional freedom techniques for anxiety: A systematic review with meta-analysis.*The Journal of Nervous and Mental Disease*, 204(5), 388–395. DOI: 10.1097/NMD.0000000000000483 PMID: 26894319

Coll, S. Y., Eustache, F., Doidy, F., Fraisse, F., Peschanski, D., Dayan, J., Gagnepain, P., & Laisney, M. (2022). Avoidance behaviour generalizes to eye processing in posttraumatic stress disorder.*European Journal of Psychotraumatology*, 13(1), 2044661. DOI: 10.1080/20008198.2022.2044661 PMID: 35479300

Conrad, C. D. (2008). Chronic stress-induced hippocampal vulnerability: The glucocorticoid vulnerability hypothesis.*Reviews in the Neurosciences*, 19(6), 395–412. DOI: 10.1515/REVNEURO.2008.19.6.395 PMID: 19317179

Contractor, A. A., Weiss, N. H., Dolan, M., & Mota, N. (2020). Examination of the structural relations between posttraumatic stress disorder symptoms and reckless/self-destructive behaviors.*International Journal of Stress Management*, 27(1), 35–44. DOI: 10.1037/str0000133 PMID: 33776397

Cooper, O., Bonert, V., Moser, F., Mirocha, J., & Melmed, S. (2017). Altered pituitary gland structure and function in posttraumatic stress disorder.*Journal of the Endocrine Society*, 1(6), 577–587. DOI: 10.1210/js.2017-00069 PMID: 29264511

Courtois, C. A. (2015). First, do no more harm: Ethics of attending to spiritual issues in trauma treatment. In Walker, D. F., Courtois, C. A., & Aten, J. D. (Eds.), *Spiritually oriented psychotherapy for trauma* (pp. 55–75). American Psychological Association. DOI: 10.1037/14500-004

Creamer, M., Bell, R., & Failla, S. (2003). Psychometric properties of the impact of event scale - Revised.*Behaviour Research and Therapy*, 41(12), 1489–1496. DOI: 10.1016/j.brat.2003.07.010 PMID: 14705607

Crombie, K. M., Adams, T. G., Dunsmoor, J. E., Greenwood, B. N., Smits, J. A., Nemeroff, C. B., & Cisler, J. M. (2023). Aerobic exercise in the treatment of PTSD: An examination of preclinical and clinical laboratory findings, potential mechanisms, clinical implications, and future directions.*Journal of Anxiety Disorders*, 94, 102680. DOI: 10.1016/j.janxdis.2023.102680 PMID: 36773486

Crouthamel, J. (2001). *Trauma, Religion, and Spirituality in Germany during the First World War*. Bloomsbury Academic.

Cruz, D., Lichten, M., Berg, K., & George, P. (2022). Developmental trauma: Conceptual framework, associated risks and comorbidities, and evaluation and treatment.*Frontiers in Psychiatry*, 13, 800687. DOI: 10.3389/fpsyt.2022.800687 PMID: 35935425

Cummings, K. J., & Leiter, J. C. (2020). Take a deep breath and wake up: The protean role of serotonin preventing sudden death in infancy.*Experimental Neurology*, 326, 113165. DOI: 10.1016/j.expneurol.2019.113165 PMID: 31887304

Cusack, K., Jonas, D. E., Forneris, C. A., Wines, C., Sonis, J., Middleton, J. C., Feltner, C., Brownley, K. A., Olmsted, K. R., Greenblatt, A., Weil, A., & Gaynes, B. N. (2016). Psychological treatments for adults with posttraumatic stress disorder: A systematic review and meta-analysis.*Clinical Psychology Review*, 43, 128–141. DOI: 10.1016/j.cpr.2015.10.003 PMID: 26574151

D'Souza, D. (1995). Post-traumatic stress disorder – A scar for life.*The British Journal of Clinical Practice*, 49(Suppl 6), 309–313. DOI: 10.1111/j.1742-1241.1995.tb09994.x PMID: 8554955

Daskalakis, N. P., Lehrner, A., & Yehuda, R. (2013). Endocrine aspects of post-traumatic stress disorder and implications for diagnosis and treatment.*Endocrinology and Metabolism Clinics of North America*, 42(3), 503–513. DOI: 10.1016/j.ecl.2013.05.004 PMID: 24011883

Datta, N., Matheson, B. E., Citron, K., Van Wye, E. M., & Lock, J. D. (2023). Evidence based update on psychosocial treatments for eating disorders in children and adolescents.*Journal of Clinical Child and Adolescent Psychology*, 52(2), 159–170. DOI: 10.1080/15374416.2022.2109650 PMID: 35950931

David, J. P., Ladd, K., & Spilka, B. (1992). *The multidimensionality of prayer and its roles as a source of secondary control.* Paper presented at the meeting of the American Psychological Association, Washington, DC.

Davidson, J. R., Hughes, D., Blazer, D. G., & George, L. K. (1991). Post-traumatic stress disorder in the community: An epidemiological study.*Psychological Medicine*, 21(Suppl 3), 713–721. DOI: 10.1017/S0033291700022352 PMID: 1946860

Davidson, J., Swartz, M., Storck, M., Krishnan, R. R., & Hammett, E. (1985). A diagnostic and family study of posttraumatic stress disorder.*The American Journal of Psychiatry*, 142(1), 90–93. DOI: 10.1176/ajp.142.1.90 PMID: 3966591

Davidson, K. W., Mangione, C. M., Barry, M. J., Nicholson, W. K., Cabana, M. D., Caughey, A. B., Davis, E. M., Donahue, K. E., Doubeni, C. A., Kubik, M., Li, L., Ogedegbe, G., Pbert, L., Silverstein, M., Stevermer, J., Tseng, C.-W., & Wong, J. B.US Preventive Services Task Force. (2022). Collaboration and Shared Decision-Making Between Patients and Clinicians in Preventive Health Care Decisions and US Preventive Services Task Force Recommendations.*Journal of the American Medical Association*, 327(12), 1171–1176. DOI: 10.1001/jama.2022.3267 PMID: 35315879

Davidson, P., & Parker, K. (2001). Eye movement desensitization and reprocessing (EMDR): A meta-analysis.*Journal of Consulting and Clinical Psychology*, 69(2), 305–316. DOI: 10.1037/0022-006X.69.2.305 PMID: 11393607

Davis, L. W., Schmid, A. A., Daggy, J. K., & Yang, Z. (2023). Mediators of improved PTSD symptoms in veterans and civilians following a yoga program.*Acta Neuropsychiatrica*, 35(4), 1–9. DOI: 10.1017/neu.2023.5 PMID: 36710002

de Jongh, A., de Roos, C., & El-Leithy, S. (2024). State of the science: Eye movement desensitization and reprocessing (EMDR) therapy.*Journal of Traumatic Stress*, 37(2), 205–216. DOI: 10.1002/jts.23012 PMID: 38282286

de Vernejoul, P., Albarède, P., & Darras, J. C. (1992). Nuclear medicine and acupuncture message transmission. *Journal of Nuclear Medicine: Official publication, Society of Nuclear Medicine, 33*(3), 409–412.

Delahanty, D. L., Nugent, N. R., Christopher, N. C., & Walsh, M. (2005). Initial urinary epinephrine and cortisol levels predict acute PTSD symptoms in child trauma victims.*Psychoneuroendocrinology*, 30(2), 121–128. DOI: 10.1016/j.psyneuen.2004.06.004 PMID: 15471610

Delanerolle, G., Zeng, Y., Shi, J. Q., Yeng, X., Goodison, W., Shetty, A., Shetty, S., Haque, N., Elliot, K., Ranaweera, S., Ramakrishnan, R., Raymont, V., Rathod, S., & Phiri, P. (2022). Mental health impact of the Middle East respiratory syndrome, SARS, and COVID-19: A comparative systematic review and meta-analysis.*World Journal of Psychiatry*, 12(5), 739–765. DOI: 10.5498/wjp.v12.i5.739 PMID: 35663292

Deuel, L. M., & Seeberger, L. C. (2020). Complementary Therapies in Parkinson Disease: A Review of Acupuncture, Tai Chi, Qi Gong, Yoga, and Cannabis.*Neurotherapeutics; the Journal of the American Society for Experimental NeuroTherapeutics*, 17(4), 1434–1455. DOI: 10.1007/s13311-020-00900-y PMID: 32785848

Deutch, A. Y., & Roth, R. H. (1991). The determinants of stress-induced activation of the prefrontal cortical dopamine system.*Progress in Brain Research*, 85, 367–403. DOI: 10.1016/S0079-6123(08)62691-6 PMID: 2094906

Di Rienzo, F., Saruco, E., Church, D., Daligault, S., Delpuech, C., Gurret, J. M., & Guillot, A. (2019). Neuropsychological correlates of an energy psychology intervention on flight phobia: A MEG single-case study.*OSF Preprints*,https://doi.org/ DOI: 10.31234/osf.io/s3hce

Dienstmann, G. (2018). Practical meditation: A simple step-by-step guide. New York, NY: DK.

Dikanović, M., Demarin, V., Kadojić, D., Kadojić, M., Trkanjec, Z., Titlić, M., Bitunjac, M., & Soldo-Butković, S. (2011). Effect of elevated catecholamine levels on cerebral hemodynamics in patients with chronic post-traumatic stress disorder. *Collegium Antropologicum*, 35(2), 471–475. PMID: 21755720

Dixon, M. L., Thiruchselvam, R., Todd, R., & Christoff, K. (2017). Emotion and the prefrontal cortex: An integrative review. *Psychological Bulletin*, 143(10), 1033–1081. DOI: 10.1037/bul0000096 PMID: 28616997

Dominique, J.-F. (2007). Glucocorticoid-induced reduction of traumatic memories: Implications for the treatment of PTSD. *Progress in Brain Research*, 167, 239–247. DOI: 10.1016/S0079-6123(07)67017-4 PMID: 18037019

Dominique, J.-F., Aerni, A., Schelling, G., & Roozendaal, B. (2009). Glucocorticoids and the regulation of memory in health and disease. *Frontiers in Neuroendocrinology*, 30(3), 358–370. DOI: 10.1016/j.yfrne.2009.03.002 PMID: 19341764

Do-Monte, F. H., Manzano-Nieves, G., Quiñones-Laracuente, K., Ramos-Medina, L., & Quirk, G. J. (2015). Revisiting the role of infralimbic cortex in fear extinction with optogenetics. *The Journal of Neuroscience : The Official Journal of the Society for Neuroscience*, 35(8), 3607–3615. DOI: 10.1523/JNEUROSCI.3137-14.2015 PMID: 25716859

Drew, R. (2001, September 20). A Day of Terror. https://archive.nytimes.com/www.nytimes.com/slideshow/2001/09/20/12DEST.9.slideshow_4.html

Drissi, N., Ouhbi, S., Idtissi, M. A. J., & Ghogho, M. (2019). Gamification-based apps for PTSD: An analysis of functionality and characteristics. 2019 IEEE/ACS 16th International Conference on Computer Systems and Applications (AICCSA), Abu Dhabi, United Arab Emirates, pp. 1-6.

DuBois, H. M. (2023). Empowerment and Transformation: Correlating John of the Cross and Judith Herman for Trauma Healing. *International Journal of Practical Theology*, 27(1), 99–113. DOI: 10.1515/ijpt-2022-0013

Duek, O., Seidemann, R., Pietrzak, R. H., & Harpaz-Rotem, I. (2023). Distinguishing emotional numbing symptoms of posttraumatic stress disorder from major depressive disorder. *Journal of Affective Disorders*, 324, 294–299. DOI: 10.1016/j.jad.2022.12.105 PMID: 36586605

Dunsmoor, J. E., Kroes, M. C. W., Li, J., Daw, N. D., Simpson, H. B., & Phelps, E. A. (2019). Role of human ventromedial prefrontal cortex in learning and recall of enhanced extinction. *The Journal of Neuroscience : The Official Journal of the Society for Neuroscience*, 39(17), 3264–3276. DOI: 10.1523/JNEUROSCI.2713-18.2019 PMID: 30782974

Eckart, C., Stoppel, C., Kaufmann, J., Tempelmann, C., Hinrichs, H., Elbert, T., Heinze, H.-J., & Kolassa, I.-T. (2011). Structural alterations in lateral prefrontal, parietal and posterior midline regions of men with chronic posttraumatic stress disorder.*Journal of Psychiatry & Neuroscience*, 36(3), 176–186. DOI: 10.1503/jpn.100010 PMID: 21118656

Eder-Moreau, E., Zhu, X., Fisch, C. T., Bergman, M., Neria, Y., & Helpman, L. (2022). Neurobiological alterations in females with PTSD: A systematic review.*Frontiers in Psychiatry*, 13, 862476. DOI: 10.3389/fpsyt.2022.862476 PMID: 35770056

Ehlers, A., & Clark, D. (2000). A cognitive model of posttraumatic stress disorder.*Behaviour Research and Therapy*, 38(4), 319–345. DOI: 10.1016/S0005-7967(99)00123-0 PMID: 10761279

Ehlers, A., Hackmann, A., & Michael, T. (2004). Intrusive re-experiencing in post-traumatic stress disorder: Phenomenology, theory, and therapy.*Memory (Hove, England)*, 12(4), 403–415. DOI: 10.1080/09658210444000025 PMID: 15487537

Ehrenstein, M. R., & Shipa, M. (2023). SLE is not a one-size-fits-all disease.*The Journal of Experimental Medicine*, 220(6), e20230559. DOI: 10.1084/jem.20230559 PMID: 37097613

Ehret, M. (2019). Treatment of posttraumatic stress disorder: Focus on pharmacotherapy.*The Mental Health Clinician*, 9(6), 373–382. DOI: 10.9740/mhc.2019.11.373 PMID: 31857933

Eissazade, N., Mosavari, H., Eghdami, S., Boroon, M., Ashrafi, F., & Shalbafan, M. (2023). Efficacy and safety of 5-hydroxytryptamine-3 (5-HT3) receptor antagonists in augmentation with selective serotonin reuptake inhibitors (SSRIs) in the treatment of moderate to severe obsessive-compulsive disorder: A systematic review and meta-analysis of randomized clinical trials.*Scientific Reports*, 13(1), 20837. DOI: 10.1038/s41598-023-47931-x PMID: 38012263

Emerson, D., & Hopper, E. (2011). *Overcoming trauma through yoga: Reclaiming your body*. North Atlantic Books.

Emmanouilidou, L. (2020, December 17). Arab uprisings: What role did social media really play? The World from PRX. https://theworld.org/stories/2020/12/17/arab-uprisings-what-role-did-social-media-really-play

Ernst, A., & Frisén, J. (2015). Adult neurogenesis in humans-common and unique traits in mammals.*PLoS Biology*, 13(1), e1002045. DOI: 10.1371/journal.pbio.1002045 PMID: 25621867

Eshel, N., Maron-Katz, A., Wu, W., Abu-Amara, D., Marmar, C. R., & Etkin, A. (2021). Neural correlates of anger expression in patients with PTSD.*Neuropsychopharmacology*, 46(9), 1635–1642. DOI: 10.1038/s41386-020-00942-y PMID: 33500557

Exline, J. J., Kaplan, K. J., & Grubbs, J. B. (2012). Anger, exit, and assertion: Do people see protest toward God as morally acceptable?*Psychology of Religion and Spirituality*, 4(4), 264–277. DOI: 10.1037/a0027667

Eyni, S., & Musavi, S. E. (2024). Social Isolation of War Veterans with Post-Traumatic Stress Disorder Based on Emotional Inhibition: The Mediating Role of Rejection Sensitivity. *We are a service founded by Vietnam Veterans, now for all veterans and families., 32*(1).

Fantasia, A. T., Prybutok, G., & Prybutok, V. (2023). The Impact of Post-Traumatic Stress Disorder on Addiction to Information over Searching and Information Avoidance.

Fatafta, M. (2024, March 20). Genocide in the digital age: What role do social media companies play? Association for Progressive Communications. https://www.apc.org/en/blog/genocide-digital-age-what-role-do-social-media-companies-play

Feinstein, D. (2022a). The energy of energy psychology.*OBM Integrative and Complimentary Medicine*, 7(2), 1–32. DOI: 10.21926/obm.icm.2202015 PMID: 35548526

Feinstein, D. (2022b). Uses of energy psychology following catastrophic events. *Frontiers in Psychology*, 13, 856209. DOI: 10.3389/fpsyg.2022.856209 PMID: 35548526

Feinstein, D. (2023). Integrating the manual stimulation of acupuncture points into psychotherapy: A systematic review with clinical recommendations.*Journal of Psychotherapy Integration*, 33(1), 47–67. Advance online publication. DOI: 10.1037/int0000283

Fink, G. (2009). Stress: definition and history. *Encyclopedia of Neuroscience*. 549-555.

First, M. B., Gaebel, W., Maj, M., Stein, D. J., Kogan, C. S., Saunders, J. B., Poznyak, V. B., Gureje, O., Lewis-Fernández, R., Maercker, A., Brewin, C. R., Cloitre, M., Claudino, A., Pike, K. M., Baird, G., Skuse, D., Krueger, R. B., Briken, P., Burke, J. D., & Reed, G. M. (2021). An organization- and category-level comparison of diagnostic requirements for mental disorders in ICD-11 and DSM-5.*World Psychiatry; Official Journal of the World Psychiatric Association (WPA)*, 20(1), 34–51. DOI: 10.1002/wps.20825 PMID: 33432742

Fisher, C. (2023). Trauma-Informed Nature Therapy: A Case Study.*Ecopsychology*, 15(3), 214–221. DOI: 10.1089/eco.2022.0064

Foa, E. B., Hembree, E. A., & Rothbaum, B. O. (2007). *Prolonged exposure therapy for PTSD: Emotional process of traumatic experiences-Therapist guide*. Oxford University Press. DOI: 10.1093/med:psych/9780195308501.001.0001

Foa, E. B., Keane, T. M., & Friedman, M. J. (2000). *Effective treatments for PTSD*.

Foa, E. B., Keane, T., & Friedman, M. (2000). *Effective treatments for post traumatic stress disorder: practice guidelines from the International Society for Traumatic Stress Studies*. Guilford Press.

Foa, E., Carmen, P., Capaldi, S., & Rosenfield, D. (2013). Prolonged exposure vs supportive counseling for sexual abuse–related PTSD in adolescent girls. A randomized clinical trial.*Journal of the American Medical Association*, 310(24), 650–2657. DOI: 10.1001/jama.2013.282829 PMID: 24368465

Foa, E., Rothbaum, B., & Furr, J. (2003). Augmenting exposure therapy with other CBT procedures.*Psychiatric Annals*, 33(1), 47–53. DOI: 10.3928/0048-5713-20030101-08

Fonzo, G. A., Simmons, A. N., Thorp, S. R., Norman, S. B., Paulus, M. P., & Stein, M. B. (2010). Exaggerated and disconnected insular-amygdalar blood oxygenation level-dependent response to threat-related emotional faces in women with intimate-partner violence posttraumatic stress disorder.*Biological Psychiatry*, 68(5), 433–441. DOI: 10.1016/j.biopsych.2010.04.028 PMID: 20573339

Ford, J. D., Grasso, D. J., Elhai, J. D., & Courtois, C. A. (2015). Social, cultural, and other diversity issues in the traumatic stress field. Posttraumatic Stress Disorder, 503-546.

Ford, J. D., & Courtois, C. A. (2021). Complex PTSD and borderline personality disorder.*Borderline Personality Disorder and Emotion Dysregulation*, 8(1), 16. DOI: 10.1186/s40479-021-00155-9 PMID: 33958001

Forkey, H. (2019). Putting Your Trauma Lens On.*Pediatric Annals*, 48(7), e269–e273. DOI: 10.3928/19382359-20190618-01 PMID: 31305944

Forman-Hoffman, V., Middleton, J. C., Feltner, C., Gaynes, B. N., Weber, R. P., Bann, C., Viswanathan, M., Lohr, K. N., Baker, C., & Green, J. (2018). Psychological and pharmacological treatments for adults with posttraumatic stress disorder: a systematic review update. AHRQ Comparative Effectiveness Reviews, Rockville (MD): Agency for Healthcare Research and Quality (US), Report No.: 18-EHC011-EFReport No.: 2018-SR-01. DOI: 10.23970/AHRQEPCCER207

Fournier, J. C., DeRubeis, R. J., Hollon, S. D., Dimidjian, S., Amsterdam, J. D., Shelton, R. C., & Fawcett, J. (2010). Antidepressant drug effects and depression severity: A patient-level meta-analysis.*Journal of the American Medical Association*, 303(1), 47–53. DOI: 10.1001/jama.2009.1943 PMID: 20051569

Francati, V., Vermetten, E., & Bremner, J. D. (2007). Functional neuroimaging studies in posttraumatic stress disorder: Review of current methods and findings. *Depression and Anxiety*, 24(3), 202–218. DOI: 10.1002/da.20208 PMID: 16960853

Frank, D. L., Khorshid, L., Kiffer, J. F., Moravec, C. S., & McKee, M. G. (2010). Biofeedback in medicine: Who, when, why and how?*Mental Health in Family Medicine*, 7(2), 85–91. PMID: 22477926

Frankl, V. E. (1963). *Man's search for meaning*. Simon and Schuster.

Freedom, J., Hux, M., & Warner, J. (2022). Research on acupoint tapping therapies proliferating around the world.*Energy Psychology*, 4(1), 22–37. Advance online publication. DOI: 10.9769/EPJ.2022.14.1.JF

Freese, J. B. (2023). Towards Trauma-Informed Buddhist Spiritual Care: A Mutual Critical Correlation of Vipassana Meditation and Somatic Experiencing.*Pastoral Psychology*, 72(3), 447–464. DOI: 10.1007/s11089-023-01065-z

Freud, S. (2002). *The Psychopathology of Everyday Life* (Bell, A. L., Trans.). Penguin Modern Classics. Penguin Classics.

Friedman, S. B., Chodoff, P., Mason, J. W., & Hamburg, D. A. (1963). Behavioral observations on parents anticipating the death of a child. *Pediatrics*, 32(4), 610–625. DOI: 10.1542/peds.32.4.610 PMID: 14069103

Frijling, J. L. (2017). Preventing PTSD with oxytocin: Effects of oxytocin administration on fear neurocircuitry and PTSD symptom development in recently trauma-exposed individuals.*European Journal of Psychotraumatology*, 8(1), 1302652. DOI: 10.1080/20008198.2017.1302652 PMID: 28451068

Fuchs, E., & Gould, E. (2000). Mini-review: in vivo neurogenesis in the adult brain: regulation and functional implications.*The European Journal of Neuroscience*, 12(7), 2211–2214. DOI: 10.1046/j.1460-9568.2000.00130.x PMID: 10947799

Furtado, M., & Katzman, M. A. (2015). Examining the role of neuroinflammation in major depression.*Psychiatry Research*, 229(1–2), 27–36. DOI: 10.1016/j.psychres.2015.06.009 PMID: 26187338

Fu, T. (2023). New Interventions for the Treatment of PTSD. *Journal of Education. Humanities and Social Sciences*, 8, 848–855.

Ganzel, B. L., Kim, P., Glover, G. H., & Temple, E. (2008). Resilience after 9/11: Multimodal neuroimaging evidence for stress-related change in the healthy adult brain.*NeuroImage*, 40(2), 788–795. DOI: 10.1016/j.neuroimage.2007.12.010 PMID: 18234524

Garfinkel, S. N., Abelson, J. L., King, A. P., Sripada, R. K., Wang, X., Gaines, L. M., & Liberzon, I. (2014). Impaired contextual modulation of memories in PTSD: An fMRI and psychophysiological study of extinction retention and fear renewal. *The Journal of Neuroscience : The Official Journal of the Society for Neuroscience*, 34(40), 13435–13443. DOI: 10.1523/JNEUROSCI.4287-13.2014 PMID: 25274821

Geracioti, T. D.Jr, Baker, D. G., Ekhator, N. N., West, S. A., Hill, K. K., Bruce, A. B., Schmidt, D., Rounds-Kugler, B., Yehuda, R., Keck, P. E.Jr, & Kasckow, J. W. (2001). CSF norepinephrine concentrations in posttraumatic stress disorder. *The American Journal of Psychiatry*, 158(8), 1227–1230. DOI: 10.1176/appi.ajp.158.8.1227 PMID: 11481155

Gersons, B. P. R., Carlier, I. V. E., Lamberts, R. D., & van der Kolk, B. (2000). A randomized clinical trial of brief eclectic psychotherapy in police officers with posttraumatic stress disorder.*Journal of Traumatic Stress*, 13(2), 333–437. DOI: 10.1023/A:1007793803627 PMID: 10838679

Gharib, M. (2023, November 24). Watching war unfold is distressing—Here's how to protect your mental health. NPR. https://www.npr.org/sections/health-shots/2023/11/24/1214534579/images-war-gaza-israel-vicarious-trauma-stress

Gillespie, P. G., & Walker, R. G. (2001). Molecular basis of mechanosensory transduction.*Nature*, 413(6852), 194–202. DOI: 10.1038/35093011 PMID: 11557988

Gilmartin, M. R., Balderston, N. L., & Helmstetter, F. J. (2014). Prefrontal cortical regulation of fear learning.*Trends in Neurosciences*, 37(8), 455–464. DOI: 10.1016/j.tins.2014.05.004 PMID: 24929864

Glover, D. A., Powers, M. B., Bergman, L., Smits, J. A. J., Telch, M. J., & Stuber, M. (2003). Urinary dopamine and turn bias in traumatized women with and without PTSD symptoms.*Behavioural Brain Research*, 144(1–2), 137–141. DOI: 10.1016/S0166-4328(03)00074-3 PMID: 12946604

Goetter, E. M., Blackburn, A. M., Stasko, C., Han, Y., Brenner, L. H., Lejeune, S., Tanev, K. S., Spencer, T. J., & Wright, E. C. (2021). Comparative effectiveness of prolonged exposure and cognitive processing therapy for military service members in an intensive treatment program.*Psychological Trauma: Theory, Research, Practice, and Policy*, 13(6), 632–640. DOI: 10.1037/tra0000956 PMID: 32915044

Golier, J. A., Yehuda, R., De Santi, S., Segal, S., Dolan, S., & de Leon, M. J. (2005). Absence of hippocampal volume differences in survivors of the Nazi Holocaust with and without posttraumatic stress disorder.*Psychiatry Research: Neuroimaging*, 139(1), 53–64. DOI: 10.1016/j.pscychresns.2005.02.007 PMID: 15939577

Gómez-Revuelta, M., Pelayo-Terán, J. M., Juncal-Ruiz, M., Vázquez-Bourgon, J., Suárez-Pinilla, P., Romero-Jiménez, R., Setién Suero, E., Ayesa-Arriola, R., & Crespo-Facorro, B. (2020). Antipsychotic Treatment Effectiveness in First Episode of Psychosis: PAFIP 3-Year Follow-Up Randomized Clinical Trials Comparing Haloperidol, Olanzapine, Risperidone, Aripiprazole, Quetiapine, and Ziprasidone. *The International Journal of Neuropsychopharmacology*, 23(4), 217–229. DOI: 10.1093/ijnp/pyaa004 PMID: 31974576

Goswami, M. (2018). Social Media and Hashtag Activism. In Liberty, Dignity, and Change in Journalism (pp. 252–262). Kanishka.

Gøtzsche, C. R., & Woldbye, D. P. D. (2016). The role of NPY in learning and memory.*Neuropeptides*, 55, 79–89. DOI: 10.1016/j.npep.2015.09.010 PMID: 26454711

Graham, D. A., Green, A., Murphy, C., & Richards, P. (2019, May 13). An Oral History of Trump's Bigotry. The Atlantic. https://www.theatlantic.com/magazine/archive/2019/06/trump-racism-comments/588067/

Green, A. (2011). Art and music therapy for trauma survivors.*Canadian Art Therapy Association Journal*, 24(2), 14–19. DOI: 10.1080/08322473.2011.11415547

Green, B. L. (1982). Assessing levels of psychological impairment following disaster: Consideration of actual and methodological dimensions.*The Journal of Nervous and Mental Disease*, 170(9), 544–552. DOI: 10.1097/00005053-198209000-00005 PMID: 7108503

Gros, D. F., Flanagan, J. C., Korte, K. J., Mills, A. C., Brady, K. T., & Back, S. E. (2016). Relations between social support, PTSD symptoms, and substance use in veterans.*Psychology of Addictive Behaviors*, 30(7), 764–770. DOI: 10.1037/adb0000205 PMID: 27786511

Gross, T. (2021, August 25). In "Dopamine Nation," Overabundance Keeps Us Craving More. NPR. https://www.npr.org/sections/health-shots/2021/08/25/1030930259/in-dopamine-nation-overabundance-keeps-u-s-craving-more

Gustavson, S. M., Sandoval, D. A., Ertl, A. C., Bao, S., Raj, S. R., & Davis, S. N. (2008). Stimulation of both type I and type II corticosteroid receptors blunts counterregulatory responses to subsequent hypoglycemia in healthy man.*American Journal of Physiology. Endocrinology and Metabolism*, 294(3), E506–E512. DOI: 10.1152/ajpendo.00589.2007 PMID: 18182467

Ha, A., Wilkins, S. S., Melrose, R. J., & Lee, C. C. (2023). Depression and PTSD as Predictors of Attrition in Older Adult Exercise Programs: A Systematic Review.*Topics in Geriatric Rehabilitation*, 39(1), 31–38. DOI: 10.1097/TGR.0000000000000383

Haaker, J., Gaburro, S., Sah, A., Gartmann, N., Lonsdorf, T. B., Meier, K., Singewald, N., Pape, H.-C., Morellini, F., & Kalisch, R. (2013). Single dose of L-dopa makes extinction memories context-independent and prevents the return of fear. *Proceedings of the National Academy of Sciences of the United States of America*, 110(26), E2428–E2436. DOI: 10.1073/pnas.1303061110 PMID: 23754384

Hafeez, S. (2002). The relationship between violence-related trauma and length of exposure to PTSD in emergency medical technicians [Unpublished doctoral dissertation]. Hofstra University.

Haller, H., Mitzinger, D., & Cramer, H. (2023). The integration of yoga breathing techniques in cognitive behavioral therapy for post-traumatic stress disorder: A pragmatic randomized controlled trial.*Frontiers in Psychiatry*, 14, 1101046. DOI: 10.3389/fpsyt.2023.1101046 PMID: 37139325

Hamner, M. B., & Diamond, B. I. (1993). Elevated plasma dopamine in posttraumatic stress disorder: A preliminary report.*Biological Psychiatry*, 33(4), 304–306. DOI: 10.1016/0006-3223(93)90302-T PMID: 8471687

Hansford, M., & Jobson, L. (2021). Social support and self-construal as moderators of lifetime trauma exposure on posttraumatic stress disorder symptoms.*Traumatology*, 27(2), 205–214. DOI: 10.1037/trm0000281

Harada, K., Yamaji, T., & Matsuoka, N. (2008). Activation of the serotonin 5-HT2C receptor is involved in the enhanced anxiety in rats after single-prolonged stress.*Pharmacology, Biochemistry, and Behavior*, 89(1), 11–16. DOI: 10.1016/j.pbb.2007.10.016 PMID: 18067955

Harned, M. S., Schmidt, S. C., Korslund, K. E., & Gallop, R. J. (2021). Does Adding the Dialectical Behavior Therapy Prolonged Exposure (DBT PE) Protocol for PTSD to DBT Improve Outcomes in Public Mental Health Settings? A Pilot Nonrandomized Effectiveness Trial With Benchmarking.*Behavior Therapy*, 52(3), 639–655. DOI: 10.1016/j.beth.2020.08.003 PMID: 33990239

Harris, A., & Reece, J. (2021). Transcranial magnetic stimulation as a treatment for posttraumatic stress disorder: A meta-analysis.*Journal of Affective Disorders*, 289(15), 55–65. DOI: 10.1016/j.jad.2021.04.003 PMID: 33940319

Harrison, B. J., Fullana, M. A., Via, E., Soriano-Mas, C., Vervliet, B., Martínez-Zalacaín, I., Pujol, J., Davey, C. G., Kircher, T., Straube, B., & Cardoner, N. (2017). Human ventromedial prefrontal cortex and the positive affective processing of safety signals.*NeuroImage*, 152, 12–18. DOI: 10.1016/j.neuroimage.2017.02.080 PMID: 28254509

Harris, R. (2009). *ACT Made Simple: An Easy-To-Read Primer on Acceptance and Commitment Therapy*. New Harbinger Publications.

Haugen, M. R. G. (2011). *Does trauma lead to religiousness? A longitudinal study of the effects of traumatic events on religiousness and spirituality during the first three years at university.* (Unpublished doctoral dissertation). Bowling Green State University.

Hayes, S. C., & Lillis, J. (2012). *Acceptance and commitment therapy*. American Psychological Association. DOI: 10.1037/17335-000

Hayes, S. C., Strosahl, K. D., & Wilson, G. (2016). *Acceptance and commitment therapy: The process and practice of mindful change*. Spiegel and Grau.

Heilig, M., McLeod, S., Brot, M., Heinrichs, S. C., Menzaghi, F., Koob, G. F., & Britton, K. T. (1993). Anxiolytic-like action of neuropeptide Y: Mediation by Y1 receptors in amygdala, and dissociation from food intake effects.*Neuropsychopharmacology*, 8(4), 357–363. DOI: 10.1038/npp.1993.35 PMID: 8099792

Heim, C., & Nemeroff, C. B. (2009). Neurobiology of posttraumatic stress disorder. *CNS Spectrums*, 14(1, Suppl 1), 13–24. PMID: 19169190

Helbig, S., & Fehm, L. (2004). Problems with homework in CBT: Rare exception or rather frequent?*Behavioural and Cognitive Psychotherapy*, 32(3), 291–301. DOI: 10.1017/S1352465804001365

Helpman, L., Marin, M.-F., Papini, S., Zhu, X. I., Sullivan, G. M., Schneier, F., Neria, M., Shvil, E., Aragon, M. J. M., & Markowitz, J. C. (2016). Neural changes in extinction recall following prolonged exposure treatment for PTSD: A longitudinal fMRI study.*NeuroImage. Clinical*, 12, 715–723. DOI: 10.1016/j.nicl.2016.10.007 PMID: 27761402

Hembree, E. A., & Foa, E. B. (2000). Posttraumatic stress disorder: Psychological factors and psychosocial interventions.*The Journal of Clinical Psychiatry*, 61S, 33–39. PMID: 10795607

Hendrickson, R. C., & Raskind, M. A. (2016). Noradrenergic dysregulation in the pathophysiology of PTSD.*Experimental Neurology*, 284, 181–195. DOI: 10.1016/j.expneurol.2016.05.014 PMID: 27222130

Hendriksen, H., Prins, J., Olivier, B., & Oosting, R. S. (2010). Environmental enrichment induces behavioral recovery and enhanced hippocampal cell proliferation in an antidepressant-resistant animal model for PTSD.*PLoS One*, 5(8), e11943. DOI: 10.1371/journal.ponc.0011943 PMID: 20700523

Herman, J. L. (1992). *Trauma and Recovery*. Basic Books.

Herman, J. P., McKlveen, J. M., Ghosal, S., Kopp, B., Wulsin, A., Makinson, R., Scheimann, J., & Myers, B. (2016). Regulation of the hypothalamic-pituitary-adrenocortical stress response.*Comprehensive Physiology*, 6(2), 603–621. DOI: 10.1002/cphy.c150015 PMID: 27065163

Hikind, N., & Maroun, M. (2008). Microinfusion of the D1 receptor antagonist, SCH23390 into the IL but not the BLA impairs consolidation of extinction of auditory fear conditioning.*Neurobiology of Learning and Memory*, 90(1), 217–222. DOI: 10.1016/j.nlm.2008.03.003 PMID: 18442937

Hirschberger, G. (2018). Collective Trauma and the Social Construction of Meaning. *Frontiers in Psychology*, 9, 1441. DOI: 10.3389/fpsyg.2018.01441 PMID: 30147669

Hobbs, M. M. (2023). Healing Journeys: Veterans, Trauma, and the Return to Vietnam.*The Journal of American History*, 110(1), 82–107. DOI: 10.1093/jahist/jaad094

Hofmann, S. G., & Gomez, A. F. (2017). Mindfulness-based interventions for anxiety and depression.*The Psychiatric Clinics of North America*, 40(4), 739–749. DOI: 10.1016/j.psc.2017.08.008 PMID: 29080597

Holland, J. (2001). Medicine for the new millennium. In Holland, J. (Ed.), *Ecstasy: A complete guide-A comprehensive look at the risks and benefits of MDMA* (pp. 1–5). Park Street Press.

Hollifield, M., Sinclair-Lian, N., Warner, T. D., & Hammeschlag, R. (2007). Acupuncture for posttraumatic stress disorder: A randomized controlled pilot trial. *The Journal of Nervous and Mental Disease*, 195(6), 504–513. DOI: 10.1097/NMD.0b013e31803044f8 PMID: 17568299

Holman, E. A., Garfin, D. R., Lubens, P., & Silver, R. C. (2020). Media Exposure to Collective Trauma, Mental Health, and Functioning: Does It Matter What You See?-*Clinical Psychological Science*, 8(1), 111–124. DOI: 10.1177/2167702619858300

Holmes, E. A., Grey, N., & Young, K. A. D. (2005). Intrusive images and "hotspots" of trauma memories in Posttraumatic Stress Disorder: An exploratory investigation of emotions and cognitive themes.*Journal of Behavior Therapy and Experimental Psychiatry*, 36(1), 3–17. DOI: 10.1016/j.jbtep.2004.11.002 PMID: 15687006

Holsboer, F., & Ising, M. (2008). Central CRH system in depression and anxiety—Evidence from clinical studies with CRH1 receptor antagonists.*European Journal of Pharmacology*, 583(2–3), 350–357. DOI: 10.1016/j.ejphar.2007.12.032 PMID: 18272149

Holzer, P., Reichmann, F., & Farzi, A. (2012). Neuropeptide Y, peptide YY and pancreatic polypeptide in the gut–brain axis.*Neuropeptides*, 46(6), 261–274. DOI: 10.1016/j.npep.2012.08.005 PMID: 22979996

Hopper, J. W., Frewen, P. A., van der Kolk, B. A., & Lanius, R. A. (2007). Neural correlates of reexperiencing, avoidance, and dissociation in PTSD: Symptom dimensions and emotion dysregulation in responses to script-driven trauma imagery.*Journal of Traumatic Stress*, 20(5), 713–725. DOI: 10.1002/jts.20284 PMID: 17955540

Horn, S. R., & Feder, A. (2018). Understanding resilience and preventing and treating PTSD.*Harvard Review of Psychiatry*, 26(3), 158–174. DOI: 10.1097/HRP.0000000000000194 PMID: 29734229

Horton, A. L., Wilkins, M. M., & Wright, W. (1988). Women who ended abuse: What religious leaders and religion did for these victims. In Horton, A. L., & Williamson, J. A. (Eds.), *Abuse and religion: When praying isn't enough* (pp. 235–246). Lexington Books.

Horwath, A. O., Del Re, A. C., Fluckiger, C., & Symonds, D. (2011). Alliance in individual psychotherapy.*Psychotherapy (Chicago, Ill.)*, 48(1), 9–16. DOI: 10.1037/a0022186 PMID: 21401269

Hoskins, O. P., & Lewis, C. (2023). Post-traumatic stress disorder: Symptoms, diagnosis and treatment. *BMJ Best Practice*. Retrieved December 30, 2023, from https://bestpractice.bmj.com/topics/en-gb/430

Hoskins, M., Pearce, J., Bethell, A., Dankova, L., Barbui, C., Tol, W. A., Van Ommeren, M., De Jong, J., Seedat, S., Chen, H., & Bisson, J. I. (2015). Pharmacotherapy for post-traumatic stress disorder: Systematic review and meta-analysis.*The British Journal of Psychiatry*, 206(2), 93–100. DOI: 10.1192/bjp.bp.114.148551 PMID: 25644881

Hou, C., Liu, J., Wang, K., Li, L., Liang, M., He, Z., Liu, Y., Zhang, Y., Li, W., & Jiang, T. (2007). Brain responses to symptom provocation and trauma-related short-term memory recall in coal mining accident survivors with acute severe PTSD.*Brain Research*, 1144, 165–174. DOI: 10.1016/j.brainres.2007.01.089 PMID: 17331476

Huckins, L. M., Chatzinakos, C., Breen, M. S., Hartmann, J., Klengel, T., da Silva Almeida, A. C., Dobbyn, A., Girdhar, K., Hoffman, G. E., Klengel, C., Logue, M. W., Lori, A., Maihofer, A. X., Morrison, F. G., Nguyen, H. T., Park, Y., Ruderfer, D., Sloofman, L. G., van Rooij, S. J. H., & Daskalakis, N. P.PTSD Working Group of Psychiatric Genomics Consortium. (2020). Analysis of Genetically Regulated Gene Expression Identifies a Prefrontal PTSD Gene, SNRNP35, Specific to Military Cohorts.*Cell Reports*, 31(9), 107716. DOI: 10.1016/j.celrep.2020.107716 PMID: 32492425

Hu, J., Feng, B., Zhu, Y., Wang, W., Xie, J., & Zheng, X. (2017). Gender Differences in PTSD: Susceptibility and Resilience. In Alvinus, A. (Ed.), *Gender Differences in Different Contexts*. IntechOpen Limited. DOI: 10.5772/65287

Hunter, E. J., McCubbin, H. I., & Metres, P. J.Jr. (1974). Religion and POW/MIA wife. In McCubbin, H. I., Dahl, B. B., Metres, P. J.Jr, Hunter, E. J., & Plag, J. A. (Eds.), *Family separation and reunion: Families of prisoners of war and servicemen missing in action* (pp. 85–93). US Government Printing Office.

Inslicht, S. S., Metzler, T. J., Garcia, N. M., Pineles, S. L., Milad, M. R., Orr, S. P., Marmar, C. R., & Neylan, T. C. (2013). Sex differences in fear conditioning in posttraumatic stress disorder.*Journal of Psychiatric Research*, 47(1), 64–71. DOI: 10.1016/j.jpsychires.2012.08.027 PMID: 23107307

Iqbal, J., Huang, G.-D., Xue, Y.-X., Yang, M., & Jia, X.-J. (2023). The neural circuits and molecular mechanisms underlying fear dysregulation in posttraumatic stress disorder.*Frontiers in Neuroscience*, 17, 17. DOI: 10.3389/fnins.2023.1281401 PMID: 38116070

Ishikawa, R., Uchida, C., Kitaoka, S., Furuyashiki, T., & Kida, S. (2019). Improvement of PTSD-like behavior by the forgetting effect of hippocampal neurogenesis enhancer memantine in a social defeat stress paradigm.*Molecular Brain*, 12(1), 4–9. DOI: 10.1186/s13041-019-0488-6 PMID: 31370877

Jackson, K. (2014). Treatment for veterans with PTSD – Outside the traditional toolbox.*Social Work Today*, 14, 18.

Jacobs, J. (2022). The Intergenerational Transmission of Trauma: Religion, Spirituality, and Ritual among Children and Grandchildren of Holocaust Survivors. In *Interpreting Religion*. Bristol University Press., DOI: 10.2307/j.ctv2m7c5ks.8

Jacobson, L. (2014). Hypothalamic-pituitary-adrenocortical axis: Neuropsychiatric aspects.*Comprehensive Physiology*, 4(2), 715–738. DOI: 10.1002/cphy.c130036 PMID: 24715565

Jacques, P. L. S., Botzung, A., Miles, A., & Rubin, D. C. (2011). Functional neuroimaging of emotionally intense autobiographical memories in post-traumatic stress disorder.*Journal of Psychiatric Research*, 45(5), 630–637. DOI: 10.1016/j.jpsychires.2010.10.011 PMID: 21109253

Jamil, A., Gutlapalli, S. D., Ali, M., Oble, M. J., Sonia, S. N., George, S., Shahi, S. R., Ali, Z., Abaza, A., & Mohammed, L. (2023). Meditation and its mental and physical health benefits in 2023.*Cureus*, 15(6). Advance online publication. DOI: 10.7759/cureus.40650 PMID: 37476142

Jatzko, A., Rothenhöfer, S., Schmitt, A., Gaser, C., Demirakca, T., Weber-Fahr, W., Wessa, M., Magnotta, V., & Braus, D. F. (2006). Hippocampal volume in chronic posttraumatic stress disorder (PTSD): MRI study using two different evaluation methods.*Journal of Affective Disorders*, 94(1–3), 121–126. DOI: 10.1016/j.jad.2006.03.010 PMID: 16701903

Jayawickrene, E., & Blackie, L. E. R. (2014). Posttraumatic growth as positive personality change: Evidence, controversies, and future directions. *European Journal of Personality*, 28(4), 312–331. DOI: 10.1002/per.1963

Jericho, B., Luo, A., & Berle, D. (2022). Trauma-focused psychotherapies for post-traumatic stress disorder: A systematic review and network meta-analysis.*Acta Psychiatrica Scandinavica*, 145(2), 132–155. DOI: 10.1111/acps.13366 PMID: 34473342

Jiang, S., Postovit, L., Cattaneo, A., Binder, E. B., & Aitchison, K. J. (2019). Epigenetic modifications in stress response genes associated with childhood trauma. *Frontiers in Psychiatry*, 10, 808. DOI: 10.3389/fpsyt.2019.00808 PMID: 31780969

Johansen, A. B., Kristiansen, E., Bjelland, I., & Tavakoli, S. (2019). Secondary traumatic stress in Norwegian SUD-therapists: Symptoms and related factors. Nordisk Alkohol- & Narkotikatidskrift. *Nordisk Alkohol- & Narkotikatidskrift*, 36(6), 522–531. DOI: 10.1177/1455072519847014 PMID: 32934585

Johansen, V. A., Milde, A. M., Nilsen, R. M., Breivik, K., Nordanger, D. Ø., Stormark, K. M., & Weisæth, L. (2022). The relationship between perceived social support and PTSD symptoms after exposure to physical assault: An 8 years longitudinal study.*Journal of Interpersonal Violence*, 37(9-10), NP7679–NP7706. DOI: 10.1177/0886260520970314 PMID: 33140665

Jones, K. A., Freijah, I., Carey, L., Carleton, R. N., Devenish-Meares, P., Dell, L., Rodrigues, S., Madden, K., Johnson, L., Hosseiny, F., & Phelps, A. J. (2022). Moral Injury, Chaplaincy and Mental Health Provider Approaches to Treatment: A Scoping Review.*Journal of Religion and Health*, 61(2), 1051–1094. DOI: 10.1007/s10943-022-01534-4 PMID: 35290554

Jones, M. B., Agrawal, R., Sharafkhaneh, A., Kunik, M. E., Jorge, R. E., & Marsh, L. (2022). Dream Enactment Behaviors Associated With Posttraumatic Stress Disorder.*The Journal of Neuropsychiatry and Clinical Neurosciences*, 34(2), 124–131. DOI: 10.1176/appi.neuropsych.21050115 PMID: 34763524

Joschko, L., Palsdottir, A. M., Grahn, P., & Hinse, M. (2023). Nature-based therapy in individuals with mental health disorders, with a focus on mental well-being and connectedness to nature-a pilot study.*International Journal of Environmental Research and Public Health*, 20(3), 2167. DOI: 10.3390/ijerph20032167 PMID: 36767534

Joseph, S., Linley, P. A., Andrews, L., Harris, G., Howle, B., Woodward, C., & Shevlin, M. (2005). Assessing positive and negative changes in the aftermath of adversity: Psychometric evaluation of the Changes in Outlook Questionnaire.*Psychological Assessment*, 17(2), 70–80. DOI: 10.1037/1040-3590.17.1.70 PMID: 15769229

Joseph, S., Williams, R., & Yule, W. (1993). Changes in outlook following disaster: The preliminary development of a measure to assess positive and negative responses. *Journal of Traumatic Stress*, 6(2), 271–279. DOI: 10.1002/jts.2490060209

Jovanovic, T., Norrholm, S. D., Fennell, J. E., Keyes, M., Fiallos, A. M., Myers, K. M., Davis, M., & Duncan, E. J. (2009). Posttraumatic stress disorder may be associated with impaired fear inhibition: Relation to symptom severity.*Psychiatry Research*, 167(1–2), 151–160. DOI: 10.1016/j.psychres.2007.12.014 PMID: 19345420

Jovanovic, T., Phifer, J. E., Sicking, K., Weiss, T., Norrholm, S. D., Bradley, B., & Ressler, K. J. (2011). Cortisol suppression by dexamethasone reduces exaggerated fear responses in posttraumatic stress disorder.*Psychoneuroendocrinology*, 36(10), 1540–1552. DOI: 10.1016/j.psyneuen.2011.04.008 PMID: 21601366

Jowf, G. I. A., Ahmed, Z. T., An, N., Reijnders, R. A., Ambrosino, E., Rutten, B. P. F., De Nijs, L., & Eijssen, L. (2022, May26). *A Public Health Perspective of Post-Traumatic Stress Disorder*. International Journal of Environmental Research and Public Health. *International Journal of Environmental Research and Public Health*, 19(11), 6474. Advance online publication. DOI: 10.3390/ijerph19116474 PMID: 35682057

Kabat-Zinn, J. (1994). *Wherever you go, there you are: Mindfulness meditation in everyday life*. Hyperion.

Kaczkurkin, A. N., & Foa, E. B. (2015). Cognitive-behavioral therapy for anxiety disorders: An update on the empirical evidence.*Current Psychiatry Reports*, 17(3), 337–346. https://www.ncbi.nlm.nih.gov/pmc/articles/PMC4610618/ PMID: 26487814

Kaczkurkin, A. N., & Foa, E. B. (2015). Cognitive-behavioral therapy for anxiety disorders: An update on the empirical evidence.*Dialogues in Clinical Neuroscience*, 17(3), 337–346. DOI: 10.31887/DCNS.2015.17.3/akaczkurkin PMID: 26487814

Kaidesoja, M., Cooper, Z., & Fordham, B. (2023). Cognitive behavioral therapy for eating disorders: A map of the systematic review evidence base.*International Journal of Eating Disorders*, 56(2), 295–313. DOI: 10.1002/eat.23831 PMID: 36315392

Karatzias, T., Murphy, P., Cloitre, M., Bisson, J., Roberts, N., Shevlin, M., Hyland, P., Maercker, A., Ben-Ezra, M., Coventry, P., Mason-Roberts, S., Bradley, A., & Hutton, P. (2019). Psychological interventions for ICD-11 complex PTSD symptoms: Systematic review and meta-analysis.*Psychological Medicine*, 49(11), 1761–1775. DOI: 10.1017/S0033291719000436 PMID: 30857567

Karim, F., Oyewande, A. A., Abdalla, L. F., Chaudhry Ehsanullah, R., & Khan, S. (2020). Social Media Use and Its Connection to Mental Health: A Systematic Review.*Cureus*, 12(6), e8627. DOI: 10.7759/cureus.8627 PMID: 32685296

Karl, A., Schaefer, M., Malta, L. S., Dörfel, D., Rohleder, N., & Werner, A. (2006). A meta-analysis of structural brain abnormalities in PTSD.*Neuroscience and Biobehavioral Reviews*, 30(7), 1004–1031. DOI: 10.1016/j.neubiorev.2006.03.004 PMID: 16730374

Kar, N. (2011). Cognitive behavioral therapy for the treatment of post-traumatic stress disorder: A review.*Neuropsychiatric Disease and Treatment*, 7, 167–181. DOI: 10.2147/NDT.S10389 PMID: 21552319

Kartol, A., Üztemur, S., & Yaşar, P. (2023). 'I cannot see ahead': Psychological distress, doomscrolling and dark future among adult survivors following Mw 7.7. and 7.6 earthquakes in Türkiye.*BMC Public Health*, 23(1), 2513. DOI: 10.1186/s12889-023-17460-3 PMID: 38102569

Kask, A., Harro, J., von Hörsten, S., Redrobe, J. P., Dumont, Y., & Quirion, R. (2002). The neurocircuitry and receptor subtypes mediating anxiolytic-like effects of neuropeptide Y.*Neuroscience and Biobehavioral Reviews*, 26(3), 259–283. DOI: 10.1016/S0149-7634(01)00066-5 PMID: 12034130

Katzman, M. A., Bleau, P., Blier, P., Chokka, P., Kjernisted, K., & van Ameringen, M. (2014). Canadian clinical practice guidelines for the management of anxiety, posttraumatic stress and obsessive compulsive disorders.*BMC Psychiatry*, 14(Suppl 1), S1. DOI: 10.1186/1471-244X-14-S1-S1 PMID: 25081580

Kazantzis, N., Deane, F. P., & Ronan, K. R. (2000). Homework assignments in cognitive and behavioral therapy: A meta-analysis.*Clinical Psychology : a Publication of the Division of Clinical Psychology of the American Psychological Association*, 7(2), 189–202. DOI: 10.1093/clipsy.7.2.189

Kearns, M. C., Ressler, K. J., Zatzick, D., & Rothbaum, B. O. R. (2012). Early interventions for PTSD: A review.*Depression and Anxiety*, 29(10), 833–842. DOI: 10.1002/da.21997 PMID: 22941845

Kellner, M., Yassouridis, A., Hübner, R., Baker, D. G., & Wiedemann, K. (2003). Endocrine and cardiovascular responses to corticotropin-releasing hormone in patients with posttraumatic stress disorder: A role for atrial natriuretic peptide?*Neuropsychobiology*, 47(2), 102–108. DOI: 10.1159/000070018 PMID: 12707494

Kerig, P. K. (2019). Linking childhood trauma exposure to adolescent justice involvement: The concept of posttraumatic risk-seeking.*Clinical Psychology : a Publication of the Division of Clinical Psychology of the American Psychological Association*, 26(3), e12280. DOI: 10.1111/cpsp.12280

Kerr, J. I., Weibel, R. P., Naegelin, M., Ferrario, A., Schinazi, V. R., La Marca, R., Hoelscher, C., Nater, U. M., & von Wangenheim, F. (2023). The effectiveness and user experience of a biofeedback intervention program for stress management supported by virtual reality and mobile technology: A randomized controlled study. *BMC Digital Health*, 1(1), 42. DOI: 10.1186/s44247-023-00042-z

Kessler, R. C., Sonnega, A., Bromet, E., Hughes, M., & Nelson, C. B. (1995). Posttraumatic stress disorder in the national comorbidity survey.*Archives of General Psychiatry*, 52(12), 1048–1060. DOI: 10.1001/archpsyc.1995.03950240066012 PMID: 7492257

Kezelman, C., & Stavropoulos, P. (Eds.). (2019). *Practice guidelines for clinical treatment of complex trauma*. Blue Knot Foundation. https://aztrauma.org/wp-content/uploads/2020/11/BlueKnot_Practice_Guidelines_2019.pdf

Khatib, R., McKee, M., & Yusuf, S. (2024). Counting the dead in Gaza: Difficult but essential.*Lancet*, 0(0), 237–238. Advance online publication. DOI: 10.1016/S0140-6736(24)01169-3 PMID: 38976995

Khwaja, K., Deban, M., Iqbal, S., Alowais, J., Al Bader, B., Deckelbaum, D., & Razek, T. (2023). The McGill simulation complexity Score (MSCS): A novel complexity scoring system for simulations in trauma.*Canadian Journal of Surgery*, 66(2), E206–E211. DOI: 10.1503/cjs.002220 PMID: 37085295

Kikuchi, A., Shimizu, K., Nibuya, M., Hiramoto, T., Kanda, Y., Tanaka, T., Watanabe, Y., Takahashi, Y., & Nomura, S. (2008). Relationship between post-traumatic stress disorder-like behavior and reduction of hippocampal 5-bromo-2′-deoxyuridine-positive cells after inescapable shock in rats.*Psychiatry and Clinical Neurosciences*, 62(6), 713–720. DOI: 10.1111/j.1440-1819.2008.01875.x PMID: 19068009

Kim, J., Chesworth, B., Franchino-Olsen, H., & Macy, R. J. (2022). A scoping review of vicarious trauma interventions for service providers working with people who have experienced traumatic events.*Trauma, Violence & Abuse*, 23(5), 152483802199131. DOI: 10.1177/1524838021991310 PMID: 33685294

Kim, S. H., Schneider, S. M., Kravitz, L., Mermier, C., & Burge, M. R. (2013). Mind-body practices for posttraumatic stress disorder.*Journal of Investigative Medicine*, 61(5), 827–834. DOI: 10.2310/JIM.0b013e3182906862 PMID: 23609463

Kim, T. D., Lee, S., & Yoon, S. (2020). Inflammation in post-traumatic stress disorder (PTSD): A review of potential correlates of PTSD with a neurological perspective. *Antioxidants*, 9(2), 107. DOI: 10.3390/antiox9020107 PMID: 31991875

Kim, Y.-K., Amidfar, M., & Won, E. (2019). A review on inflammatory cytokine-induced alterations of the brain as potential neural biomarkers in post-traumatic stress disorder.*Progress in Neuro-Psychopharmacology & Biological Psychiatry*, 91, 103–112. DOI: 10.1016/j.pnpbp.2018.06.008 PMID: 29932946

Kip, K. E., & Diamond, D. M. (2018). Clinical, Empirical, and Theoretical Rationale for Selection of Accelerated Resolution Therapy for Treatment of Post-traumatic Stress Disorder in VA and DoD Facilities.*Military Medicine*, 183(9-10), e314–e321. DOI: 10.1093/milmed/usy027 PMID: 29635395

Kira, I. A., Aboumediene, S., Ashby, J. S., Odenat, L., Mohanesh, J., & Alamia, H. (2013). The dynamics of posttraumatic growth across different trauma types in a Palestinian sample.*Journal of Loss and Trauma*, 18(2), 120–139. DOI: 10.1080/15325024.2012.679129

Kira, I. A., Ashby, J. S., Lewandowski, L., Alawneh, A. W. N., Mohanesh, J., & Odenat, L. (2013). Advances in continuous traumatic stress theory: Traumatogenic dynamics and consequences of intergroup conflict: The Palestinian adolescents case.*Psychology (Irvine, Calif.)*, 4(04), 396–409. DOI: 10.4236/psych.2013.44057

Kitayama, N., Vaccarino, V., Kutner, M., Weiss, P., & Bremner, J. D. (2005). Magnetic resonance imaging (MRI) measurement of hippocampal volume in posttraumatic stress disorder: A meta-analysis.*Journal of Affective Disorders*, 88(1), 79–86. DOI: 10.1016/j.jad.2005.05.014 PMID: 16033700

Klein, T. (2024). Editor's Note: War with Hamas pushes Israelis closer to God. The Jerusalem Post.

Knox, D., Stanfield, B. R., Staib, J. M., David, N. P., DePietro, T., Chamness, M., Schneider, E. K., Keller, S. M., & Lawless, C. (2018). Using c-Jun to identify fear extinction learning-specific patterns of neural activity that are affected by single prolonged stress.*Behavioural Brain Research*, 341, 189–197. DOI: 10.1016/j.bbr.2017.12.037 PMID: 29292158

Koenig, H. G. (2021). Mechanisms: religion's impact on mental health. In Moreira-Almeida, A. (Ed.), *Spirituality and Mental Health Across Cultures*. Oxford University Press.

Korem, N., Duek, O., Ben-Zion, Z., Kaczkurkin, A. N., Lissek, S., Orederu, T., Schiller, D., Harpaz-Rotem, I., & Levy, I. (2022). Emotional numbing in PTSD is associated with lower amygdala reactivity to pain.*Neuropsychopharmacology*, 47(11), 1913–1921. DOI: 10.1038/s41386-022-01405-2 PMID: 35945274

Kosarkova, A., Malinakova, K., Koncalova, Z., Tavel, P., & van Dijk, J. P. (2020). Childhood Trauma is associated with the spirituality of non-religious respondents. *International Journal of Environmental Research and Public Health*, 17(4), 1268. DOI: 10.3390/ijerph17041268 PMID: 32079153

Kothgassner, O. D., Goreis, A., Kafka, J. X., Eickels, R. L. V., Plener, P. L., & Felnhofer, A. (2019). Virtual reality exposure therapy for posttraumatic stress disorder (PTSD): A meta-analysis.*European Journal of Psychotraumatology*, 10(1), 1654782. DOI: 10.1080/20008198.2019.1654782 PMID: 31489138

Krüger, C. (2020). Culture, trauma and dissociation: A broadening perspective for our field.*Journal of Trauma & Dissociation*, 21(1), 1–13. DOI: 10.1080/15299732.2020.1675134 PMID: 31891334

Kuhfuß, M., Maldei, T., Hetmanek, A., & Baumann, N. (2021). Somatic experiencing-effectiveness and key factors of a body-oriented trauma therapy: A scoping literature review.*European Journal of Psychotraumatology*, 12(1), 1929023. DOI: 10.1080/20008198.2021.1929023 PMID: 34290845

Kühn, S., & Gallinat, J. (2013). Gray matter correlates of posttraumatic stress disorder: A quantitative meta-analysis.*Biological Psychiatry*, 73(1), 70–74. DOI: 10.1016/j.biopsych.2012.06.029 PMID: 22840760

Kulka, R. A., Schlenger, W. E., Fairbank, J. A., Hough, R. L., Jordan, B. K., Marmar, C. R., & Weiss, D. S. (1990). *Trauma and the Vietnam War Generation: Report of findings from the National Vietnam Veterans Readjustment Study*. Brunner/Mazel.

Kumar, S. A., Brand, B. L., & Courtois, C. A. (2022). The need for trauma training: Clinicians' reactions to training on complex trauma.*Psychological Trauma: Theory, Research, Practice, and Policy*, 14(8), 1387–1394. DOI: 10.1037/tra0000515 PMID: 31580137

Kuzelova, H., Ptacek, R., & Macek, M. (2010). The serotonin transporter gene (5-HTT) variant and psychiatric disorders: Review of current literature.*Neuroendocrinology Letters*, 31(1), 4–10. PMID: 20150867

Kvetnanský, R., Pacák, K., Fukuhara, K., Viskupic, E., Hiremagalur, B., Nankova, B., Goldstein, D. S., Sabban, E. L., & Kopin, I. J. (1995). Sympathoadrenal system in stress. Interaction with the hypothalamic-pituitary-adrenocortical system.*Annals of the New York Academy of Sciences*, 771(1), 131–158. DOI: 10.1111/j.1749-6632.1995.tb44676.x PMID: 8597393

Kwon, A., Lee, H. S., & Lee, S.-H. (2021). The Mediation Effect of Hyperarousal Symptoms on the Relationship Between Childhood Physical Abuse and Suicidal Ideation of Patients With PTSD.*Frontiers in Psychiatry*, 12, 613735. Advance online publication. DOI: 10.3389/fpsyt.2021.613735 PMID: 33841200

La Greca, A. M., Taylor, C. J., & Herge, W. M. (2012). Traumatic stress disorders in children and adolescents. In Beck, J. G., & Sloan, D. M. (Eds.), *The Oxford Handbook of Traumatic Stress Disorders*. Oxford University Press. DOI: 10.1093/oxfordhb/9780195399066.013.0008

Lai, F., Wang, L., Zhang, J., Shan, S., Chen, J., & Tian, L. (2023). Relationship between Social Media Use and Social Anxiety in College Students: Mediation Effect of Communication Capacity.*International Journal of Environmental Research and Public Health*, 20(4), 3657. DOI: 10.3390/ijerph20043657 PMID: 36834357

Lamba, N., Khokhlova, O., Bhatia, A., & McHugh, C. (2023). Mental health hygiene during a health crisis: Exploring factors associated with media-induced secondary trauma in relation to the COVID-19 pandemic.*Health Psychology Open*, 10(2), 20551029231199578. Advance online publication. DOI: 10.1177/20551029231199578 PMID: 37746585

Lanctôt, N., Reid, J. A., & Laurier, C. (2020). Nightmares and flashbacks: The impact of commercial sexual exploitation of children among female adolescents placed in residential care.*Child Abuse & Neglect*, 100, 104195. DOI: 10.1016/j.chiabu.2019.104195 PMID: 31582275

Langevin, H. M., & Yandow, J. A. (2002). Relationship of acupuncture points and meridians to connective tissue planes.*The Anatomical Record*, 269(6), 257–265. DOI: 10.1002/ar.10185 PMID: 12467083

Lanius, R. A., Frewen, P. A., Girotti, M., Neufeld, R. W. J., Stevens, T. K., & Densmore, M. (2007). Neural correlates of trauma script-imagery in posttraumatic stress disorder with and without comorbid major depression: A functional MRI investigation.*Psychiatry Research: Neuroimaging*, 155(1), 45–56. DOI: 10.1016/j.pscychresns.2006.11.006 PMID: 17412567

Lanius, R. A., Williamson, P. C., Densmore, M., Boksman, K., Gupta, M. A., Neufeld, R. W., Gati, J. S., & Menon, R. S. (2001). Neural correlates of traumatic memories in posttraumatic stress disorder: A functional MRI investigation.*The American Journal of Psychiatry*, 158(11), 1920–1922. DOI: 10.1176/appi.ajp.158.11.1920 PMID: 11691703

Laplaud, N., Perrochon, A., Gallou-Guyot, M., Moens, M., Goudman, L., David, R., Rigoard, P., & Billot, M. (2023). Management of post-traumatic stress disorder symptoms by yoga: An overview.*BMC Complementary Medicine and Therapies*, 23(1), 258. DOI: 10.1186/s12906-023-04074-w PMID: 37480017

Laws, B. (2019). The return of the suppressed: Exploring how emotional suppression reappears as violence and pain among male and female prisoners.*Punishment & Society*, 21(5), 560–577. DOI: 10.1177/1462474518805071

Le Doux, J. E. (1996). *The emotional brain*. Simon and Schuster.

Lee, D. H., Lee, J., Hong, D. Y., Lee, E. C., Park, S. W., Lee, M. R., & Oh, J. S. (2022, April20). Neuroinflammation in Post-Traumatic Stress Disorder.*Biomedicines*. Advance online publication. DOI: 10.3390/biomedicines10102518 PMID: 35625690

Lee, E. E., Torous, J., De Choudhury, M., Depp, C. A., Graham, S. A., Kim, H. C., Paulus, M. P., Krystal, J. H., & Jeste, D. V. (2021). Artificial Intelligence for Mental Health Care: Clinical Applications, Barriers, Facilitators, and Artificial Wisdom. *Biological Psychiatry: Cognitive Neuroscience and Neuroimaging*, 6(9), 856–864. DOI: 10.1016/j.bpsc.2021.02.001 PMID: 33571718

Lely, J. C. G., Smid, G. E., Jongedijk, R. A., Knipscheer, J. W., & Kleber, R. J. (2019). The effectiveness of narrative exposure therapy: A review, meta-analysis and meta-regression analysis.*European Journal of Psychotraumatology*, 10(1), 1550344. DOI: 10.1080/20008198.2018.1550344 PMID: 31007868

Lerer, B., Bleich, A., Bennett, E. R., Ebstein, R. P., & Balkin, J. (1990). Platelet adenylate cyclase and phospholipase C activity in posttraumatic stress disorder. *Biological Psychiatry*, 27(7), 735–740. DOI: 10.1016/0006-3223(90)90588-S PMID: 2328269

Leuba, J. H. (1912). *A psychological study of religion*. Macmillan.

Levesque, P., Desmeules, C., Béchard, L., Huot-Lavoie, M., Demers, M.-F., Roy, M.-A., & Deslauriers, J. (2023). Sex-specific immune mechanisms in PTSD symptomatology and risk: A translational overview and perspectives.*Brain Research Bulletin*, 195, 120–129. DOI: 10.1016/j.brainresbull.2023.02.013 PMID: 36822271

Lewis, C., Roberts, N. P., Andrew, M., Starling, E., & Bisson, J. I. (2020). Psychological therapies for post-traumatic stress disorder in adults: Systematic review and meta-analysis.*European Journal of Psychotraumatology*, 11(1), 1729633. DOI: 10.1080/20008198.2020.1729633 PMID: 32284821

Lewis, H. B. (1971). *Shame and guilt in neurosis*. International Universities.

Liberzon, I., & Abelson, J. L. (2016). Context Processing and the Neurobiology of Post-Traumatic Stress Disorder.*Neuron*, 92(1), 14–30. DOI: 10.1016/j.neuron.2016.09.039 PMID: 27710783

Li, J., & Sanchez-Garcia, R. (2023). Equine-assisted interventions for veterans with posttraumatic stress disorder: A systematic review.*Frontiers in Psychiatry*, 14, 1277338. DOI: 10.3389/fpsyt.2023.1277338 PMID: 38025432

Li, J., Wang, Q., Liang, H., Dong, H., Li, Y., Ng, E. H., & Wu, X. (2012). Biophysical characteristics of meridians and acupoints: A systematic review.*Evidence-Based Complementary and Alternative Medicine*, 793841, 1–6. Advance online publication. DOI: 10.1155/2012/793841 PMID: 23346214

Li, N.-X., Hu, Y.-R., Chen, W.-N., & Zhang, B. (2022). Dose effect of psilocybin on primary and secondary depression: A preliminary systematic review and meta-analysis.*Journal of Affective Disorders*, 296, 26–34. DOI: 10.1016/j.jad.2021.09.041 PMID: 34587546

Lindauer, R. J. L., Booij, J., Habraken, J. B. A., van Meijel, E. P. M., Uylings, H. B. M., Olff, M., Carlier, I. V. E., den Heeten, G. J., van Eck-Smit, B. L. F., & Gersons, B. P. R. (2008). Effects of psychotherapy on regional cerebral blood flow during trauma imagery in patients with post-traumatic stress disorder: A randomized clinical trial.*Psychological Medicine*, 38(4), 543–554. DOI: 10.1017/S0033291707001432 PMID: 17803835

Lindauer, R. J. L., Olff, M., Van Meijel, E. L. S. P. M., Carlier, I. V. E., & Gersons, B. P. R. (2006). Cortisol, learning, memory, and attention in relation to smaller hippocampal volume in police officers with posttraumatic stress disorder.*Biological Psychiatry*, 59(2), 171–177. DOI: 10.1016/j.biopsych.2005.06.033 PMID: 16154543

Linehan, M. M. (1993). *Cognitive-behavioral treatment of borderline personality disorder*. Guilford Press.

Linehan, M. M. (2020). *Building a life worth living: a memoire*. Random House.

Linley, P. A., & Joseph, S. (2004). Positive change following trauma and adversity: A review.*Journal of Traumatic Stress*, 17(1), 11–21. DOI: 10.1023/B:JOTS.0000014671.27856.7e PMID: 15027788

Lissek, S., Powers, A. S., McClure, E. B., Phelps, E. A., Woldehawariat, G., Grillon, C., & Pine, D. S. (2005). Classical fear conditioning in the anxiety disorders: A meta-analysis.*Behaviour Research and Therapy*, 43(11), 1391–1424. DOI: 10.1016/j.brat.2004.10.007 PMID: 15885654

Li, T.-T., Wan, Q., Zhang, X., Xiao, Y., Sun, L.-Y., Zhang, Y.-R., Liu, X.-N., & Yang, W.-C. (2022). Stellate ganglion block reduces inflammation and improves neurological function in diabetic rats during ischemic stroke.*Neural Regeneration Research*, 17(9), 1991. DOI: 10.4103/1673-5374.335162 PMID: 35142688

Litvin, S., Saunders, R., Maier, M. A., & Luttke, S. (2020). Gamification as an approach to improve resilience and reduce attrition in mobile mental health interventions: A randomized controlled trial.*PLoS One*, 15(9), e0237220. DOI: 10.1371/journal.pone.0237220 PMID: 32877425

Liu, Z., Ren, L., Xiao, C., Zhang, K., & Demian, P. (2022). Virtual Reality Aided Therapy towards Health 4.0: A Two-Decade Bibliometric Analysis.*International Journal of Environmental Research and Public Health*, 19(3), 1525. DOI: 10.3390/ijerph19031525 PMID: 35162546

Li, X. M., Han, F., Liu, D. J., & Shi, Y. X. (2010). Single-prolonged stress induced mitochondrial-dependent apoptosis in hippocampus in the rat model of post-traumatic stress disorder.*Journal of Chemical Neuroanatomy*, 40(3), 248–255. DOI: 10.1016/j.jchemneu.2010.07.001 PMID: 20624456

Li, X., Han, F., Liu, D., & Shi, Y. (2010). Changes of Bax, Bcl-2 and apoptosis in hippocampus in the rat model of post-traumatic stress disorder.*Neurological Research*, 32(6), 579–586. DOI: 10.1179/016164110X12556180206194 PMID: 20092675

Li, Y., Zhou, Y., Chen, X., Fan, F., Musa, G., & Hoven, C. (2020). Post-Traumatic Stress Disorder in Children and Adolescents: Some Recent Research Findings. In Lobera, I. J. (Ed.), *Pyschosomatic Medicine*. IntechOpen Limited. DOI: 10.5772/intechopen.92284

Logue, M. W., van Rooij, S. J. H., Dennis, E. L., Davis, S. L., Hayes, J. P., Stevens, J. S., Densmore, M., Haswell, C. C., Ipser, J., Koch, S. B. J., Korgaonkar, M., Lebois, L. A. M., Peverill, M., Baker, J. T., Boedhoe, P. S. W., Frijling, J. L., Gruber, S. A., Harpaz-Rotem, I., Jahanshad, N., & Morey, R. A. (2018). Smaller hippocampal volume in posttraumatic stress disorder: a multisite ENIGMA-PGC study: subcortical volumetry results from posttraumatic stress disorder consortia.*Biological Psychiatry*, 83(3), 244–253. DOI: 10.1016/j.biopsych.2017.09.006 PMID: 29217296

Lohr, J. B., Palmer, B. W., Eidt, C. A., Aailaboyina, S., Mausbach, B. T., Wolkowitz, O. M., Thorp, S. R., & Jeste, D. V. (2015). Is post-traumatic stress disorder associated with premature senescence? A review of the literature.*The American Journal of Geriatric Psychiatry*, 23(7), 709–725. DOI: 10.1016/j.jagp.2015.04.001 PMID: 25959921

López-Castro, T., Saraiya, T., Zumberg-Smith, K., & Dambreville, N. (2019). Association between shame and posttraumatic stress disorder: A meta-analysis.*Journal of Traumatic Stress*, 32(4), 484–495. DOI: 10.1002/jts.22411 PMID: 31291483

Lopez, S. J., Pedrotti, J. T., & Snyder, C. R. (2018). *Positive psychology: the scientific practical explorations of human strengths* (4th ed.). Sage Publications.

Lord, S. A. (2008). Therapeutic Work with Trauma, Revictimization, and Perpetration: Bearing Witness, Offering Hope, Embracing Despair.*Psychoanalytic Social Work*, 15(2), 110–131. DOI: 10.1080/15228870802103671

Lowe, H., Toyang, N., Steele, B., Grant, J., Ali, A., Gordon, L., & Ngwa, W. (2022). Psychedelics: Alternative and potential therapeutic options for treating mood and anxiety disorders.*Molecules (Basel, Switzerland)*, 27(8), 2520. DOI: 10.3390/molecules27082520 PMID: 35458717

MacLeish, K. (2018). On 'moral injury': Psychic fringes and war violence.*History of the Human Sciences*, 31(2), 128–146. DOI: 10.1177/0952695117750342

Maeng, L. Y., & Shors, T. J. (2013). The stressed female brain: Neuronal activity in the prelimbic but not infralimbic region of the medial prefrontal cortex suppresses learning after acute stress.*Frontiers in Neural Circuits*, 7, 198. DOI: 10.3389/fncir.2013.00198 PMID: 24391548

Maercker, A., & Horn, A. B. (2013). A socio-interpersonal perspective on PTSD: The case for environments and interpersonal processes.*Clinical Psychology & Psychotherapy*, 20(6), 465–481. DOI: 10.1002/cpp.1805 PMID: 22730216

Maercker, A., & Zoellner, T. (2004). The Janus face of self-perceived growth: Toward a two-component model of posttraumatic growth. *Psychological Inquiry*, 15(1), 41–48.

Magill, M., Kiluk, B. D., & Ray, L. A. (2023). Efficacy of Cognitive Behavioral Therapy for Alcohol and Other Drug Use Disorders: Is a One-Size-Fits-All Approach Appropriate?*Substance Abuse and Rehabilitation*, 14, 1–11. DOI: 10.2147/SAR.S362864 PMID: 36844999

Maharaj, M. (2016). Differential gene expression after Emotional Freedom Techniques (EFT) treatment: A novel pilot protocol for salivary mRNA assessment. *Energy Psychology*, 8(1), 17–32. DOI: 10.9769/EPJ.2016.8.1.MM

Maihofer, A. X., Choi, K. W., Coleman, J. R. I., Daskalakis, N. P., Denckla, C. A., Ketema, E., Morey, R. A., Polimanti, R., Ratanatharathorn, A., Torres, K., Wingo, A. P., Zai, C. C., Aiello, A. E., Almli, L. M., Amstadter, A. B., Andersen, S. B., Andreassen, O. A., Arbisi, P. A., Ashley-Koch, A. E., & Nievergelt, C. M. (2022). Enhancing Discovery of Genetic Variants for Posttraumatic Stress Disorder Through Integration of Quantitative Phenotypes and Trauma Exposure Information.*Biological Psychiatry*, 91(7), 626–636. DOI: 10.1016/j.biopsych.2021.09.020 PMID: 34865855

Mak, T. (2019, October 8). Senate Report: Russians Used Social Media Mostly To Target Race In 2016. NPR. https://www.npr.org/2019/10/08/768319934/senate-report-russians-used-used-social-media-mostly-to-target-race-in-2016

Makhdoomi, S. M., Rakhra, M., Singh, D., & Singh, A. (2022). Artificial-Intelligence based Prediction of Post-Traumatic Stress Disorder (PTSD) using EEG reports. 2022 5th International Conference on Contemporary Computing and Informatics (IC3I)

Malaktaris, A. L., & Lynn, S. J. (2019). The Phenomenology and Correlates of Flashbacks in Individuals With Posttraumatic Stress Symptoms.*Clinical Psychological Science*, 7(2), 249–264. DOI: 10.1177/2167702618805081

Malberg, J. E. (2004). Implications of adult hippocampal neurogenesis in antidepressant action.*Journal of Psychiatry & Neuroscience*, 29(3), 196–205. PMID: 15173896

Malgaroli, M., & Schultebraucks, K. (2021). Artificial intelligence and posttraumatic stress disorder.*European Psychologist*, 25(4), 272–282. DOI: 10.1027/1016-9040/a000423

Manger, T. A., & Motta, R. W. (2005). The impact of an exercise program on posttraumatic stress disorder, anxiety, and depression.*International Journal of Emergency Mental Health*, 7, 49–57. PMID: 15869081

Mann, J. J., Stanley, M., McBride, P. A., & McEwen, B. S. (1986). Increased serotonin2 and β-adrenergic receptor binding in the frontal cortices of suicide victims.*Archives of General Psychiatry*, 43(10), 954–959. DOI: 10.1001/archpsyc.1986.01800100048007 PMID: 3019268

Mann, S. K., & Marwaha, R. (2023). Posttraumatic Stress Disorder. [Updated 2023 Jan 30] In *StatPearls* [Internet]. StatPearls Publishing., Available from https://www.ncbi.nlm.nih.gov/books/NBK559129/

Mansbart, F., Kienberger, G., Sönnichsen, A., & Mann, E. (2022). Efficacy and safety of adrenergic alpha-1 receptor antagonists in older adults: A systematic review and meta-analysis supporting the development of recommendations to reduce potentially inappropriate prescribing.*BMC Geriatrics*, 22(1), 771. DOI: 10.1186/s12877-022-03415-7 PMID: 36171560

Marchand, W. R., Sandoval, K., Lackner, R., Parker, S. C., Herrmann, T., Yabko, B., Velasquez, T., Lewis, L., & Butler, J. (2021). Mindfulness-based interventions for military veterans: A systematic review and analysis of the literature.*Complementary Therapies in Clinical Practice*, 42, 101274. DOI: 10.1016/j.ctcp.2020.101274 PMID: 33276226

Martínez, V., Iriondo De-Hond, A., Borrelli, F., Capasso, R., Del Castillo, M. D., & Abalo, R. (2020). Cannabidiol and other non-psychoactive cannabinoids for prevention and treatment of gastrointestinal disorders: Useful nutraceuticals?*International Journal of Molecular Sciences*, 21(9), 3067.

Marwit, S. J. (2003). Post-Traumatic Stress Disorder. *Encyclopedia of Death and Dying, Table 1*, 364–366. DOI: 10.1056/NEJMra1612499

Maslow, A. H. (1943). A theory of human motivation.*Psychological Review*, 50(4), 370–396. DOI: 10.1037/h0054346

Masoumian Hosseini, M., Masoumian Hosseini, S. T., Qayumi, K., Ahmady, S., & Koohestani, H. R. (2023). The Aspects of Running Artificial Intelligence in Emergency Care; a Scoping Review.*Archives of Academic Emergency Medicine*, 11(1), e38. DOI: 10.22037/aaem.v11i1.1974 PMID: 37215232

Mate, G., & Hollington-Sawyer, S. (2014, July 28). Israel: The Beautiful Dream has become a Nightmare. https://drgabormate.com/beautiful-dream-israel-become-nightmare/

Matheson, K., Asokumar, A., & Anisman, H. (2020). Resilience: Safety in the aftermath of traumatic stressor experiences.*Frontiers in Behavioral Neuroscience*, 14, 596919. DOI: 10.3389/fnbeh.2020.596919 PMID: 33408619

Matsuoka, Y. (2011). Clearance of fear memory from the hippocampus through neurogenesis by omega-3 fatty acids: A novel preventive strategy for posttraumatic stress disorder?*BioPsychoSocial Medicine*, 5(February), 3. Advance online publication. DOI: 10.1186/1751-0759-5-3 PMID: 21303552

Mattson, E., James, L., & Engdahl, B. (2018). Personality factors and their impact on PTSD and post-traumatic growth is mediated by coping style among OIF/OEF veterans.*Military Medicine*, 183(9-10), e475–e480. DOI: 10.1093/milmed/usx201 PMID: 29590428

Mausbach, B. T., Moore, R., Roesch, S., Cardenas, V., & Patterson, T. L. (2010). The relationship between homework compliance and therapy outcomes: An updated meta-analysis.*Cognitive Therapy and Research*, 34(5), 429–438. DOI: 10.1007/s10608-010-9297-z PMID: 20930925

Mavranezouli, I., Megnin-Viggars, O., Daly, C., Dias, S., Stockton, S., Meiser-Stedman, R., Trickey, D., & Pilling, S. (2019). Psychological and psychosocial treatments for children and young people with post-traumatic stress disorder: A network meta-analysis.*Journal of Child Psychology and Psychiatry, and Allied Disciplines*, 61(1), 18–29. DOI: 10.1111/jcpp.13094 PMID: 31313834

Mavranezouli, I., Megnin-Viggars, O., Daly, C., Dias, S., Welton, N. J., Stockton, S., Bhutani, G., Grey, N., Leach, J., Greenberg, N., Katona, C., El Leithy, S., & Pilling, S. (2020). Psychological treatments for post-traumatic stress disorder in adults: A network meta-analysis.*Psychological Medicine*, 50(4), 542–555. DOI: 10.1017/S0033291720000070 PMID: 32063234

Mavranezouli, I., Megnin-Viggars, O., Grey, N., Bhutani, G., Leach, J., Daly, C., Dias, S., Welton, N. J., Katona, C., El-Leithy, S., Greenberg, N., Stockton, S., & Pilling, S. (2020). Cost-effectiveness of psychological treatments for post-traumatic stress disorder in adults.*PLoS One*, 15(4), e0232245. DOI: 10.1371/journal.pone.0232245 PMID: 32353011

McCann, I. L., & Pearlman, L. A. (1990). Vicarious traumatization: A framework for understanding the psychological effects of working with victims.*Journal of Traumatic Stress*, 3(1), 131–149. DOI: 10.1007/BF00975140

McCurry, K. L., Frueh, B. C., Chiu, P. H., & King-Casas, B. (2020). Opponent Effects of Hyperarousal and Re-experiencing on Affective Habituation in Posttraumatic Stress Disorder.*Biological Psychiatry: Cognitive Neuroscience and Neuroimaging*, 5(2), 203–212. DOI: 10.1016/j.bpsc.2019.09.006 PMID: 31759868

McEwen, B. S. (2000). Allostasis and allostatic load: Implications for neuropsychopharmacology.*Neuropsychopharmacology*, 22(2), 108–124. DOI: 10.1016/S0893-133X(99)00129-3 PMID: 10649824

McFall, M. E., Murburg, M. M., Ko, G. N., & Veith, R. C. (1990). Autonomic responses to stress in Vietnam combat veterans with posttraumatic stress disorder. *Biological Psychiatry*, 27(10), 1165–1175. DOI: 10.1016/0006-3223(90)90053-5 PMID: 2340325

McFarland, C., & Alvaro, C. (2000). The impact of motivation of temporal comparisons: Coping with traumatic events by perceiving personal growth.*Journal of Personality and Social Psychology*, 79(3), 327–343. DOI: 10.1037/0022-3514.79.3.327 PMID: 10981837

McGeary, D. D., Resick, P. A., Penzien, D. B., McGeary, C. A., Houle, T. T., Eapen, B. C., Jaramillo, C. A., Nabity, P. S., Reed, D. E.II, Moring, J. C., Bira, L. M., Hansen, H. R., Young-McCaughan, S., Cobos, B. A., Mintz, J., Keane, T. M., & Peterson, A. L. (2022). Cognitive Behavioral Therapy for Veterans With Comorbid Posttraumatic Headache and Posttraumatic Stress Disorder Symptoms: A Randomized Clinical Trial.*JAMA Neurology*, 79(8), 746–757. DOI: 10.1001/jamaneurol.2022.1567 PMID: 35759281

McGorrill, S. (2023). The Benefits of Sensory Exploration in Art Therapy with Children with Social, Emotional and Behavioral Difficulties Through a Trauma Informed Lens.

McHugh, B. C., Wisniewski, P., Rosson, M. B., & Carroll, J. M. (2018). When social media traumatizes teens: The roles of online risk exposure, coping, and post-traumatic stress. *Internet Research*, 28(5), 1169–1188. DOI: 10.1108/IntR-02-2017-0077

McLean, C. P., Levy, H. C., Miller, M. L., & Tolin, D. F. (2022). Exposure therapy for PTSD in military populations: A systematic review and meta-analysis of randomized clinical trials.*Journal of Anxiety Disorders*, 90, 102607. DOI: 10.1016/j.janxdis.2022.102607 PMID: 35926254

McLean, C. P., Levy, H. C., Miller, M. L., & Tolin, D. F. (2022). Exposure therapy for PTSD: A meta-analysis.*Clinical Psychology Review*, 91, 102115. DOI: 10.1016/j.cpr.2021.102115 PMID: 34954460

McMillen, J. C., Smith, E. M., & Fisher, R. H. (1997). Perceived benefit and mental health after three types of disaster.*Journal of Consulting and Clinical Psychology*, 65(5), 733–739. DOI: 10.1037/0022-006X.65.5.733 PMID: 9337492

McRae, E. M., Stoppelbein, L., O'Kelley, S. E., Fite, P., & Smith, S. B. (2021). An Examination of Post-Traumatic Stress Symptoms and Aggression among Children with a History of Adverse Childhood Experiences.*Journal of Psychopathology and Behavioral Assessment*, 43(3), 657–670. DOI: 10.1007/s10862-021-09884-1

Meewisse, M.-L., Reitsma, J. B., De Vries, G.-J., Gersons, B. P. R., & Olff, M. (2007). Cortisol and post-traumatic stress disorder in adults: Systematic review and meta-analysis.*The British Journal of Psychiatry*, 191(5), 387–392. DOI: 10.1192/bjp.bp.106.024877 PMID: 17978317

Mellon, S. H., Gautam, A., Hammamieh, R., Jett, M., & Wolkowitz, O. M. (2018). Metabolism, metabolomics, and inflammation in posttraumatic stress disorder. *Biological Psychiatry*, 83(10), 866–875. DOI: 10.1016/j.biopsych.2018.02.007 PMID: 29628193

Menninger, K. (1963). *The vital balance: The life process in mental health and illness*. Viking.

Mentis, A. F. A., Lee, D., & Roussos, P. (2023). Applications of artificial intelligence-machine learning for detection of stress: A critical overview.*Molecular Psychiatry*. Advance online publication. DOI: 10.1038/s41380-023-02047-6 PMID: 37020048

Merkley, T. L., Esopenko, C., Zizak, V. S., Bilder, R. M., Strutt, A. M., Tate, D. F., & Irimia, A. (2023). Challenges and opportunities for harmonization of cross-cultural neuropsychological data.*Neuropsychology*, 37(3), 237–246. DOI: 10.1037/neu0000818 PMID: 35549387

Mestrovic, A. H., Tudor, L., Perkovic, M. N., Erjavec, G. N., Petrovic, Z. K., Strac, D. S., Konjevod, M., & Pivac, N. (2018). Significant association between catechol-O-methyltransferase (COMT) Val158/108Met polymorphism and cognitive function in veterans with PTSD.*Neuroscience Letters*, 666, 38–43. DOI: 10.1016/j.neulet.2017.12.033 PMID: 29248614

Metcalf, O., Finlayson-Short, L., Forbes, D., O'Donnell, M., & Varker, T. (2023). A systematic review of treatments for problem anger in veteran and military populations with PTSD.*Aggression and Violent Behavior*, 70, 101837. DOI: 10.1016/j.avb.2023.101837

Michopoulos, V., Rothbaum, A. O., Jovanovic, T., Almli, L. M., Bradley, B., Rothbaum, B. O., Gillespie, C. F., & Ressler, K. J. (2015). Association of CRP genetic variation and CRP level with elevated PTSD symptoms and physiological responses in a civilian population with high levels of trauma.*The American Journal of Psychiatry*, 172(4), 353–362. DOI: 10.1176/appi.ajp.2014.14020263 PMID: 25827033

Midgley, N. (2007). Anna Freud: The Hampstead War Nurseries and the role of the direct observation of children for psychoanalysis.*The International Journal of Psycho-Analysis*, 88(4), 939–959. DOI: 10.1516/V28R-J334-6182-524H PMID: 17681901

Midyett, L. K. (2023). One Size Fits All Versus Individualized Medicine in Type 1 Diabetes Management.*Diabetes Technology & Therapeutics*, 25(S3), S-42–S-47. DOI: 10.1089/dia.2023.0109 PMID: 37306440

Milad, M. R., Pitman, R. K., Ellis, C. B., Gold, A. L., Shin, L. M., Lasko, N. B., Zeidan, M. A., Handwerger, K., Orr, S. P., & Rauch, S. L. (2009). Neurobiological basis of failure to recall extinction memory in posttraumatic stress disorder. *Biological Psychiatry*, 66(12), 1075–1082. DOI: 10.1016/j.biopsych.2009.06.026 PMID: 19748076

Miles, S. R., Hale, W. J., Mintz, J., Wachen, J. S., Litz, B. T., Dondanville, K. A., Yarvis, J. S., Hembree, E. A., Young-McCaughan, S., Peterson, A. L., & Resick, P. A. (2023). Hyperarousal symptoms linger after successful PTSD treatment in active duty military.*Psychological Trauma: Theory, Research, Practice, and Policy*, 15(8), 1398–1405. DOI: 10.1037/tra0001292 PMID: 35901423

Ming, G., & Song, H. (2011). Adult neurogenesis in the mammalian brain: Significant answers and significant questions.*Neuron*, 70(4), 687–702. DOI: 10.1016/j.neuron.2011.05.001 PMID: 21609825

Mitrovica, A. (2023, December 7). Volodymyr Zelenskyy: The forgotten man. Al Jazeera. https://www.aljazeera.com/opinions/2023/12/7/volodymyr-zelenskyy-the-forgotten-man

Mohamed, A., Touheed, S., Ahmed, M., Hor, M., & Fatima, S. (2022). The efficacy of psychedelic-assisted therapy in managing post-traumatic stress disorder (PTSD): A new frontier? *Cureus*, 14(10), e30919. DOI: 10.7759/cureus.30919 PMID: 36465766

Mohammed, A. A. (2022). Trauma and Recovery: A Psychoanalytic Study of Gharbi Mustafa's When Mountains Weep. *Journal of University of Human Development*, 8(2), 2. Advance online publication. DOI: 10.21928/juhd.v8n2y2022.pp28-36

Monane, R., Sanchez, G. J., Kronish, I. M., Edmondson, D., & Diaz, K. M. (2018). Post-traumatic stress disorder symptoms and aversive cognitions regarding physical activity in patients evaluated for acute coronary syndrome. *European Journal of Preventive Cardiology*, 25(4), 402–403. DOI: 10.1177/2047487317746255 PMID: 29198138

Monson, C. M., Schnurr, P. P., Resick, P. A., Friedman, M. J., Young-Xu, Y., & Stevens, S. P. (2006). Cognitive processing therapy for veterans with military-related posttraumatic stress disorder. *Journal of Consulting and Clinical Psychology*, 74(5), 898–907. DOI: 10.1037/0022-006X.74.5.898 PMID: 17032094

Moreira, A., Moreira, A. C., & Rocha, J. C. (2022). Randomized Controlled Trial: Cognitive-Narrative Therapy for IPV Victims. *Journal of Interpersonal Violence*, 37(5–6), NP2998–NP3014. DOI: 10.1177/0886260520943719 PMID: 32755265

Morey, R. A., Dolcos, F., Petty, C. M., Cooper, D. A., Hayes, J. P., LaBar, K. S., & McCarthy, G. (2009). The role of trauma-related distractors on neural systems for working memory and emotion processing in posttraumatic stress disorder. *Journal of Psychiatric Research*, 43(8), 809–817. DOI: 10.1016/j.jpsychires.2008.10.014 PMID: 19091328

Morina, N., Kampmann, I., Emmelkamp, P., Barbui, C., & Hoppen, T. H. (2023). Meta-analysis of virtual reality exposure therapy for social anxiety disorder. *Psychological Medicine*, 53(5), 2176–2178. DOI: 10.1017/S0033291721001690 PMID: 34001293

Morina, N., Schnyder, U., Klaghofer, R., Müller, J., & Martin-Soelch, C. (2018). Trauma exposure and the mediating role of posttraumatic stress on somatic symptoms in civilian war victims. *BMC Psychiatry*, 18(1), 92. DOI: 10.1186/s12888-018-1680-4 PMID: 29631551

Morland, L. A., Butler, L. D., & Leskin, G. A. (2008). Resilience and thriving in a time of terrorism. In Joseph, S., & Linley, P. A. (Eds.), *Trauma, Recovery, and Growth: Positive Psychological Perspectives on Posttraumatic Stress* (pp. 39–61). John Wiley & Sons, Inc.DOI: 10.1002/9781118269718.ch3

Morland, L. A., Greene, C. J., Rosen, C. S., Kuhn, E., Hoffman, J., & Sloan, D. M. (2017). Telehealth and eHealth interventions for posttraumatic stress disorder. *Current Opinion in Psychology*, 14, 102–108. DOI: 10.1016/j.copsyc.2016.12.003 PMID: 28813306

Moser, D. A., Graf, S., Glaus, J., Urben, S., Jouabli, S., Perrizolo, V. P., Suardi, F., Robinson, J., Serpa, S. R., & Plessen, K. J. (2023). On the complex and dimensional relationship of maternal posttraumatic stress disorder during early childhood and child outcomes at school-age.*European Psychiatry*, 66(1), e20. DOI: 10.1192/j.eurpsy.2023.8 PMID: 36734250

Motlagh, H. (2010). Impact of event scale revised.*Journal of Physiotherapy*, 56(3), 203. DOI: 10.1016/S1836-9553(10)70029-1 PMID: 20795930

Motta, R.W. (2013, Winter). PTSD and secondary traumatization: A comprehensive review. *Mental Health News,* pp. 1, 6, 14, 16, 22, 26, 27, 30.

Motta, R. W. (2018). The role of exercise in reducing PTSD and negative emotional states. In Taukeni, S. G. (Ed.), *Psychology of health-Biopsychosocial approach.* InTech Open.

Motta, R. W. (2020). *Alternative therapies for PTSD: The science of mind-body treatments.* American Psychological Association. DOI: 10.1037/0000186-000

Motta, R. W. (2023). *Secondary trauma: Silent suffering and its treatment.* Springer. DOI: 10.1007/978-3-031-44308-4

Motta, R. W., Kefer, J. M., Hertz, M. D., & Hafeez, S. (1999). Initial evaluation of the Secondary Trauma Questionnaire.*Psychological Reports*, 85(3 Pt 1), 997–1002. DOI: 10.2466/pr0.1999.85.3.997 PMID: 10672764

Motta, R., Hafeez, S., Sciancalepore, R., & Diaz, A. (2001). Discriminant Validation of the Modified Secondary Trauma Questionnaire.*Journal of Psychotherapy in Independent Practice*, 24(4), 17–25. DOI: 10.1300/J288v02n04_02

Muehlhausen, B. L. (2020). Spirituality and vicarious trauma among trauma clinicians: A qualitative study.[Published online.]. *International Journal of Environmental Research and Public Health*, 17(4), 1268. PMID: 32079153

Mueller, J., Orth, U., Wang, J., & Maercker, A. (2009). Disclosure attitudes and social acknowledgement as predictors of posttraumatic stress disorder symptom severity in Chinese and German crime victims.*Canadian Journal of Psychiatry*, 54(8), 547–556. DOI: 10.1177/070674370905400807 PMID: 19726007

Mulholland, J. M. Tara. (2019, March 15). How the Christchurch terrorist attack was made for social media | CNN Business. CNN. https://www.cnn.com/2019/03/15/tech/christchurch-internet-radicalization-intl/index.html

Muzaale, A. D., Daubresse, M., Bae, S., Chu, N. M., Lentine, K. L., Segev, D. L., & McAdams-DeMarco, M. (2020). Benzodiazepines, Codispensed Opioids, and Mortality among Patients Initiating Long-Term In-Center Hemodialysis.*Clinical Journal of the American Society of Nephrology; CJASN*, 15(6), 794–804. DOI: 10.2215/CJN.13341019 PMID: 32457228

Nacasch, N., Avni, C., & Toren, P. (2023). Medical cannabis for treatment-resistant combat PTSD.*Frontiers in Psychiatry*, 13, 1014630. DOI: 10.3389/fpsyt.2022.1014630 PMID: 36741572

Namisango, E., Matovu, L., Harding, R., & Berger, A. (2022). Existentialism and spirituality in the healing processes of cancer patients. In (Ed.). in *Global Perspectives in Cancer Care: Religion, Spirituality, and Cultural Diversity in Health and Healing*. Oxford University Press.

Nandi, C., Crombach, A., Elbert, T., Bambonye, M., Pryss, R., Schobel, J., & Weierstall-Pust, R. (2020). The cycle of violence as a function of PTSD and appetitive aggression: A longitudinal study with Burundian soldiers.*Aggressive Behavior*, 46(5), 391–399. DOI: 10.1002/ab.21895 PMID: 32363661

National Institute for Clinical Excellence. (2005). *The management of post traumatic stress disorder in primary and secondary care*. NICE.

National Institute for Health and Care Excellence. (2018). Post-traumatic stress disorder (NICE Quality Standard NG116) [Internet]. Available from: https://www.nice.org.uk.guidance/ng116/evidenc.

National Institutes of Health. (2021). *Post-traumatic stress disorder (PTSD) 2023*. Retrieved 23rd December 2023, https://hr.nih.gov/working-nih/civil/post-traumatic-stress-disorder-ptsd-2023

Nelms, J. A., & Castel, L. (2016). A systematic review and meta-analysis of randomized and nonrandomized trials of clinical emotional freedom techniques (EFT) for the treatment of depression.*Explore (New York, N.Y.)*, 12(6), 416–426. DOI: 10.1016/j.explore.2016.08.001 PMID: 27843054

Nelson, C., Dossett, K., & Walker, D. L. (2022). Equine-assisted therapy for post-traumatic stress disorder among first responders.*Psychological Reports*. Advance online publication. DOI: 10.1177/00332941221146707 PMID: 36542680

Neuner, F. (2023). Physical and social trauma: Towards an integrative transdiagnostic perspective on psychological trauma that involves threats to status and belonging. *Clinical Psychology Review*, 99, 102219. DOI: 10.1016/j.cpr.2022.102219 PMID: 36395560

Newport, D. J., & Nemeroff, C. B. (2000). Neurobiology of posttraumatic stress disorder.*Current Opinion in Neurobiology*, 10(2), 211–218. DOI: 10.1016/S0959-4388(00)00080-5 PMID: 10753802

Ney, L. J., Akhurst, J., Bruno, R., Laing, P. A. F., Matthews, A., & Felmingham, K. L. (2021). Dopamine, endocannabinoids and their interaction in fear extinction and negative affect in PTSD.*Progress in Neuro-Psychopharmacology & Biological Psychiatry*, 105, 110118. DOI: 10.1016/j.pnpbp.2020.110118 PMID: 32991952

Nickerson, A., Cloitre, M., Bryant, R. A., Schnyder, U., Morina, N., & Schick, M. (2016). The factor structure of complex posttraumatic stress disorder in traumatized refugees.*European Journal ofPsychotraumatology*, 7(1), 33253. DOI: 10.3402/ejpt.v7.33253 PMID: 27989268

Nietzsche, F. (1889). *Twilight of the idols*. Penguin Classics.

Nievergelt, C. M., Maihofer, A. X., Klengel, T., Atkinson, E. G., Chen, C. Y., Choi, K. W., Coleman, J. R. I., Dalvie, S., Duncan, L. E., Gelernter, J., Levey, D. F., Logue, M. W., Polimanti, R., Provost, A. C., Ratanatharathorn, A., Stein, M. B., Torres, K., Aiello, A. E., Almli, L. M., & Koenen, K. C. (2019). International meta-analysis of PTSD genome-wide association studies identifies sex- and ancestry-specific genetic risk loci.*Nature Communications*, 10(1), 4558. DOI: 10.1038/s41467-019-12576-w PMID: 31594949

Nie, Y., Wen, L., Song, J., Wang, N., Huang, L., Gao, L., & Qu, M. (2022). Emerging trends in epigenetic and childhood trauma: Bibliometrics and visual analysis.*Frontiers in Psychiatry*, 13, 925273. DOI: 10.3389/fpsyt.2022.925273 PMID: 36458128

Nie, Y., Zhang, Y., Ren, R., Sanford, L. D., Vitiello, M. V., & Tang, X. (2023). Interventions for Trauma-Related Nightmare: Where Are We Now?*The International Journal of Neuropsychopharmacology*, 26(6), 412–414. DOI: 10.1093/ijnp/pyad022 PMID: 37226283

Niles, B. L., Mori, D. L., Polizzi, C., Pless Kaiser, A., Weinstein, E. S., Gershkovich, M., & Wang, C. (2018). A systematic review of randomized trials of mind-body interventions for PTSD.*Journal of Clinical Psychology*, 74(9), 1485–1508. DOI: 10.1002/jclp.22634 PMID: 29745422

Niles, B., Lang, A., & Olff, M. (2023). *Complementary and integrative interventions for PTSD* (Vol. 14). Taylor & Francis.

Nisar, S., Bhat, A. A., Hashem, S., Syed, N., Yadav, S. K., Uddin, S., Fakhro, K., Bagga, P., Thompson, P. M., Reddy, R., Frenneaux, M., & Haris, M. (2020, June24). Genetic and Neuroimaging Approaches to Understanding Post-Traumatic Stress Disorder.*International Journal of Molecular Sciences*, 21(12), 4503. Advance online publication. DOI: 10.3390/ijms21124503 PMID: 32599917

Nixon, R. D., Meiser-Stedman, R., Dalgleish, T., Yule, W., Clark, D. M., Perrin, S., & Smith, P. (2013). The Child PTSD Symptom Scale: An update and replication of its psychometric properties.*Psychological Assessment*, 25(3), 1025–1031. DOI: 10.1037/a0033324 PMID: 23815109

Norwitz, N. G., & Naidoo, U. (2021). Nutrition as metabolic treatment of anxiety. *Frontiers in Psychiatry*, 12, 598119. DOI: 10.3389/fpsyt.2021.598119 PMID: 33643090

Novaco, R. W. (2010). Anger and Psychopathology. In Potegal, M., Stemmler, G., & Spielberger, C. (Eds.), *International Handbook of Anger: Constituent and Concomitant Biological, Psychological, and Social Processes* (pp. 465–497). Springer., DOI: 10.1007/978-0-387-89676-2_27

O'Haire, M. E., & Rodriguez, K. E. (2018). Preliminary efficacy of service dogs as a complementary treatment for posttraumatic stress disorder in military members and veterans.*Journal of Consulting and Clinical Psychology*, 86(2), 179–188. DOI: 10.1037/ccp0000267 PMID: 29369663

O'Leary, V. E., & Ickovics, J. R. (1995). Resilience and thriving in response to challenge: An opportunity for a paradigm shift in women's health.*Women's Health: Research on Gender, Behavior, and Policy*, 1(2), 121–142. PMID: 9373376

Olff, M. (2017). Sex and gender differences in post-traumatic stress disorder: an update. Eur J Psychotraumatol, 8(sup4), 1351204.

Opendak, M., & Gould, E. (2015). Adult neurogenesis: A substrate for experience-dependent change.*Trends in Cognitive Sciences*, 19(3), 151–161. DOI: 10.1016/j.tics.2015.01.001 PMID: 25715908

Ophir, I., & Jacoby, R. (2020). "Sparks that became a little light over time": A qualitative investigation of musicking as a means of coping in adults with PTSD. *PLoS One*, 15(1), e0228050. DOI: 10.1371/journal.pone.0228050 PMID: 31999728

Orr, S. P., & Roth, W. T. (2000). Psychophysiological assessment: Clinical applications for PTSD.*Journal of Affective Disorders*, 61(3), 225–240. DOI: 10.1016/S0165-0327(00)00340-2 PMID: 11163424

Pacitto, R., Peters, C., Iadipaolo, A., & Rabinak, C. A. (2022). Cannabinoid modulation of brain activation during volitional regulation of negative affect in trauma-exposed adults.*Neuropharmacology*, 218, 109222. DOI: 10.1016/j.neuropharm.2022.109222 PMID: 35981598

Palgi, Y., Karatzias, T., Hyland, P., Shevlin, M., & Ben-Ezra, M. (2021). Can subjective perceptions of trauma differentiate between ICD-11 PTSD and complex PTSD? A cross-cultural comparison of three African countries.*Psychological Trauma: Theory, Research, Practice, and Policy*, 13(2), 142–148. DOI: 10.1037/tra0000966 PMID: 32940522

Palomar-Ciria, N., & Bello, H. J. (2023). Equine-assisted therapy in post-traumatic stress disorder: A systematic review and meta-analysis.*Journal of Equine Veterinary Science*, 128, 104871. DOI: 10.1016/j.jevs.2023.104871 PMID: 37355148

Pan, X., Kaminga, A. C., Wen, S. W., & Liu, A. (2018). Catecholamines in post-traumatic stress disorder: A systematic review and meta-analysis.*Frontiers in Molecular Neuroscience*, 11, 450. DOI: 10.3389/fnmol.2018.00450 PMID: 30564100

Pargament, K. J., & Mahoney, A. (2017). Spirituality: the search for the sacred. In C. R. Snyder, S. J. Lopez, L. Edwards, & S. C. Marques (Eds), *Oxford handbook of positive psychology* (3rd ed.) (pp. 1-27), Oxford University Press.

Pargament, K. I., & Exline, J. J. (2022). *Working with spiritual struggles in psychotherapy: From research to practice*. The Guilford Press.

Pargament, K. J. (1997). *The Psychology of Religion and Coping Theory, Research, Practice*. The Guildford Press.

Parish-Plass, N. (2008). Animal-assisted therapy with children suffering from insecure attachment due to abuse and neglect: A method to lower the risk of intergenerational transmission of abuse.*Clinical Child Psychology and Psychiatry*, 13(1), 7–30. DOI: 10.1177/1359104507086338 PMID: 18411863

Park, C. L., Cohen, L. H., & Murch, R. L. (1996). Assessment and prediction of stress-related growth.*Journal of Personality*, 6(1), 71–105. DOI: 10.1111/j.1467-6494.1996.tb00815.x PMID: 8656319

Park, C. L., & Fenster, J. R. (2004). Stress-related growth: Predictors of occurrence and correlates with psychological adjustment.*Journal of Social and Clinical Psychology*, 23(2), 195–215. DOI: 10.1521/jscp.23.2.195.31019

Paulus, E. V., & Mintz, E. M. (2016). Circadian rhythms of clock gene expression in the cerebellum of serotonin-deficient Pet-1 knockout mice.*Brain Research*, 1630, 10–17. DOI: 10.1016/j.brainres.2015.10.044 PMID: 26529643

Pederson, C. L., Maurer, S. H., Kaminski, P. L., Zander, K. A., Peters, C. M., Stokes-Crowe, L. A., & Osborn, R. E. (2004). Hippocampal volume and memory performance in a community-based sample of women with posttraumatic stress disorder secondary to child abuse.*Journal of Traumatic Stress*, 17(1), 37–40. DOI: 10.1023/B:JOTS.0000014674.84517.46 PMID: 15027791

Peng, Z., Zhang, R., Wang, H., Chen, Y., Xue, F., Wang, L., Yang, F., Chen, Y., Liu, L., Kuang, F., & Tan, Q. (2013). Ziprasidone ameliorates anxiety-like behaviors in a rat model of PTSD and up-regulates neurogenesis in the hippocampus and hippocampus-derived neural stem cells.*Behavioural Brain Research*, 244, 1–8. DOI: 10.1016/j.bbr.2013.01.032 PMID: 23384713

Penner, S. B., Smyth, D. D., & Glavin, G. B. (1993). Effects of neuropeptide Y and [Leu31, Pro34] neuropeptide Y on experimental gastric lesion formation and gastric secretion in the rat.*The Journal of Pharmacology and Experimental Therapeutics*, 266(1), 339–343. PMID: 8101219

Perez Alday, E. A., Da Poian, G., Levantsevych, O., Murrah, N., Shallenberger, L., Alkhalaf, M., Haffar, A., Kaseer, B., Ko, Y. A., Goldberg, J., Smith, N., Lampert, R., Bremner, J. D., Clifford, G. D., Vaccarino, V., & Shah, A. J. (2023). Association of Autonomic Activation with traumatic reminder challenges in posttraumatic stress disorder: A co-twin control study.*Psychophysiology*, 60(2), e14167. DOI: 10.1111/psyp.14167 PMID: 35959570

Perrin, S., Meiser-Stedman, R., & Smith, P. (2005). The Children's Revised Impact of Event Scale (CRIES): Validity as a screening instrument for PTSD.*Behavioural and Cognitive Psychotherapy*, 33(4), 487–498. DOI: 10.1017/S1352465805002419

Perrotta, G. (2020). The state of consciousness: From perceptual alterations to dissociative forms. Analysis of neurobiological and clinical profiles. *Journal of Neurology, Neurological Science and Disorders*, 7(1), 006–018. https://doi.org/ DOI: 10.17352/jnnsd.000042

Pert, C. (1999). *Molecules of emotion: The science behind mind-body medicine*. Scribner.

Petty, F., Kramer, G. L., & Wu, J. (1997). Serotonergic modulation of learned helplessness.*Annals of the New York Academy of Sciences*, 821(1), 538–541. DOI: 10.1111/j.1749-6632.1997.tb48324.x PMID: 9238247

Petty, F., Kramer, G., & Wilson, L. (1992). Prevention of learned helplessness: In vivo correlation with cortical serotonin.*Pharmacology, Biochemistry, and Behavior*, 43(2), 361–367. DOI: 10.1016/0091-3057(92)90163-A PMID: 1438477

Phan, K. L., Britton, J. C., Taylor, S. F., Fig, L. M., & Liberzon, I. (2006). Corticolimbic blood flow during nontraumatic emotional processing in posttraumatic stress disorder.*Archives of General Psychiatry*, 63(2), 184–192. DOI: 10.1001/archpsyc.63.2.184 PMID: 16461862

Phelps, A. J., Forbes, D., & Creamer, M. (2008). Understanding posttraumatic nightmares: An empirical and conceptual review.*Clinical Psychology Review*, 28(2), 338–355. DOI: 10.1016/j.cpr.2007.06.001 PMID: 17629384

Pietrzak, R. H., Galea, S., Southwick, S. M., & Gelernter, J. (2013). Examining the relation between the serotonin transporter 5-HTTPLR genotype x trauma exposure interaction on a contemporary phenotypic model of posttraumatic stress symptomatology: A pilot study.*Journal of Affective Disorders*, 148(1), 123–128. DOI: 10.1016/j.jad.2012.11.003 PMID: 23183127

Pitman, R. K., Shin, L. M., Ph, D., & Rauch, S. L. (2001). *Posttraumatic Stress Disorder With Neuroimaging rig ht a du. 62*(suppl 17).

Pitman, R. K., Rasmusson, A. M., Koenen, K. C., Shin, L. M., Orr, S. P., Gilbertson, M. W., Milad, M. R., & Liberzon, I. (2012). Biological studies of post-traumatic stress disorder.*Nature Reviews. Neuroscience*, 13(11), 769–787. DOI: 10.1038/nrn3339 PMID: 23047775

Pitman, R. K., Shin, L. M., & Rauch, S. L. (2001). Investigating the pathogenesis of posttraumatic stress disorder with neuroimaging.*The Journal of Clinical Psychiatry*, 62(Suppl 17), 47–54. PMID: 11495097

Popoli, M., Yan, Z., McEwen, B. S., & Sanacora, G. (2012). The stressed synapse: The impact of stress and glucocorticoids on glutamate transmission.*Nature Reviews. Neuroscience*, 13(1), 22–37. DOI: 10.1038/nrn3138 PMID: 22127301

Porcheret, K., Iyadurai, L., Bonsall, M. B., Goodwin, G. M., Beer, S. A., Darwent, M., & Holmes, E. A. (2020). Sleep and intrusive memories immediately after a traumatic event in emergency department patients.*Sleep (Basel)*, 43(8), zsaa033. Advance online publication. DOI: 10.1093/sleep/zsaa033 PMID: 32133531

Poulsen, D. V., Stigsdotter, U. K., & Refshage, A. D. (2015). Whatever happened to the soldiers? Nature-assisted therapies for veterans diagnosed with post- traumatic stress disorder: A literature review.*Urban Forestry & Urban Greening*, 14(2), 438–445. DOI: 10.1016/j.ufug.2015.03.009

Pourhamzeh, M., Moravej, F. G., Arabi, M., Shahriari, E., Mehrabi, S., Ward, R., Ahadi, R., & Joghataei, M. T. (2022). The roles of serotonin in neuropsychiatric disorders.*Cellular and Molecular Neurobiology*, 42(6), 1671–1692. DOI: 10.1007/s10571-021-01064-9 PMID: 33651238

Prange, A. J. (1999). Thyroid axis sustaining hypothesis of posttraumatic stress disorder.*Psychosomatic Medicine*, 61(2), 139–140. DOI: 10.1097/00006842-199903000-00002 PMID: 10204963

Prasad, R. (2019, November 29). How Trump talks about women—And does it matter? https://www.bbc.com/news/world-us-canada-50563106

Prasad, A., Chaichi, A., Kelley, D. P., Francis, J., & Gartia, M. R. (2019). Current and future functional imaging techniques for post-traumatic stress disorder.*RSC Advances*, 9(42), 24568–24594. DOI: 10.1039/C9RA03562A PMID: 35527877

Preston, J. D., O'Neal, J. H., & Talaga, M. C. (2002). *Handbook of clinical psychopharmacology for therapists* (3rd ed.). New Harbinger.

Pries, J., Niecke, A., Vetter, A., & Schultz-Venrath, U. (2022). More than one way home - Student raters' impressions of interventions and group processes in mentalisation based group psychotherapy and group analytic psychotherapy.*Research in Psychotherapy*, 25(3), 642. DOI: 10.4081/ripppo.2022.642 PMID: 36629759

Pringle, G., Boddy, J., Slattery, M., & Harris, P. (2023). Adventure Therapy for Adolescents with Complex Trauma: A Scoping Review and Analysis.*Journal of Experiential Education*, 46(4), 433–454. DOI: 10.1177/10538259221147195

Pringle, G., Boddy, J., Slattery, M., & Harris, P. (2023). Adventure therapy for adolescents with complex trauma: A scoping review and analysis.*Journal of Experimental Education*, 46(4), 433–454.

Pro-Palestine student protests spread to Japan. (2024, May 3). Middle East Monitor. https://www.middleeastmonitor.com/20240503-pro-palestine-student-protests-spread-to-japan/

PTSD & the Brain. (n.d.). PTSD. https://ptsdvietnam1.weebly.com/ptsd--the-brain.html

Puchalski, C., & Romer, A. L. (2000). Taking a spiritual history allows clinicians to understand patients more fully.*Journal of Palliative Medicine*, 3(1), 129–137. DOI: 10.1089/jpm.2000.3.129 PMID: 15859737

Punski-Hoogervorst, J. L., Avital, A., & Engel-Yeger, B. (2023). Challenges in basic and instrumental activities of daily living among adults with posttraumatic stress disorder: A scoping review.*Occupational Therapy in Mental Health*, 39(2), 184–210. DOI: 10.1080/0164212X.2022.2094523

Purgato, M., Prina, E., Ceccarelli, C., Cadorin, C., Abdulmalik, J. O., Amaddeo, F., Arcari, L., Churchill, R., Jordans, M. J., Lund, C., Papola, D., Uphoff, E., van Ginneken, N., Tol, W. A., & Barbui, C. (2023). Primary-level and community worker interventions for the prevention of mental disorders and the promotion of well-being in low- and middle-income countries.*Cochrane Database of Systematic Reviews*, 10(10), CD014722. Advance online publication. DOI: 10.1002/14651858.CD014722.pub2 PMID: 37873968

Putri, V. S. I. S., Wijayanti, L. R., & Hidayati, I. N. (2023). The Positive Effect of The Forest Environment in The Ecotherapy Healing Forest Program on The Physical and Mental Health After COVID-19. BIO Web of Conferences

Radley, J. J., & Sawchenko, P. E. (2011). A common substrate for prefrontal and hippocampal inhibition of the neuroendocrine stress response.*The Journal of Neuroscience : The Official Journal of the Society for Neuroscience*, 31(26), 9683–9695. DOI: 10.1523/JNEUROSCI.6040-10.2011 PMID: 21715634

Radley, J. J., Williams, B., & Sawchenko, P. E. (2008). Noradrenergic innervation of the dorsal medial prefrontal cortex modulates hypothalamo-pituitary-adrenal responses to acute emotional stress.*The Journal of Neuroscience : The Official Journal of the Society for Neuroscience*, 28(22), 5806–5816. DOI: 10.1523/JNEUROSCI.0552-08.2008 PMID: 18509042

Raghuraman, S., Stuttard, N., & Hunt, N. (2021). Evaluating narrative exposure therapy for post-traumatic stress disorder and depression symptoms: A meta-analysis of the evidence base.*Clinical Psychology & Psychotherapy*, 28(1), 1–23. DOI: 10.1002/cpp.2486 PMID: 32525597

Ragnhildstveit, A., Kaiyo, M., Snyder, M. B., Jackson, L. K., Lopez, A., Mayo, C., Miranda, A. C., August, R. J., Seli, P., Robison, R., & Averill, L. A. (2023). Cannabis-assisted psychotherapy for complex dissociative posttraumatic stress disorder: A case report.*Frontiers in Psychiatry*, 14, 1051542. DOI: 10.3389/fpsyt.2023.1051542 PMID: 36846226

Ramachandran, V. (1995). Mirror neurons and imitation learning as the driving force behind the great leap forward in human evolution. Retrieved f2nd March 2024 from https://www.edge.org/conversation/vilayanur_ramachandran-mirror-neurons -and-imitation-learning-as-the-driving-force

Ramirez de Arellano, M. A., Lyman, D. R., Jobe-Shields, L., George, P., Dougherty, R. H., Daniels, A. S., Ghose, S. S., Huang, L., & Delphin-Rittmon, M. E. (2014). Trauma-Focused Cognitive-Behavioral Therapy for Children and Adolescents: Assessing the Evidence.*Psychiatric Services (Washington, D.C.)*, 65(5), 591–602. DOI: 10.1176/appi.ps.201300255 PMID: 24638076

Rasmusson, A. M., Hauger, R. L., Morgan, C. A.III, Bremner, J. D., Charney, D. S., & Southwick, S. M. (2000). Low baseline and yohimbine-stimulated plasma neuropeptide Y (NPY) levels in combat-related PTSD.*Biological Psychiatry*, 47(6), 526–539. DOI: 10.1016/S0006-3223(99)00185-7 PMID: 10715359

Rasmusson, A. M., Lipschitz, D. S., Wang, S., Hu, S., Vojvoda, D., Bremner, J. D., Southwick, S. M., & Charney, D. S. (2001). Increased pituitary and adrenal reactivity in premenopausal women with posttraumatic stress disorder.*Biological Psychiatry*, 50(12), 965–977. DOI: 10.1016/S0006-3223(01)01264-1 PMID: 11750893

Rauch, S. L., Shin, L. M., Segal, E., Pitman, R. K., Carson, M. A., McMullin, K., Whalen, P. J., & Makris, N. (2003). Selectively reduced regional cortical volumes in post-traumatic stress disorder.*Neuroreport*, 14(7), 913–916. PMID: 12802174

Regier, D. A., Kuhl, E. A., & Kupfer, D. J. (2013). The DSM-5: Classification and criteria changes.*World Psychiatry; Official Journal of the World Psychiatric Association (WPA)*, 12(2), 92–98. DOI: 10.1002/wps.20050 PMID: 23737408

Reichmann, F., & Holzer, P. (2016). Neuropeptide Y: A stressful review.*Neuropeptides*, 55, 99–109. DOI: 10.1016/j.npep.2015.09.008 PMID: 26441327

Reis, R., & Ortega, F. (2021). Neuroscientific perspectives for a theory of trauma: A critical review of integrative models of biology and culture.*Cadernos de Saude Publica*, 37, e00352820. DOI: 10.1590/0102-311x00352820 PMID: 34495102

Resick, P. A. (2001). Cognitive processing therapy: Generic version. University of Missouri: St. Lewis.

Ressler, K. J. (2010). Amygdala activity, fear, and anxiety: Modulation by stress. *Biological Psychiatry*, 67(12), 1117–1119. DOI: 10.1016/j.biopsych.2010.04.027 PMID: 20525501

Ressler, K. J., Berretta, S., Bolshakov, V. Y., Rosso, I. M., Meloni, E. G., Rauch, S. L., & Carlezon, W. A.Jr. (2022). Post-traumatic stress disorder: Clinical and translational neuroscience from cells to circuits.*Nature Reviews. Neurology*, 18(5), 273–288. DOI: 10.1038/s41582-022-00635-8 PMID: 35352034

Rivers, W. H. R. (1918). The repression of war experience.*Lancet*, 1, 73–177. PMID: 19980290

Roeder, S. S., Burkardt, P., Rost, F., Rode, J., Brusch, L., Coras, R., Englund, E., Håkansson, K., Possnert, G., Salehpour, M., Primetzhofer, D., Csiba, L., Molnár, S., Méhes, G., Tonchev, A. B., Schwab, S., Bergmann, O., & Huttner, H. B. (2022). Evidence for postnatal neurogenesis in the human amygdala.*Communications Biology*, 5(1), 1–8. DOI: 10.1038/s42003-022-03299-8 PMID: 35440676

Rosenstock, I. M. (1974). Historical origins of the Health Belief Model.*Health Education Monographs*, 2(4), 328–335. DOI: 10.1177/109019817400200403

Rowe, J. (2005). The effects of EFT on long-term psychological symptoms.*Counseling and Clinical Psychology Journal*, 2(3), 104.

Rutt, B. T., Oehlert, M. E., Krieshok, T. S., & Lichtenberg, J. W. (2018). Effectiveness of Cognitive Processing Therapy and Prolonged Exposure in the Department of Veterans Affairs.*Psychological Reports*, 121(2), 282–302. DOI: 10.1177/0033294117727746 PMID: 28886664

Saboory, E., Ghasemi, M., & Mehranfard, N. (2020). Norepinephrine, neurodevelopment and behavior.*Neurochemistry International*, 135, 104706. DOI: 10.1016/j.neuint.2020.104706 PMID: 32092327

Sadeghi, M., McDonald, A. D., & Sasangohar, F. (2022). Posttraumatic stress disorder hyperarousal event detection using smartwatch physiological and activity data. *PLoS One*, 17(5), e0267749. DOI: 10.1371/journal.pone.0267749 PMID: 35584096

Salome, G., Vignaud, P., Galia, P., Prieto, N., & Chauliac, N. (2023). Determinants of care pathways for C-PTSD patients in French psychotrauma centers: A qualitative study.[PubMed]. *International Journal of Environmental Research and Public Health*, 20(13), 6278.

Saraiya, T., & Lopez-Castro, T. (2016). Ashamed and Afraid: A Scoping Review of the Role of Shame in Post-Traumatic Stress Disorder (PTSD).*Journal of Clinical Medicine*, 5(11), 11. Advance online publication. DOI: 10.3390/jcm5110094 PMID: 27809274

Sareen, J. (2014). Posttraumatic stress disorder in adults: Impact, comorbidity, risk factors, and treatment.*Canadian Journal of Psychiatry*, 59(9), 460–467. DOI: 10.1177/070674371405900902 PMID: 25565692

Saudia, T. L., Kinney, M. R., Brown, K. C., & Yong-Ward, L. (1991). Health locus of control and helpfulness of prayer.*Heart & Lung*, 20, 60–65. PMID: 1988394

Scelles, C., & Bulnes, L. C. (2021). EMDR as Treatment Option for Conditions Other Than PTSD: A Systematic Review.*Frontiers in Psychology*, 12, 644369. Advance online publication. DOI: 10.3389/fpsyg.2021.644369 PMID: 34616328

Schäfer, S. K., Lüder, C. C., Porcheret, K., Hu, X., Margraf, J., Michael, T., Holmes, E. A., Werner, G. G., Wilhelm, I., Woud, M. L., Zeng, S., Friesen, E., Haim-Nachum, S., Lass-Hennemann, J., Lieb, K., Kunzler, A. M., Wirth, B. E., & Sopp, M. R. (2023). To sleep or not to sleep, that is the question: A systematic review and meta-analysis on the effect of post-trauma sleep on intrusive memories of analog trauma. *Behaviour Research and Therapy*, 167, 104359. DOI: 10.1016/j.brat.2023.104359 PMID: 37422952

Schelling, G., Kilger, E., Roozendaal, B., Dominique, J.-F., Briegel, J., Dagge, A., Rothenhäusler, H.-B., Krauseneck, T., Nollert, G., & Kapfhammer, H.-P. (2004). Stress doses of hydrocortisone, traumatic memories, and symptoms of posttraumatic stress disorder in patients after cardiac surgery: A randomized study.*Biological Psychiatry*, 55(6), 627–633. DOI: 10.1016/j.biopsych.2003.09.014 PMID: 15013832

Schmeltzer, S. N., Herman, J. P., & Sah, R. (2016). Neuropeptide Y (NPY) and posttraumatic stress disorder (PTSD): A translational update.*Experimental Neurology*, 284, 196–210. DOI: 10.1016/j.expneurol.2016.06.020 PMID: 27377319

Schnurr, P. P., Chard, K. M., Ruzek, J. I., Chow, B. K., Resick, P. A., Foa, E. B., Marx, B. P., Friedman, M. J., Bovin, M. J., Caudle, K. L., Castillo, D., Curry, K. T., Hollifield, M., Huang, G. D., Chee, C. L., Astin, M. C., Dickstein, B., Renner, K., Clancy, C. P., & Shih, M.-C. (2022). Comparison of Prolonged Exposure vs Cognitive Processing Therapy for Treatment of Posttraumatic Stress Disorder Among US Veterans: A Randomized Clinical Trial.*JAMA Network Open*, 5(1), e2136921. DOI: 10.1001/jamanetworkopen.2021.36921 PMID: 35044471

Schrader, C., & Ross, A. (2021). A review of PTSD and current treatment strategies. *Annals of Clinical Psychiatry*, 33(6), 546–551. https://www.ncbi.nlm.nih.gov/pmc/articles/PMC8672952/ PMID: 34924624

Schrader, C., & Ross, A. (2021). A Review of PTSD and Current Treatment Strategies.*Missouri Medicine*, 118(6), 546–551. PMID: 34924624

Schubert, C. F., Schmidt, U., & Rosner, R. (2015). PTSD growth in populations with posttraumatic stress disorder-a systematic review on growth-related psychological constructs and biological variables.*Clinical Psychology & Psychotherapy*, •••, 1985. PMID: 26514236

Schulz, K. M. (2007). Integrating energy psychology into treatment for adult survivors of childhood sexual abuse: An exploratory clinical study from the therapist's perspective.*Dissertation Abstracts International. B, The Sciences and Engineering*, 68(1-B), 635.

Schweitzer, R., Melville, F., Steel, Z., & Lacherez, P. (2006). Trauma, Post-Migration Living Difficulties, and Social Support as Predictors of Psychological Adjustment in Resettled Sudanese Refugees.*The Australian and New Zealand Journal of Psychiatry*, 40(2), 179–187. DOI: 10.1080/j.1440-1614.2006.01766.x PMID: 16476137

Sciarrino, N. A., & Myers, U. S. (2023). If it's offered, will they come? Practical considerations when offering intensive PTSD treatment in an outpatient Veterans Affairs PTSD clinic.*Bulletin of the Menninger Clinic*, 87(1), 46–62. DOI: 10.1521/bumc.2023.87.1.46 PMID: 36856477

Scott, M. (2023, December 14). Does social media favor Palestine over Israel? POLITICO. https://www.politico.eu/newsletter/digital-bridge/does-social-media-favor-palestine-over-israel/

Seal, K. H., Cohen, G., Waldrop, A., Cohen, B. E., Maguen, S., & Ren, L. (2011). Substance use disorders in Iraq and Afghanistan veterans in VA healthcare, 2001–2010: Implications for screening, diagnosis and treatment.*Drug and Alcohol Dependence*, 116(1–3), 93–101. DOI: 10.1016/j.drugalcdep.2010.11.027 PMID: 21277712

Sebastian, B., & Nelms, J. (2017). The effectiveness of emotional freedom techniques in the treatment of posttraumatic stress disorder: A meta- analysis.*Explore (New York, N.Y.)*, 13(1), 16–25. DOI: 10.1016/j.explore.2016.10.001 PMID: 27889444

Shafia, S., Ghadirzadeh, E., Fayyaz Shahandashti, A. S., & Ehsani Vostacolaee, S. (2023). Comparing the Effects of High and Moderate Intensity Exercise on Male and Female Rats with and without PTSD: A Behavioral and Biochemical Study. *Journal of Mazandaran University of Medical Sciences*, 32(216), 20–33.

Shafranske, E. P., & Cummings, J. P. (2013). Religious and spiritual beliefs, affirmations, and practices of psychologist. In Pargament, K. I., Mahoney, A., & Shafranske, E. P. (Eds.), APA handbook of psychology, religion, and spirituality: Vol. 2. *An applied psychology of religion and spirituality. (* (pp. 23–42). American Psychological Association.

Shapiro, F. (1989). Eye movement desensitization: A new treatment for post-traumatic stress disorder.*Journal of Behavior Therapy and Experimental Psychiatry*, 20(3), 211–217. DOI: 10.1016/0005-7916(89)90025-6 PMID: 2576656

Shapiro, F. (2014). The role of eye movement desensitization and reprocessing (EMDR) therapy in medicine: Addressing the psychological and physical symptoms stemming from adverse life experiences.*The Permanente Journal*, 18(1), 71–77. DOI: 10.7812/TPP/13-098 PMID: 24626074

Sherin, J. E., & Nemeroff, C. B. (2011). Post-traumatic stress disorder: The neurobiological impact of psychological trauma.*Dialogues in Clinical Neuroscience*, 13(3), 263–278. DOI: 10.31887/DCNS.2011.13.2/jsherin PMID: 22034143

Shin, L. M., Lasko, N. B., Macklin, M. L., Karpf, R. D., Milad, M. R., Orr, S. P., Goetz, J. M., Fischman, A. J., Rauch, S. L., & Pitman, R. K. (2009). Resting metabolic activity in the cingulate cortex and vulnerability to posttraumatic stress disorder.*Archives of General Psychiatry*, 66(10), 1099–1107. DOI: 10.1001/archgenpsychiatry.2009.138 PMID: 19805700

Shin, L. M., McNally, R. J., Kosslyn, S. M., Thompson, W. L., Rauch, S. L., Alpert, N. M., Metzger, L. J., Lasko, N. B., Orr, S. P., & Pitman, R. K. (1999). Regional cerebral blood flow during script-driven imagery in childhood sexual abuse-related PTSD: A PET investigation.*The American Journal of Psychiatry*, 156(4), 575–584. DOI: 10.1176/ajp.156.4.575 PMID: 10200737

Shin, L. M., Orr, S. P., Carson, M. A., Rauch, S. L., Macklin, M. L., Lasko, N. B., Peters, P. M., Metzger, L. J., Dougherty, D. D., Cannistraro, P. A., Alpert, N. M., Fischman, A. J., & Pitman, R. K. (2004). Regional cerebral blood flow in the amygdala and medial prefrontalcortex during traumatic imagery in male and female vietnam veterans with ptsd.*Archives of General Psychiatry*, 61(2), 168–176. DOI: 10.1001/archpsyc.61.2.168 PMID: 14757593

Shin, L. M., Whalen, P. J., Pitman, R. K., Bush, G., Macklin, M. L., Lasko, N. B., Orr, S. P., McInerney, S. C., & Rauch, S. L. (2001). An fMRI study of anterior cingulate function in posttraumatic stress disorder.*Biological Psychiatry*, 50(12), 932–942. DOI: 10.1016/S0006-3223(01)01215-X PMID: 11750889

Shin, L. M., Wright, C. I., Cannistraro, P. A., Wedig, M. M., McMullin, K., Martis, B., Macklin, M. L., Lasko, N. B., Cavanagh, S. R., Krangel, T. S., Orr, S. P., Pitman, R. K., Whalen, P. J., & Rauch, S. L. (2005). A functional magnetic resonance imaging study of amygdala and medial prefrontal cortex responses to overtly presented fearful faces in posttraumatic stress disorder.*Archives of General Psychiatry*, 62(3), 273–281. DOI: 10.1001/archpsyc.62.3.273 PMID: 15753240

Shubina, I. (2015). Cognitive-behavioral Therapy of Patients with PTSD: Literature Review.*Procedia: Social and Behavioral Sciences*, 165, 208–216. DOI: 10.1016/j.sbspro.2014.12.624

Siebner, H. R., Funke, K., Aberra, A. S., Antal, A., Bestmann, S., Chen, R., Classen, J., Davare, M., Di Lazzaro, V., Fox, P. T., Hallett, M., Karabanov, A. N., Kesselheim, J., Beck, M. M., Koch, G., Liebetanz, D., Meunier, S., Miniussi, C., Paulus, W., & Ugawa, Y. (2022). Transcranial magnetic stimulation of the brain: What is stimulated? - A consensus and critical position paper.*Clinical Neurophysiology*, 140, 59–97. DOI: 10.1016/j.clinph.2022.04.022 PMID: 35738037

Sihvonen, R., Paavola, M., Itala, A., Joukainen, A., Nurmi, H., & Jarvinen, T. L. N. (2013). Arthros.copic partial meniscectomy versus sham surgery for a degenerative meniscal tear. *The New England Journal of Medicine*, 369(26), 2515–2524. DOI: 10.1056/NEJMoa1305189 PMID: 24369076

Simmons, A. N., & Matthews, S. C. (2012). Neural circuitry of PTSD with or without mild traumatic brain injury: A meta-analysis.*Neuropharmacology*, 62(2), 598–606. DOI: 10.1016/j.neuropharm.2011.03.016 PMID: 21420986

Simmons, A. N., Paulus, M. P., Thorp, S. R., Matthews, S. C., Norman, S. B., & Stein, M. B. (2008). Functional activation and neural networks in women with post-traumatic stress disorder related to intimate partner violence.*Biological Psychiatry*, 64(8), 681–690. DOI: 10.1016/j.biopsych.2008.05.027 PMID: 18639236

Skolariki, K., Vrahatis, A. G., Krokidis, M. G., Exarchos, T. P., & Vlamos, P. (2023). Assessing and modelling of post-traumatic stress disorder using molecular and functional biomarkers.*Biology (Basel)*, 12(8), 1050. DOI: 10.3390/biology12081050 PMID: 37626936

Sloan, D. M., Marx, B. P., Resick, P. A., Young-McCaughan, S., Dondanville, K. A., Mintz, J., Litz, B. T., & Peterson, A. L.STRONG STAR Consortium. (2019). Study design comparing written exposure therapy to cognitive processing therapy for PTSD among military service members: A noninferiority trial.*Contemporary Clinical Trials Communications*, 17, 100507. DOI: 10.1016/j.conctc.2019.100507 PMID: 31890987

Smith, B. W., Oritz, J. A., Wiggins, K. T., Bernard, J. F., & Dalen, J. (2012). Spirituality, resilience, and positive emotions. In Miller, A. (Ed.), *The Oxford Handbook of Psychology and Spirituality*. Oxford University Press.

Smith, P., Perrin, S., Yule, W., & Rabe-Hesketh, S. (2001). War exposure and maternal reactions in the psychological adjustment of children from Bosnia-Hercegovina. *Journal of Child Psychology and Psychiatry, and Allied Disciplines*, 42(3), 395–404. DOI: 10.1111/1469-7610.00732 PMID: 11321208

Sommer, J. L., El-Gabalawy, R., Contractor, A. A., Weiss, N. H., & Mota, N. (2020). PTSD's risky behavior criterion: Associated risky and unhealthy behaviors and psychiatric correlates in a nationally representative sample.*Journal of Anxiety Disorders*, 73, 102247. DOI: 10.1016/j.janxdis.2020.102247 PMID: 32502805

Somvanshi, P. R., Mellon, S. H., Flory, J. D., Abu-Amara, D., Wolkowitz, O. M., Yehuda, R., Jett, M., Hood, L., Marmar, C., & Doyle, F. J. (2019). Mechanistic inferences on metabolic dysfunction in PTSD from an integrated model and multiomic analysis: Role of glucocorticoid receptor sensitivity.*American Journal of Physiology. Endocrinology and Metabolism.* Advance online publication. DOI: 10.1152/ajpendo.00065.2019

Song, S. Y., Ko, Y. B., Kim, H., Lee, G. W., Yang, J. B., Chang, H. K., Kwak, S. M., Jung, J., Lee, S., Lee, S. Y., & Yoo, H. J. (2020). Effect of serotonin-norepinephrine reuptake inhibitors for patients with chemotherapy-induced painful peripheral neuropathy: A meta-analysis.*Medicine*, 99(1), e18653. DOI: 10.1097/MD.0000000000018653 PMID: 31895829

Song, X., & Vilares, I. (2021). Assessing the relationship between the human learned helplessness depression model and anhedonia.*PLoS One*, 16(3), e0249056. DOI: 10.1371/journal.pone.0249056 PMID: 33784324

Sonnenschein, S. F., Gomes, F. V., & Grace, A. A. (2020). Dysregulation of midbrain dopamine system and the pathophysiology of schizophrenia.*Frontiers in Psychiatry*, 11, 613. DOI: 10.3389/fpsyt.2020.00613 PMID: 32719622

Southwick, S. M., Bremner, J. D., Rasmusson, A., Morgan, C. A.III, Arnsten, A., & Charney, D. S. (1999). Role of norepinephrine in the pathophysiology and treatment of posttraumatic stress disorder.*Biological Psychiatry*, 46(9), 1192–1204. DOI: 10.1016/S0006-3223(99)00219-X PMID: 10560025

Stapleton, P., Buchan, C., Mitchell, I., McGrath, Y., Gorton, P., & Carter, B. (2019). An initial investigation of neural changes in overweight adults with food cravings after emotional freedom techniques. *OBM Integrative and Complementary Medicine*, *4*(1), 010. DOI: 10.21926/obm.icm.1901010

Stapleton, P., Baumann, O., O'Keefe, T., & Bhuta, S. (2022). Neural changes after emotional freedom techniques treatment for chronic pain sufferers.*Complementary Therapies in Clinical Practice*, 53, 101653. DOI: 10.1016/j.ctcp.2022.101653 PMID: 35933806

Stapleton, P., Crighton, G., Sabot, D., & O'Neill, H. M. (2020). Reexamining the effect of emotional freedom techniques on stress biochemistry: A randomized controlled trial.*Traumatology*, 26(12), 869–877. DOI: 10.1037/tra0000563 PMID: 32162958

Stapleton, P., Kip, K., Church, D., Toussaint, L., Footman, J., Ballantyne, P., & O'Keefe, T. (2023). Emotional freedom techniques for treating posttraumatic stress disorder: An updated systematic review and meta-analysis.*Frontiers in Psychology*, 14, 1195286. DOI: 10.3389/fpsyg.2023.1195286 PMID: 37637920

Steenkamp, M. M., Litz, B. T., Hoge, C. W., & Marmar, C. R. (2015). Psychotherapy for military-related PTSD: A review of randomized clinical trials.*Journal of the American Medical Association*, 314(5), 489–500. DOI: 10.1001/jama.2015.8370 PMID: 26241600

Stefanov, M., Potroz, M., Kim, J., Lim, J., Cha, R., & Nam, M.-H. (2013). The primo vascular system as a new anatomical system.*Journal of Acupuncture and Meridian Studies*, 6(6), 331–338. DOI: 10.1016/j.jams.2013.10.001 PMID: 24290797

Steinberg, A. M., Brymer, M. J., Decker, K. B., & Pynoos, R. S. (2004). The University of California at Los Angeles posttraumatic stress disorder reaction index. *Current Psychiatry Reports*, 6(2), 96–100. DOI: 10.1007/s11920-004-0048-2 PMID: 15038911

Stein, D. J., Harris, M. G., Vigo, D. V., Tat Chiu, W., Sampson, N., Alonso, J., Altwaijri, Y., Bunting, B., Caldas-de-Almeida, J. M., Cía, A., Ciutan, M., Degenhardt, L., Gureje, O., Karam, A., Karam, E. G., Lee, S., Medina-Mora, M. E., Mneimneh, Z., Navarro-Mateu, F., & Kessler, R. C.WHO World Mental Health Survey Collaborators. (2020). Perceived helpfulness of treatment for posttraumatic stress disorder: Findings from the World Mental Health Surveys.*Depression and Anxiety*, 37(10), 972–994. DOI: 10.1002/da.23076 PMID: 32667096

Stevens, J. S., Jovanovic, T., Fani, N., Ely, T. D., Glover, E. M., Bradley, B., & Ressler, K. J. (2013). Disrupted amygdala-prefrontal functional connectivity in civilian women with posttraumatic stress disorder.*Journal of Psychiatric Research*, 47(10), 1469–1478. DOI: 10.1016/j.jpsychires.2013.05.031 PMID: 23827769

Steward, T., Das, P., Malhi, G. S., Bryant, R. A., & Felmingham, K. L. (2020). Dysfunctional coupling of the parahippocampal cortex and inferior frontal gyrus during memory suppression in posttraumatic stress disorder.*European Neuropsychopharmacology*, 41, 146–151. DOI: 10.1016/j.euroneuro.2020.09.634 PMID: 32967787

Stouffer, S. A., Consadaine, A. A., Consadaine, M. H., Willians, R. W., Jr., & Smith, M. B., Janis, J. L., Star, S. A., & Cottrell, L. S., Jr. (1963). *The American soldier: Combat and its aftermath* (Vol. 2). Wiley.

Streeter, C. C., Gerbarg, P. L., Saper, R. B., Ciraulo, D. A., & Brown, R. P. (2012). Effects of yoga on the autonomic nervous system, gamma-aminobutyric-acid, and allostasis in epilepsy, depression, and post-traumatic stress disorder.*Medical Hypotheses*, 78(5), 571–579. DOI: 10.1016/j.mehy.2012.01.021 PMID: 22365651

Summerfield, D. (2001). The invention of post-traumatic stress disorder and the social usefulness of a psychiatric category.*BMJ (Clinical Research Ed.)*, 322(7278), 95–98. DOI: 10.1136/bmj.322.7278.95 PMID: 11154627

Sun, L., Cui, K., Xing, F., & Liu, X. (2020). Akt dependent adult hippocampal neurogenesis regulates the behavioral improvement of treadmill running to mice model of post-traumatic stress disorder. *Behavioural Brain Research, 379*(October 2019), 112375. DOI: 10.1016/j.bbr.2019.112375

Sussman, D., Pang, E. W., Jetly, R., Dunkley, B. T., & Taylor, M. J. (2016). Neuroanatomical features in soldiers with post-traumatic stress disorder.*BMC Neuroscience*, 17(1), 1–11. DOI: 10.1186/s12868-016-0247-x PMID: 27029195

Swinton, J., & Vanderport, L. (2017). The unforeseen relationship between spirituality and psychiatric medication: A hermeneutic phenomenological study. *Journal of Spirituality in Mental Health*. Advance online publication. DOI: 10.1080/19349637.2017.1297692

Szoke, D., Putnam, A., & Hazlett-Stevens, H. (2021). Mindfulness-Based Interventions for Traumatic Stress. In Hazlett-Stevens, H. (Ed.), *Biopsychosocial Factors of Stress, and Mindfulness for Stress Reduction* (pp. 177–200). Springer International Publishing., DOI: 10.1007/978-3-030-81245-4_8

Taguchi, K., Numata, N., Takanashi, R., Takemura, R., Yoshida, T., Kutsuzawa, K., Yoshimura, K., & Shimizu, E. (2021). Integrated cognitive behavioral therapy for chronic pain: An open labeled prospective single-arm trial.*Medicine*, 100(6), e23859. DOI: 10.1097/MD.0000000000023859 PMID: 33578513

Takemura, N. U. (2005). Evidence for neurogenesis within the white matter beneath the temporal neocortex of the adult rat brain.*Neuroscience*, 134(1), 121–132. DOI: 10.1016/j.neuroscience.2005.04.033 PMID: 15964698

Takemura, N. U., & Kato, N. (2007). Adult neurogenesis and systemic adaptation: Animal experiments and clinical perspectives for PTSD.*Progress in Brain Research*, 167(07), 99–109. DOI: 10.1016/S0079-6123(07)67007-1 PMID: 18037009

Tang, X., Lin, S., Fang, D., Lin, B., Yao, L., Wang, L., Xu, Q., Lu, L., & Xu, N. (2023). Efficacy and underlying mechanisms of acupuncture therapy for PTSD: Evidence from animal and clinical studies.*Frontiers in Behavioral Neuroscience*, 17, 1163718. DOI: 10.3389/fnbeh.2023.1163718 PMID: 37200784

Tasan, R. O., Verma, D., Wood, J., Lach, G., Hörmer, B., de Lima, T. C. M., Herzog, H., & Sperk, G. (2016). The role of Neuropeptide Y in fear conditioning and extinction.*Neuropeptides*, 55, 111–126. DOI: 10.1016/j.npep.2015.09.007 PMID: 26444585

Taylor-Desir, M. (2022, November). What is post-traumatic stress disorder (PTSD)? Psychiatry.org; American Psychiatric Association. https://www.psychiatry.org/patients-families/ptsd/what-is-ptsd

Tedeschi, R. G., & Calhoun, L. G. (1995). Trauma and Transformation: Growing in the Aftermath of Suffering.*Sage (Atlanta, Ga.)*. Advance online publication. DOI: 10.4135/9781483326931

Tedeschi, R. G., & Calhoun, L. G. (1996). The Posttraumatic Growth Inventory: Measuring the positive legacy of trauma.*Journal of Traumatic Stress*, 9(3), 455–472. DOI: 10.1002/jts.2490090305 PMID: 8827649

Tedeschi, R. G., & Calhoun, L. G. (2004). Posttraumatic growth: Conceptual foundations and empirical evidence.*Psychological Inquiry*, 15(1), 1–18. DOI: 10.1207/s15327965pli1501_01

Tedla, J. S., Sangadala, D. R., Reddy, R. S., Gular, K., & Dixit, S. (2023). High-definition trans cranial direct current stimulation and its effects on cognitive function: A systematic review.*Cerebral Cortex (New York, N.Y.)*, 33(10), 6077–6089. DOI: 10.1093/cercor/bhac485 PMID: 36533541

Temoney, K. E. (2021). The War Came Alive Inside of Them.*The Journal of Religious Ethics*, 49(3), 479–494. DOI: 10.1111/jore.12366

Terranova, J. I., Ogawa, S. K., & Kitamura, T. (2019). Adult hippocampal neurogenesis for systems consolidation of memory.*Behavioural Brain Research*, 372(June), 112035. DOI: 10.1016/j.bbr.2019.112035 PMID: 31201874

The Onion Editorial Board. (2023, October 13). 'The Onion' Stands With Israel Because It Seems Like You Get In Less Trouble For That. The Onion. https://www.theonion.com/the-onion-stands-with-israel-because-it-seems-like-yo-1850922505

Thorsell, A., Michalkiewicz, M., Dumont, Y., Quirion, R., Caberlotto, L., Rimondini, R., Mathe, A. A., & Heilig, M. (2000). Behavioral insensitivity to restraint stress, absent fear suppression of behavior and impaired spatial learning in transgenic rats with hippocampal neuropeptide Y overexpression.*Proceedings of the National Academy of Sciences of the United States of America*, 97(23), 12852–12857. DOI: 10.1073/pnas.220232997 PMID: 11058155

Tian, X., Yi, L. J., Liang, C. S., Gu, L., Peng, C., Chen, G. H., & Jiménez-Herrera, M. F. (2022). The Impact of Mindfulness-Based Stress Reduction (MBSR) on Psychological Outcomes and Quality of Life in Patients With Lung Cancer: A Meta-Analysis.*Frontiers in Psychology*, 13, 901247. DOI: 10.3389/fpsyg.2022.901247 PMID: 35837627

Tolentino, J. C., Gjorup, A. L. T., Mello, C. R., de Assis, S. G., Marques, A., Filho, A. C., Salazar, H. R. M., van Duinkerken, E., & Schmidt, S. L. (2022). Spirituality as a protective factor for chronic and acute anxiety in Brazilian healthcare workers during the COVID-19 outbreak.*PLoS One*, 17(5), e0267556. DOI: 10.1371/journal.pone.0267556 PMID: 35503766

Torrisi, S. A., Leggio, G. M., Drago, F., & Salomone, S. (2019). Therapeutic challenges of post-traumatic stress disorder: Focus on the dopaminergic system.*Frontiers in Pharmacology*, 10, 404. DOI: 10.3389/fphar.2019.00404 PMID: 31057408

Tovote, P., Fadok, J. P., & Lüthi, A. (2015). Neuronal circuits for fear and anxiety. *Nature Reviews. Neuroscience*, 16(6), 317–331. DOI: 10.1038/nrn3945 PMID: 25991441

Trajkov, I. (2023). Stress, Trauma and Post-Traumatic Stress Disorder (PTSD). *The Annual of the Faculty of Philosophy in Skopje*, 76, 629–639. DOI: 10.37510/godzbo2376629t

Tripathi, K. D. (2013). Essentials of Medical Pharmacology. Jaypee Brothers Medical Publishers (P) Ltd. Seventh edition.

Trottier, K., & Monson, C. M. (2021). Integrating cognitive processing therapy for posttraumatic stress disorder with cognitive behavioral therapy for eating disorders in PROJECT RECOVER.*Eating Disorders*, 29(3), 307–325. DOI: 10.1080/10640266.2021.1891372 PMID: 33656976

Trundle, G., & Hutchinson, R. (2021). The phased model of adventure therapy: Trauma-focussed, low arousal, & positive behavioural support.*Journal of Adventure Education and Outdoor Learning*, 21(1), 82–92. DOI: 10.1080/14729679.2020.1736109

Tsai, J., El-Gabalawy, R., Sledge, W. H., Southwick, S. M., & Pietrzak, R. H. (2015). Post-traumatic growth among veterans in the USA: Results from the National Health and Resilience in Veterans Study.*Psychological Medicine*, 45(1), 165–179. DOI: 10.1017/S0033291714001202 PMID: 25065450

Turner, S., Beidel, D., & Frueh, B. (2005). Multicomponent behavioral treatment for chronic combat-related posttraumatic stress disorder: Trauma management therapy.*Behavior Modification*, 29(1), 39–69. DOI: 10.1177/0145445504270872 PMID: 15557478

Tyson, P. (2009). Child Development and Child Psychoanalysis: Research and Education.*Journal of the American Psychoanalytic Association*, 57(4), 871–879. DOI: 10.1177/0003065109342097 PMID: 19724068

Ursin, H., & Olff, M. (1993). Psychobiology of coping and defence strategies. *Neuropsychobiology*, 28(1–2), 66–71. DOI: 10.1159/000119002 PMID: 8255412

van der Kolk, B. (2000a). Posttraumatic stress disorder and the nature of trauma. *Dialogues in Clinical Neuroscience*, 2(1), 7–22. DOI: 10.31887/DCNS.2000.2.1/bvdkolk PMID: 22034447

van der Kolk, B. (2000b). The diagnosis and treatment of Complex PTSD. In Yehuda, R. (Ed.), *Current Treatment of PTSD*. American Psychiatric Press.

van der Kolk, B. (2014). *The body keeps the score*. Viking.

van der Kolk, B. A., van der Hart, O., & Marmar, C. R. (1996). Dissociation and information processing in posttraumatic stress disorder. In van der Kolk, B. A., McFarlane, A. C., & Weisaeth, L. (Eds.), *Traumatic Stress: The Effects of Overwhelming Experience on Mind, Body and Society* (pp. 303–327). Guilford Press.

van Ginneken, N., Chin, W. Y., Lim, Y. C., Ussif, A., Singh, R., Shahmalak, U., Purgato, M., Rojas-García, A., Uphoff, E., McMullen, S., Foss, H. S., Thapa Pachya, A., Rashidian, L., Borghesani, A., Henschke, N., Chong, L.-Y., & Lewin, S. (2021). Primary-level worker interventions for the care of people living with mental disorders and distress in low- and middle-income countries.*Cochrane Database of Systematic Reviews*, 8(8), CD009149. Advance online publication. DOI: 10.1002/14651858.CD009149.pub3 PMID: 34352116

Van Minnen, A., Voorendonk, E. M., Rozendaal, L., & de Jongh, A. (2020). Sequence matters: Combining Prolonged Exposure and EMDR therapy for PTSD.*Psychiatry Research*, 290, 113032. DOI: 10.1016/j.psychres.2020.113032 PMID: 32454314

Van Praag, H. M., Asnis, G. M., Kahn, R. S., Brown, S. L., Korn, M., Friedman, J. M., & Wetzler, S. (1990). Nosological tunnel vision in biological psychiatry. A plea for a functional psychopathology.*Annals of the New York Academy of Sciences*, 600(1), 501–510. DOI: 10.1111/j.1749-6632.1990.tb16905.x PMID: 2252329

vanBruggen-Rufi, M., & van der Stouw, G. (2023). Music Therapy and Korsakoff'sSyndrome: The State of the Art.*Journal of Clinical Medicine*, 12(14), 4609. DOI: 10.3390/jcm12144609 PMID: 37510723

Vancampfort, D., De Soir, E., van Winkel, R., Louw, Q. A., McKeon, G., Rosenbaum, S., Seedat, S., & Pelayo Ramos-Sanchez, C. (2023). Physical activity, sedentary behaviour and mental health outcomes in firefighters: A cross-sectional study.*Journal of Workplace Behavioral Health*, •••, 1–18.

Vasileva, L. V., Ivanovska, M. V., Murdjeva, M. A., Saracheva, K. E., & Georgiev, M. I. (2019). Immunoregulatory natural compounds in stress-induced depression: An alternative or an adjunct to conventional antidepressant therapy?*Food and Chemical Toxicology*, 127, 81–88. DOI: 10.1016/j.fct.2019.03.004 PMID: 30858105

Veith, I. (1965). Hysteria. The history of a disease. Chicago University: Press of Chicago, pp. 1-301.

Vella, E. J., Lyman, T., & Lovering, T. (2023). Pilot Study: The Effects of a Mountain Wilderness Experience on Combat Veteran Psychosocial Wellness.*Military Behavioral Health*, 11(1-2), 1–12. DOI: 10.1080/21635781.2023.2221463

Vermetten, E., & Bremner, J. D. (2002). Circuits and systems in stress. I. Preclinical studies.*Depression and Anxiety*, 15(3), 126–147. DOI: 10.1002/da.10016 PMID: 12001181

Vermetten, E., Schmahl, C., Southwick, S. M., & Bremner, J. D. (2007). A positron tomographic emission study of olfactory induced emotional recall in veterans with and without combat-related posttraumatic stress disorder.*Psychopharmacology Bulletin*, 40(1), 8. PMID: 17285093

Veterans Affairs. (n.d.). Retrieved December 30, 2023, from https://www.ptsd.va.gov/understand/common/common_adults.asp

Veterans Health Administration, Department of Defense. (2017). *VA/DoD clinical practice guideline for the management of posttraumatic stress*. Veterans Health Administration, Department of Defense.

Wagner, C., & Cáceres-Melillo, R. (2023). Mindfulness-Based Cognitive Therapy (MBCT) and Mindfulness-Based Stress Reduction (MBSR) in the treatment of Post-Traumatic Stress Disorder (PTSD): A literature review.*Salud Mental*, 46(1), 35–42. DOI: 10.17711/SM.0185-3325.2023.005

Wahid, H., Ghazi, M., & Lashari, A. (2023). Impact of Meditation on the Level of Post-traumatic Stress in Flood Victims of Sindh.*Global Educational Studies Review, VIII*, 8(I), 272–278. DOI: 10.31703/gesr.2023(VIII-I).23

Wamser-Nanney, R., Walker, H. E., & Nanney, J. T. (2021). Trauma Exposure, Post-traumatic Stress Disorder, and Aggression Among Civilian Females.*Journal of Interpersonal Violence*, 36(17–18), NP9649–NP9669. DOI: 10.1177/0886260519860894 PMID: 31286814

Watanabe, Y., Sakai, R. R., McEwen, B. S., & Mendelson, S. (1993). Stress and antidepressant effects on hippocampal and cortical 5-HT1A and 5-HT2 receptors and transport sites for serotonin.*Brain Research*, 615(1), 87–94. DOI: 10.1016/0006-8993(93)91117-B PMID: 8364729

Waters, L. M. (2018). *Factors influencing the vicarious effects of trauma in hotline volunteers.* (Unpublished doctoral dissertation). Hofstra University, New York.

Watson, J. B. (1913). Psychology as the behaviorist views it.*Psychological Review*, 20(2), 158–177. DOI: 10.1037/h0074428

Weathers, F. W., & Ford, J. (1996). Psychometric review of PTSD Checklist (PCL-C, PCL-S, PCL-M, PCL-PR). In Stamm, B. H. (Ed.), *measurement of stress, trauma, and adaptation* (pp. 250–251). Sidran Press.

Weintraub, A. (2012). *Yoga skills for therapists: Effective practices for mood management.* Norton.

Werner, N. S., Meindl, T., Engel, R. R., Rosner, R., Riedel, M., Reiser, M., & Fast, K. (2009). Hippocampal function during associative learning in patients with post-traumatic stress disorder.*Journal of Psychiatric Research*, 43(3), 309–318. DOI: 10.1016/j.jpsychires.2008.03.011 PMID: 18490028

Whalley, M. G., Rugg, M. D., Smith, A. P. R., Dolan, R. J., & Brewin, C. R. (2009). Incidental retrieval of emotional contexts in post-traumatic stress disorder and depression: An fMRI study.*Brain and Cognition*, 69(1), 98–107. DOI: 10.1016/j.bandc.2008.05.008 PMID: 18614265

Wilde, L. (2022). Trauma: Phenomenological causality and implication.*Phenomenology and the Cognitive Sciences*, 21(3), 689–705. DOI: 10.1007/s11097-020-09725-8

Williams, L. M., Kemp, A. H., Felmingham, K., Barton, M., Olivieri, G., Peduto, A., Gordon, E., & Bryant, R. A. (2006). Trauma modulates amygdala and medial prefrontal responses to consciously attended fear. *NeuroImage*, 29(2), 347–357. DOI: 10.1016/j.neuroimage.2005.03.047 PMID: 16216534

Williston, S. K., Grossman, D., Mori, D. L., & Niles, B. L. (2021). Mindfulness interventions in the treatment of posttraumatic stress disorder. *Professional Psychology, Research and Practice*, 52(1), 46–57. DOI: 10.1037/pro0000363

Wilson, E. O. (1984). *Biophilia*. Harvard University Press. DOI: 10.4159/9780674045231

Wilson, M. A., Liberzon, I., Lindsey, M. L., Lokshina, Y., Risbrough, V. B., Sah, R., Wood, S. K., Williamson, J. B., & Spinale, F. G. (2019). Common pathways and communication between the brain and heart: Connecting post-traumatic stress disorder and heart failure. *Stress (Amsterdam, Netherlands)*, 22(5), 530–547. DOI: 10.1080/10253890.2019.1621283 PMID: 31161843

Winkler, O., Dhaliwal, R., Greenshaw, A., O'Shea, K., Abba-Aji, A., Chima, C., Purdon, S. E., & Burback, L. (2021). Web-Based Eye Movement Desensitization and Reprocessing for Adults With Suicidal Ideation: Protocol for a Randomized Controlled Trial. *JMIR Research Protocols*, 10(11), e30711. DOI: 10.2196/30711 PMID: 34734835

Wittfoth, D., Beise, J., Manuel, J., Bohne, M., & Wittfoth, M. (2022). Bifocal emotion regulation through acupoint tapping in fear of flying. *NeuroImage. Clinical*, 34, 102996. DOI: 10.1016/j.nicl.2022.102996 PMID: 35378497

Wittfoth, D., Pfeiffer, A., Bohne, M., Lanfermann, H., & Wittfoth, M. (2020). Emotion regulation through bifocal processing of fear-inducing and disgust-inducing stimuli. *BMC Neuroscience*, 21(1), 47. DOI: 10.1186/s12868-020-00597-x PMID: 33225884

Wolfgang, A. S., & Hoge, C. W. (2023). Cannabis and cannabinoids for pain and posttraumatic stress disorder in military personnel and veterans. *JAMA Psychiatry*, 80(9), 869–870. DOI: 10.1001/jamapsychiatry.2023.1685 PMID: 37436761

Wolpe, J. (1969). *The practice of behavior therapy*. Pergamon Press.

Wolpe, J., & Lazarus, A. A. (1966). *Behavior therapy techniques: A guide to the treatment of neuroses*. Pergamon Press.

Wampold, B. E. (2015). How important are common factors in psychotherapy? An update. *World Psychiatry; Official Journal of the World Psychiatric Association (WPA)*, 14(3), 270–277. DOI: 10.1002/wps.20238 PMID: 26407772

World Health Organization. (2002). *Acupuncture: Review and analysis of reports on controlled clinical trials*. Author.

Wu, J., Kramer, G. L., Kram, M., Steciuk, M., Crawford, I. L., & Petty, F. (1999). Serotonin and learned helplessness: A regional study of 5-HT1A, 5-HT2A receptors and the serotonin transport site in rat brain.*Journal of Psychiatric Research*, 33(1), 17–22. DOI: 10.1016/S0022-3956(98)00041-7 PMID: 10094235

Wylde, M. C., Mahrer, E. N., Meyer, M. L. R., & Gold, I. J. (2017). Mindfulness for Novice Pediatric Nurses: Smartphone Application Versus Traditional Intervention.*Journal of Pediatric Nursing*, 36, 205–212. DOI: 10.1016/j.pedn.2017.06.008 PMID: 28888505

Yalom, L. D. (1980). *Existential psychotherapy*. Basic Books.

Yehuda, R. (2009). Status of glucocorticoid alterations in post-traumatic stress disorder.*Annals of the New York Academy of Sciences*, 1179(1), 56–69. DOI: 10.1111/j.1749-6632.2009.04979.x PMID: 19906232

Yehuda, R. (2015). Is the glucocorticoid receptor a therapeutic target for the treatment of PTSD.*Psychoneuroendocrinology*, 61, 2. DOI: 10.1016/j.psyneuen.2015.07.391

Yehuda, R., Brand, S., & Yang, R.-K. (2006). Plasma neuropeptide Y concentrations in combat exposed veterans: Relationship to trauma exposure, recovery from PTSD, and coping.*Biological Psychiatry*, 59(7), 660–663. DOI: 10.1016/j.biopsych.2005.08.027 PMID: 16325152

Yehuda, R., Hoge, C. W., McFarlane, A. C., Vermetten, E., Lanius, R. A., Nievergelt, C. M., Hobfoll, S. E., Koenen, K. C., Neylan, T. C., & Hyman, S. E. (2015). Post-traumatic stress disorder.*Nature Reviews. Disease Primers*, 1(1), 1–22. DOI: 10.1038/nrdp.2015.57 PMID: 27189040

Yehuda, R., & LeDoux, J. (2007). Response variation following trauma: A translational neuroscience approach to understanding PTSD.*Neuron*, 56(1), 19–32. DOI: 10.1016/j.neuron.2007.09.006 PMID: 17920012

Yehuda, R., & Seckl, J. (2011). Minireview: stress-related psychiatric disorders with low cortisol levels: a metabolic hypothesis.*Endocrinology*, 152(12), 4496–4503. DOI: 10.1210/en.2011-1218 PMID: 21971152

Yeung, D. (2023, November 3). I can't help but follow graphic images from Israel-Hamas war. I should know better. USA TODAY. https://www.usatoday.com/story/opinion/voices/2023/11/03/israel-hamas-war-images-trauma-mental-health/71334176007/

Yoneda, Y., Tamaki, K., & Kakuda, T. (2008). Disturbance of adult neurogenesis by PTSD.*The International Journal of Neuropsychopharmacology*, 11, 50.

Youngren, W. A., Hamilton, N. A., & Preacher, K. (2020). Assessing Triggers of Posttrauma Nightmares.*Journal of Traumatic Stress*, 33(4), 511–520. DOI: 10.1002/jts.22532 PMID: 32521086

Yount, G., Church, D., Rachlin, K., Blickheuser, K., & Cardonna, I. (2019). Do non-coding RNAs mediate the efficacy of energy psychology?*Global Advances in Health and Medicine : Improving Healthcare Outcomes Worldwide*, 8, 2164956119832500. DOI: 10.1177/2164956119832500 PMID: 30828482

Zabik, N., Iadipaolo, A., Peters, C., & Rabinak, C. A. (2022). P654. Varying Doses of THC Rescue Neural Fear Circuitry Dysfunction in Trauma-Exposed Adults. *Biological Psychiatry*, 91(9), S354–S355. DOI: 10.1016/j.biopsych.2022.02.891

Zaccari, B., Loftis, J. M., Haywood, T., Hubbard, K., Clark, J., & Kelly, U. A. (2022). Synchronous telehealth yoga and cognitive processing group therapies for women veterans with posttraumatic stress disorder: A multisite randomized controlled trial adapted for COVID-19.*Telemedicine Journal and e-Health*, 28(11), 1642–1650. DOI: 10.1089/tmj.2021.0612 PMID: 35357957

Zaleski, K. L., Johnson, D. K., & Klein, J. T. (2016). Grounding Judith Herman's Trauma Theory within Interpersonal Neuroscience and Evidence-Based Practice Modalities for Trauma Treatment.*Smith College Studies in Social Work*, 86(4), 377–393. DOI: 10.1080/00377317.2016.1222110

Zhang, L., Deng, L., Ma, C., Zhang, H., & Dang, Y. (2023). Brain-Derived Neurotrophic Factor Delivered Intranasally Relieves Post-Traumatic Stress Disorder Symptoms Caused by a Single Prolonged Stress in Rats.*Neuropsychobiology*, 82(1), 40–50. DOI: 10.1159/000528755 PMID: 36630922

Zhang, S. L., Hilton, L., & Gordon, W. (2015). Effects of integrative PTSD treatment in a military health setting.*Energy Psychology Journal*, 7(2). Advance online publication. DOI: 10.9769/EPJ.2015.11.1.SL

Zikopoulos, B., Höistad, M., John, Y., & Barbas, H. (2017). Posterior orbitofrontal and anterior cingulate pathways to the amygdala target inhibitory and excitatory systems with opposite functions.*The Journal of Neuroscience : The Official Journal of the Society for Neuroscience*, 37(20), 5051–5064. DOI: 10.1523/JNEUROSCI.3940-16.2017 PMID: 28411274

Zohar, J., Yahalom, H., Kozlovsky, N., Cwikel-Hamzany, S., Matar, M. A., Kaplan, Z., Yehuda, R., & Cohen, H. (2011). High dose hydrocortisone immediately after trauma may alter the trajectory of PTSD: Interplay between clinical and animal studies.*European Neuropsychopharmacology*, 21(11), 796–809. DOI: 10.1016/j.euroneuro.2011.06.001 PMID: 21741804

About the Contributors

Robert W. Motta, Ph.D., ABPP, is a Professor Emeritus of Psychology and founder of the Child and Family Trauma Institute at Hofstra University, New York. There he served as the chairperson of the Psychology Department and founded an American Psychological Association (APA) accredited PsyD psychology doctoral program. He has published more than 100 scientific papers and book chapters as well as three books: Alternative Therapies for PTSD The Science of Mind-Body Treatments; Altered: A Trauma and PTSD Casebook; and Suicide. Dr. Motta is board certified in cognitive-behavioral psychology and behavior therapy. He is the former president of the School Division of the New York Psychological Association and is licensed as a clinical psychologist and certified as a school psychologist. Robert W. Motta

***

Jitendra Binwal is working as a Professor & Dean, School of Liberal Arts and Sciences, Mody University of Science and Technology, Laxmangarh-332311, Sikar, Rajasthan, India since April 2022. He has done Ph.D. (Mathematics) in the year 2010, M.Sc. (Mathematics) in 1998, and B.Sc. in 1996 from Government Holkar Science College, DAVV, Indore (M.P.), India. In total, he has more than 24.5 years teaching, research, and administrative experience at Undergraduate, Postgraduate, and Ph.D. levels in University. His areas of research include graph theory, discrete mathematics, and modeling and simulation. Dr. Binwal has published more than 44 research papers in journals of national and international reputes. He has guided 04 Ph.D., 10 PG and 12 UG Dissertations. He has published 04 Books, 01 book Chapter, 06 Patents and 01 copyright at national and international levels. He has received InSc Academic Excellence Award. He is a life member of Indian Academy of Mathematics, India, Academy of Discrete Mathematics and Its Applications, Mysore; Honorary Life Membership of Vigyan Bharati Malwa Prant(VIBHA,

India), and Indian Society for Magnetic Fluid Research, Gujrat. Dr. Binwal was selected as a member of Executive Committee for 2018 – 2025 at Indian Academy of Mathematics, Indore. He has participated in many Conferences, Seminars, Workshops, and FDP at national and International levels.

Tilak Ram Chandrakar is an accomplished forensic educationists with extensive experience in both academia and applied forensic science. He holds undergraduate honour's and postgraduate degrees in Forensic Science. His professional journey began with a role as a Scientific Assistant at the State Forensic Science Laboratory in Rohini, Delhi. Dr. Chandrakar further advanced his expertise by completing a Ph.D. in Molecular Forensics, specializing in Wildlife Forensics, from Rani Durgavati University in Jabalpur, Madhya Pradesh. In his academic career, Dr. Chandrakar has served as an Assistant Professor and Head of the Department of Forensic Science at Medi-Caps University, Indore. Currently, he holds the position of Assistant Professor and Head of Forensic Science at the School of Liberal Arts and Sciences, Mody University in Laxmangarh-Sikar, Rajasthan. Dr. Chandrakar is renowned for his deep command and knowledge in Forensic Biological Science, contributing significantly to both academic and research domains having numbers of Research Papers, Book Chapters and Patents.

Hanane El Fatimi is a PhD student in Neurosciences and Cellular Physiology research team, Interdisciplinary Laboratory of Biotechnology and Health, Mohammed VI University of Health and Sciences (UM6SS), Casablanca, Morocco

El Hiba Omar is professor of physiopathology, neuroscience and histology, Faculty of Sciences, Chouaib Doukkali University, He was born in 12 September 1985 in Marrakech-Safi state (Morocco) and was graduated in 2007 from Cadi Ayyad University (Morocco) with a bachelor degree in Biology. In 2009, hewas graduated from the same university with Master's degree in Life and Health Sciences. He obtained his PhD in 2015 on the "Physiopathology of Hepatic Encephalopathy" from Cadi Ayyad University. He is, since 2014, member of the International Parkinson and Movement Disorders Society (MDS), USA and the vice-President of the Moroccan Society of Ethics and Animal Research (MoSEAR).

Bilal El-Mansoury is a researcher in Neuroscience. His research focuses mainly on glial cells dysfunction in Hepatic encephalopathy and neurodegenerative disorders.

Sanam Hafeez, received her doctorate from Hofstra University, with a research interest in PTSD and secondary trauma, and completed her post-doctoral work in neuro-developmental Psychology at Coney Island Hospital in Brooklyn,

NY. Dr. Hafeez is a New York State licensed psychologist and a New York State certified school psychologist. Dr. Sanam Hafeez is a pioneer in neuropsychological assessments, reshaping its clinical model and best practices. She founded Comprehend the Mind in 2006 and continues to serve as the director of her neuropsychological assessment center. Dr. Sanam Hafeez is also a trusted media expert, and has appeared on CNN, MSNBC, ABCNews, and Fox News. Dr. Hafeez has contributed to the New York Times, The Washington Post, The Wall Street Journal, Harper's Bazaar, WebMD, Yahoo, Psychology Today, and serves on multiple boards as an expert in mental health and education. Dr. Hafeez is also co-authoring a book on trauma and substance abuse. Dr. Hafeez greatest role is that of 'Mama' to her twin boys. She enjoys traveling and would have been a movie critic in another life.

Divya Nair is presently serving as an Assistant Professor at the School of Education and Research, MIT Art, Design and Technology University, amassing 7 years of experience in this role. Additionally, she holds key responsibilities as the IQAC, NAAC, UTSAH, and AISHE coordinator within her department. Her educational background includes a Master's degree in Microbiology from Pune University, an M.Ed. from S.N.DT. University, Pune, and a master's degree in Psychology from IGNOU. Furthermore, she completed a Post Graduate Diploma in Mass Media from Pune University and achieved UGC NET with JRF in Education. Currently, she is pursuing her Ph.D. at Adarsha Comprehensive College of Education and Research, SPPU. Her research is titled as "Developing a strength-based program and studying its effectiveness for enhancing critical and creative thinking among teacher trainees." She excelled in various courses, earning a National level gold medal in the "Great Experiments in Psychology" offered by IIT Kharagpur through the NPTEL platform, and a national level silver medal in the "Design Thinking – A Primer" course offered by IIT Madras through NPTEL. She holds three copyrights to her name. She achieved first rank in the 167th General Orientation Program course of UGC HRDC at SPPU with 90% marks. Her academic achievements also include completing two refresher courses with outstanding results - "Advanced Research Methodology – Tools and Techniques" and "Pedagogical Innovations and Research Methodology [ARPIT]," earning A+ and 93%, respectively. Miss. Divya actively engages in various academic activities, participating in numerous FDPs, and contributing to book chapters and research papers. Her works have been published in esteemed international publications such as CRC Press Taylor and Francis, USA; Emerald Insight, England; Wiley, US; Springer, New-York; Springer-Nature, London; IGI-Global, Pennsylvania, among others. She has received accolades for her research, winning the best research paper award at both national and state levels. Miss Divya's accolades further include a Gold medal in a State-level poster competition organized by the Dept. of Microbiology, Modern College. She received the editor's choice award and outstanding entry award in the International Creative Writing Contest, judged by Chetan Bhagat. Beyond academics, her interests span Classical Dance and Classical Singing, where she holds the title of Nritya Visharad in Bharatnatyam and Mohiniattam. She has authored numerous poems and short stories in English and Hindi, earning several awards for her literary contributions.

Sameer Saharan is a dedicated researcher in Forensic Science, specializing in fingerprint analysis, cyber forensics, and DNA fingerprinting. He holds a Ph.D. in Forensic Science from Amity University, Haryana, and has authored several research papers and book chapters. With a passion for continuous learning, Dr. Saharan actively contributes to the advancement of forensic science through his expertise and knowledge. He is committed to nurturing the next generation of forensic scientists and making a positive impact in the field.

Mridu Sharma is currently working as an Assistant professor in Department of Forensic Science, School of Liberal Arts and Sciences at Mody University of Science and Technology. She has completed her Ph.D. in Forensic Science from Amity University. She has a specialization in Fingerprints and crime scene investigation.

Peta Stapleton is a registered clinical and health Psychologist and Professor, Bond University (Australia) who embraces evidence-based and innovative techniques. Peta is a world-leading researcher in Emotional Freedom Techniques and has been awarded many achievements including the Harvey Baker Research Award for meticulous research (Association of Comprehensive Energy Psychology, USA), and the 2019 Psychologist of the Year (Australian Allied Health Awards).

Rati Kailash Prasad Tripathi is currently working as an Assistant Professor at Assam Central University, Silchar, Assam, India. She received her M. Pharm. (2011) and Ph.D. (2016) degrees from the Indian Institute of Technology, Banaras Hindu University, Varanasi (India); where she specialized in Pharmaceutical Chemistry with peculiar interest in synthetic medicinal chemistry, computational chemistry and molecular modelling. She has to her credit many scientific publications in journals of international repute. She has also authored 02 books and several book chapters. She is also a recipient of several research grants and prestigious awards like Senior Research Fellowship from the Indian Council of Medical Research, Government of India and Shri C. Subramaniam Award for Excellence in Character from Bhartiya Vidya Bhavan, Mumbai. She is an active member of many scientific Indian associations viz. Indian Pharmacy Graduates' Association (IPGA) and The Association of Pharmaceutical Teachers of India (APTI). She serves as a mentor to several graduate, post graduate and PhD students. She is also an editorial board member and reviewer for many international journals of repute.

Index

H

I

M

N

P

S

T

W

www.ingramcontent.com/pod-product-compliance
Lightning Source LLC
LaVergne TN
LVHW081537300926
849161LV00006B/1462